Terrorism and Public Health

Terrorism and Public Health

A Balanced Approach to Strengthening Systems and Protecting People

Edited by

BARRY S. LEVY

VICTOR W. SIDEL

*Published in Cooperation with
the American Public Health Association*

2007

OXFORD
UNIVERSITY PRESS

Oxford University Press, Inc., publishes works that further
Oxford University's objective of excellence
in research, scholarship, and education

Oxford   New York
Auckland   Cape Town   Dar es Salaam   Hong Kong   Karachi
Kuala Lumpur   Madrid   Melbourne   Mexico City   Nairobi
New Delhi   Shanghai   Taipei   Toronto

With offices in
Argentina   Austria   Brazil   Chile   Czech Republic   France   Greece
Guatemala   Hungary   Italy   Japan   Poland   Portugal   Singapore
South Korea   Switzerland   Thailand   Turkey   Ukraine   Vietnam

Published by Oxford University Press, Inc.
198 Madison Avenue, New York, New York, 10016
http://www.oup-usa.org

Library of Congress Cataloging-in-Publication Data
Terrorism and public health : a balanced approach to strengthening systems and
protecting people/
edited by Barry S. Levy, Victor W. Sidel.
p. cm.   Includes bibliographical references and index.
ISBN-13 978-0-19-532525-6
ISBN 0-19-532525-7
1. Terrorism—Health aspects.   2. Disaster medicine.
3. Emergency medical services.   4. Weapons of mass destruction—Health aspects.
5. Emergency management.   6. Terrorism—Prevention.
7. Health planning.   8. Public health.
I. Levy, Barry S.   II. Sidel, Victor W.
RA645.5 .T477 2003   362.18—dc21   2002072672

1 2 3 4 5 6 7 8 9

Printed in the United States of America
on acid-free paper

*This book is dedicated
to public health professionals,
who help protect society
from the health consequences of terrorism
while continuing to provide
essential programs and services
to assure the conditions
in which people can be healthy.*

Foreword

The terrorist attacks of September 11 and the subsequent assaults with anthrax through the postal system underscored both strengths and weaknesses in the U.S. public health system. These events created a sense of urgency to perform a long-overdue critical reassessment of our system. *Terrorism and Public Health* provides such an assessment. It addresses how individuals, government agencies, and health care and other organizations can be more effective in responding to and preventing future acts of terrorism while at the same time meeting other essential health needs and protecting human rights.

Given the number and variety of weapons that can be used, terrorism creates unique challenges for the public health system in planning, response, and prevention efforts. Human-made and highly unpredictable, bioterrorism in particular is a special kind of terrorism that can create unusual epidemics.

Globally, public health has brought humankind together in a spirit of cooperation and mutual support. The eradication of smallpox and the near-eradication of polio are perhaps the best examples of this spirit. Terrorism represents a different kind of force as people attempt to use infectious diseases and related agents as weapons against other people. Public health has a critical role to play in responding to terrorism and preventing or reducing its impact, but it must work in conjunction with the criminal justice system and other parts of society to be truly effective in this endeavor.

This book is a strong example of the type of interdisciplinary collaboration that is needed as we move forward in planning a terrorism response and prevention effort. It has brought together experts from the fields of medicine and public health, weapons systems experts, lawyers, social scientists, civil libertarians, leaders in human rights, and others to provide a balanced approach to strengthening our systems and protecting people's health and safety.

This volume details the necessary steps we must take to prepare ourselves as a nation in the face of a new and emerging threat. One vital component of strengthening the public health infrastructure to ensure a state of readiness is a well-functioning U.S. Public Health Service. Agencies of the U.S. Department of Health and Human Services, such as the Centers for Disease Control and Prevention (CDC), need funding and other support for programs that train and educate health care providers and the public, for provision of critical tools and training to state health departments to enhance their capacity to respond effectively to terrorism, and for the myriad other responsibilities federal agencies have in preparing for a national response to terrorism.

In addition, clinicians, other front-line health care workers, and public health professionals need information and education about potential terrorist scenarios, including which infectious and other agents may be used as weapons, and training to recognize unusual clinical cases. Communication between those on the front lines and state and federal officials also needs to be enhanced to create a system that works efficiently during crises. Moreover, the general public needs to be educated to notice and report unusual illnesses or symptoms and to practice good public health habits. Healthy lifestyles are a key part of a strong public health infrastructure.

In light of these needs, the terrorist attacks have reinforced the idea that public health and medicine can no longer function independently of each other. Going back to the late 1980s, the Institute of Medicine (IOM) found the U.S. public health system to be deteriorating, poorly understood or co-ordinated, and inadequately supported and funded. While we have the most sophisticated medical care in the world, we are penny-wise and pound-foolish when it comes to promoting health and preventing disease. Creating a more balanced community health system—one that balances health promotion, disease prevention, early detection, and universal access—will not only help us save lives in the event of a terrorist attack, it also will reduce premature mortality and improve the quality of life for those suffering from chronic diseases such as diabetes, heart disease, cancer, and other illnesses. In addition, over time, we can realize tremendous economic savings through such efforts and even redirect these savings to provide access to quality health care for those who have not been able to afford it. One of the greatest lessons of the tragic events of 2001 is that we must build a stronger partnership between medicine and public health.

As we move to strengthen our ability to prepare for and respond to the health consequences of terrorism, we also cannot forget or ignore other major health problems. It would probably create more suffering if we diverted resources from existing public health programs and services in order to support new efforts to address the health aspects of terrorism. Many of our most pressing health concerns are likely to continue to cause far more morbidity and mortality than will terrorism. We can reap tremendous synergies by addressing the goals of community-based prevention and terrorism preparedness in concert, instead of creating competing efforts.

Finally, this book reminds us that as we make progress in protecting our nation from terrorist attacks, we must always be cognizant of the most vulnerable among us and strive to protect the individual liberties that are at the core of our values.

—David Satcher, M.D., Ph.D.
Former United States Surgeon General

Preface

Public health is a critical element in responding to terrorist incidents and in reducing or preventing threats of future terrorism. It is also a critical element in reducing or preventing inappropriate or hazardous responses to threats of future terrorism, such as diversion of resources and attention from other urgent public health needs, adverse health effects from misuse of antibiotics and ill-conceived immunization programs, and abrogation of civil rights and human rights. This book addresses terrorism and public health, and presents a balanced approach to strengthening systems and protecting people. It is designed to assist public health professionals and their agencies and organizations by providing up-to-date, science-based expert information on, and a systematic practical approach to, a wide range of relevant public health issues as they relate to terrorism. While there are and will be many books on terrorism and some on its public-health aspects, we believe this is the first book that addresses terrorism from a public-health perspective that is both comprehensive and balanced.

Many public health professionals have become engaged in responding to terrorist acts and the threats of future terrorism, ranging from epidemiologists to health educators, from mental health specialists to vaccine developers, from occupational and environmental health specialists to those who focus on human rights and social justice issues. There are ongoing needs to help these individuals—and the government agencies, academic institutions, health-care organizations, and civil society (nongovernmental) organizations they are affiliated with—become more effective in (a) responding to terrorist acts and reducing or preventing threats of future terrorism; and (b) reducing or preventing inappropriate responses to the threats of future terrorism. This book is designed to meet these needs. While *Terrorism and Public Health* is directed primarily at public health professionals and others in the United States, we hope it will be useful to those in other countries as well.

The public health professionals who wrote the chapters that follow drew on their expertise and experience in dealing with terrorism and closely related issues. In addition to providing information and insights into improving preparedness against terrorism, they also discuss some pitfalls we face.

The book is organized into three parts. The first describes the public health response to September 11, 2001, and its aftermath. Part II describes terrorist weapons and their use. Part III describes, in practical detail, the challenges and opportunities that terrorism presents to public health.

This book arose, in part, from scientific sessions that we planned and participated in at the Annual Meeting of the American Public Health Association in Atlanta in October 2001. It is designed to complement *War and Public Health*, which we edited and which was published by Oxford University Press in cooperation with the American Public Health Association (APHA) in 1997 (with an updated edition published by APHA in 2000).

Emergency preparedness for responding to potential terrorist acts, prevention of terrorism and its adverse health effects, and avoidance of inappropriate responses to terrorist threats need to be incorporated into the work of public health practitioners and into the curricula of schools of public health, medical schools, and other schools for health professionals. In addition, more research is needed with a focus on the health consequences of terrorist acts and terrorist weapons and those of anti-terrorism measures. We hope that this book will stimulate these initiatives in public health practice, education, and research.

Sherborn, Massachusetts   B.S.L.
The Bronx, New York   V.W.S.

Acknowledgments

Developing *Terrorism and Public Health* involved the combined skills and resources of many people, to whom we are profoundly grateful.

We greatly appreciate the guidance, assistance, and support of Jeffrey House, Vice-President and Executive Editor, Medicine; Lynda Crawford, Production Editor for this book; Edith Barry, Associate Editor; and their colleagues at Oxford University Press.

We acknowledge all of the contributors to this book, who worked on short deadlines to write chapters and boxes that reflect their observations, insights, and expertise.

We express our deep appreciation to Heather L. Merrell for her excellent work in preparing multiple drafts of the manuscript and coordinating the acquisition of photographs and other materials for this book.

Finally, we express our gratitude and appreciation to Nancy Levy and Ruth Sidel for their continuing encouragement, support, and love.

Contents

Part II Terrorist Weapons

Part III Challenges and Opportunities

Contributors

CAROL EASLEY ALLEN, PH.D.,
  R.N.
Professor and Chair
Department of Nursing
Oakwood College
Huntsville, AL

SHARON BALTER, M.D.
Medical Epidemiologist
Communicable Disease Program
New York City Department of Health
New York, NY

JEFFREY B. BENDER, D.V.M.,
  M.S.
Assistant Professor
Department of Veterinary Public Health
University of Minnesota, College of
  Veterinary Medicine
St. Paul, MN

SUSAN BLANK, M.D., M.P.H.
Assistant Commissioner
Sexually Transmitted Disease Control
  Program
New York City Department of Health
New York, NY
and
Division of Sexually Transmitted Disease
  Prevention
Centers for Disease Control and
  Prevention
Atlanta, GA

ANNALIES BORREL, M.SC.
Lecturer and Public Nutrition Research
  Fellow
Feinstein International Famine Center
Friedman School of Nutrition Science and
  Policy
Tufts University
Medford, MA

PHILIP S. BRACHMAN, M.D.
Professor
Department of International Health
The Rollins School of Public Health of
  Emory University
Atlanta, GA

MUIREANN BRENNAN, M.D.,
  M.P.H.
Medical Epidemiologist
International Emergency and Refugee
  Health Branch
Centers for Disease Control and
  Prevention
Atlanta, GA

ANTOINE CHAPDELAINE, M.D.,
  L.C.M.C., M.P.H., C.S.P.Q.,
  F.R.C.P.(C)
Physician
Centre Hospitalier Universitaire de
  Quebec (CHUQ)
Quebec City, Quebec, Canada

LUZ CLAUDIO, PH.D.
Associate Professor
Department of Community and Preventive
  Medicine
Mount Sinai School of Medicine
New York, NY

J. LYLE CONRAD, M.D., M.P.H.
Consultant
Atlanta, GA

WENDY CUKIER, M.A., M.B.A.,
  PH.D., D.U.(HON.), LL.D.
  (HON.), M.S.C.
Professor, Information Technology
  Management and Justice Studies
Ryerson University
and
Coordinator, Small Arms Firearms
  Education and Research Network
  (SAFER-Net)
Toronto, Ontario, Canada

MERAV DATAN, J.D.
Director, UN Office
Physicians for Social Responsibility &
  International Physicians for the
  Prevention of Nuclear War
New York, NY

CHERYL E. EASLEY, PH.D., R.N.
Dean and Professor
Crystal M. Lange College of Nursing &
  Health Sciences
Saginaw Valley State University
University Center, MI

MARGUERITE A. ERME, D.O.,
  M.P.H.
Disease Control Medical Officer
Akron Health Department
Akron, OH

ANJALI GARG, B.S.
Research Assistant
Department of Community and Preventive
  Medicine
Mount Sinai School of Medicine
New York, NY

H. JACK GEIGER, M.D., M.SCI.HYG.
Arthur C. Logan Professor of Community
  Medicine, Emeritus
Department of Community Health and
  Social Medicine
City University of New York Medical
  School
City College of New York
New York, NY

KATIE GENTILE, PH.D.
Assistant Professor of Counseling
John Jay College
City University of New York
New York, NY

KAY S. GOLAN
Director of Media Relations
Office of Communication
Centers for Disease Control and
  Prevention
Atlanta, GA

LAWRENCE O. GOSTIN, J.D., LL.D.
  (HON.)
Professor of Law
Georgetown University
Washington, DC
and
Professor of Public Health
Johns Hopkins University
Baltimore, MD

ROBERT M. GOULD, M.D.
President-Elect
Physicians for Social Responsibility
Washington, DC

CRAIG W. HEDBERG, PH.D.
Associate Professor
Division of Environmental and
*   Occupational Health*
University of Minnesota School of Public
*   Health*
Minneapolis, MN

TIMOTHY H. HOLTZ, M.D., M.P.H.
Preventive Medicine Fellow
Assigned to: New York City Department
*   of Health*
Division of Applied Public Health
*   Training*
and
Epidemiology Program Office
Centers for Disease Control and
*   Prevention*
Atlanta, GA

NIMMI KAPOOR
Medical Student
Weill Medical College of Cornell
*   University*
New York, NY

C. WILLIAM KECK, M.D., M.P.H.
Director of Health
Akron Health Department
Akron, OH

OXANA KHABIB, M.D.
Neurologist and Research Fellow
Scientific Research Group of
*   Academicians Yu. Isakov*
Russian Academy of Medical Sciences
Bakulev Scientific Center for
*   Cardiovascular Surgery*
Moscow, Russia

CHERYL LACKEY, M.P.H.,
   C.H.E.S.
Health Communication Specialist
Office of Communication
Centers for Disease Control and
*   Prevention*
Atlanta, GA

PHILIP J. LANDRIGAN, M.D.
Professor and Chairman
Department of Community and Preventive
*   Medicine*
Mount Sinai School of Medicine
New York, NY

SUE LAUTZE, M.P.A.
Director
Livelihoods Initiatives Program
Feinstein International Famine Center
Friedman School of Nutrition Science and
*   Policy*
Tufts University
Medford, MA

JENNIFER LEANING, M.D., S.M.H.
Professor of International Health
Harvard School of Public Health
Boston, MA

JESSICA LEIGHTON, PH.D.
Assistant Commissioner
Office of Environmental Disease
*   Prevention*
New York City Department of Health
New York, NY

BARRY S. LEVY, M.D., M.P.H.
Adjunct Professor
Department of Family Medicine and
*   Community Health*
Tufts University School of Medicine
Boston, MA
and
Consultant
Sherborn, MA

BRUCE LIPPY, C.I.H., C.S.P.
Director of Research and Special Projects
Operating Engineers National Hazmat
*   Program*
International Union of Operating
*   Engineers*
Beckley, WV

DOROTHY MARGOLSKEE, M.D.
Founder and Principal
SYNERGEE LLC
Upper Montclair, NJ

JAMES L. PEARSON, DR.P.H.,
  M.P.H.
State Laboratory Director
Virginia State Health Department
Richmond, VA

PETER SALAMA, M.D., M.P.H.
Chief, Health and Nutrition
UNICEF Afghanistan
Kabul, Afghanistan

MONICA SCHOCH-SPANA, PH.D.
Senior Fellow
Center for Civilian Biodefense Studies
Johns Hopkins University
Baltimore, MD

VICTOR W. SIDEL, M.D.
Distinguished University Professor of
  Social Medicine
Montefiore Medical Center
Albert Einstein College of Medicine
Bronx, NY
and
Adjunct Professor of Public Health
Weill Medical College of Cornell
  University
New York, NY

HERMAN SPANJAARD, M.D.
Occupational Health Specialist
Arboconsultancy
Amsterdam, The Netherlands

CHARLES B. STROZIER, PH.D.
Professor of History
John Jay College and the Graduate Center
City University of New York
New York, NY

PATRICE M. SUTTON, M.P.H.
Research Scientist
Public Health Institute
Oakland, CA

ZEBULON TAINTOR, M.D.
Professor and Vice Chairman
Department of Psychiatry
New York University School of Medicine
and
Chair, Public Health Committee
New York County Medical Society
New York, NY

DONALD VESLEY, PH.D.
Professor
Division of Environmental and
  Occupational Health
University of Minnesota School of Public
  Health
Minneapolis, MN

ISAAC WEISFUSE, M.D., M.P.H.
Associate Commissioner
Bureau of Disease Intervention Services
New York City Department of Health
New York, NY

DON WEISS, M.D., M.P.H.
Medical Director, Surveillance Unit
Communicable Disease Program
New York City Department of Health
New York, NY

PETER WEISS, J.D.
President, Lawyers Committee on Nuclear
  Policy
and
Vice President, Center for Constitutional
  Rights
New York, NY

Frequently Used Abbreviations

APHA	American Public Health Association
APHL	Association of Public Health Laboratories
AHERA	Asbestos Hazard Emergency Response Act
BWC	Biological Weapons Convention
CDC	Centers for Disease Control and Prevention
CWC	Chemical Weapons Convention
DDC	Department of Design and Construction
DOE	Department of Energy
DHHS	Department of Health and Human Services
DMATs	Disaster Medical Assistance Teams
EIS	Epidemic Intelligence Service
EOC	Emergency Operations Center
EPA	Environmental Protection Agency
FBI	Federal Bureau of Investigation
FEMA	Federal Emergency Management Agency
FRP	Federal Response Plan
GNYHA	Greater New York Hospital Association
HAZWOPER	Hazardous Waste and Emergency Response Standard
IAEA	International Atomic Energy Agency
ICS	Incident command system
IED	Improvised explosive device
IOM	Institute of Medicine
LRN	Laboratory Response Network

MIS	Management information system
MMWR	*Morbidity and Mortality Weekly Report*
NGO	Non-governmental organization (civil-society organization)
NIEHS	National Institute of Environmental Health Sciences
NIOSH	National Institute for Occupational Safety and Health
NPS	National Pharmaceutical Stockpile
NYC DEP	New York City Department of Environmental Protection
NYC DOH	New York City Department of Health
NYS DEC	New York State Department of Environmental Conservation
NYS DOH	New York State Department of Health
OPCW	Office for the Prohibition of Chemical Weapons
OSHA	Occupational Safety and Health Administration
PHA	Public health advisory
PHL	Public health laboratory
PPE	Personal protective equipment
PTSD	Post-traumatic stress disorder
SAMHSA	Substance Abuse and Mental Health Services Administration
START	Strategic Arms Reduction Treaties
WHO	World Health Organization
WMD	Weapons of mass destruction
WTC	World Trade Center

Terrorism and Public Health

The public health response to September 11 and its aftermath

1

Challenges that terrorism poses to public health

BARRY S. LEVY AND VICTOR W. SIDEL

Terrorism adversely affects health in many ways. Public health professionals can do much both to minimize and to prevent the health consequences of terrorist acts and threats.

In Chinese, the word for "crisis" has two symbols: one stands for danger; the other, for opportunity. The "crisis" of terrorism presents not only dangers, but also opportunities in public health for strengthening systems and protecting people.

Terrorism can cause injury, illness, and death; create fear, anxiety, and other psychological reactions; destroy the physical infrastructure and social fabric of communities; and cause profound, adverse economic and political impacts on individuals, communities, nations, and our global society. Some responses to terrorism, however, can be harmful as well. Vengeful responses to terrorist acts or threats may hurt innocent people (see Box 3–2 in Chapter 3). Attempts to locate, interrogate, and punish suspected terrorists may threaten civil liberties domestically and international justice abroad (Chapters 17 and 19). And the U.S. government's diversion of resources from essential public health programs for homeland defense or the "war on terrorism" may lead to a worsening of health problems in the United States and to a reduction in U.S. health-program assistance to less-developed countries.

DEFINITIONS

Public health has been defined in many ways. In a particularly appropriate characterization, the Institute of Medicine, in its 1988 report *The Future of Public Health*, defined public health as "what we, as a society, do collectively to assure the conditions in which people can be healthy."[1] It takes a society to practice public health.

Terrorism has also been defined in many ways. In this book, we define *terrorism* as politically motivated violence or the threat of violence, especially against civilians, with the intent to instill fear. [We define *bioterrorism* as the use of, or threat to use, biological weapons for this purpose (Chapter 10).] Terrorism is intended to have psychological effects that reach beyond the immediate victims to intimidate a wider population, such as a rival ethnic or religious group, a national government or political party, or an entire country.[2] It is often designed to establish power where there is none or to consolidate power where there is little. While many countries, including the United States, differentiate terrorism from war—particularly a war formally declared by a nation–state, we see little difference between terrorism and a war directed in large part against civilian populations.

The term *terrorism* is "generally applied to one's enemies and opponents, or to those with whom one disagrees and would otherwise prefer to ignore."[2] What is called terrorism depends on one's point of view. The term implies a moral judgment; if one group can attach the term to its opponent, then it may have persuaded others to adopt its moral perspective.[3] In civil wars, revolutions, and other conflicts, those considered terrorists by one side are often considered "freedom fighters" by the other. In these situations, groups that have been relatively powerless, in comparison with very powerful foes, have often utilized terrorist tactics, believing these represented their only effective weapon against superior force. An analysis of 109 definitions of the term *terrorism* revealed that the most frequent definitional elements were the words *violence, force, political*, and *fear*. (Table 1–1).[4] Because of ambiguity in the use of the term, some organizations avoid its use in formal communication. (See also Chapter 19.)

Terrorism can be construed to encompass the use by nations of weapons designed to cause casualties among civilian populations. Examples include the bombing of Guernica, Spain, by Nazi forces in 1937, and, during World War II, the bombing of Warsaw, Rotterdam, London, Coventry, and other cities by Germany; the bombing of Dresden, Hamburg, and other cities by the Allies; the bombing of Tokyo and other Japanese cities by the United States; and the detonation of nuclear weapons at Hiroshima and Nagasaki by the United States (Chapter 12). There is controversy about whether these "acts of war" should also be considered terrorism.[5]

TABLE 1–1. Frequencies of Definitional Elements in 109 Definitions of Terrorism

ELEMENT	FREQUENCY (PERCENT)
Violence, force	84
Political	65
Fear, terror emphasized	51
Threat	47
(Psychological) effects and (anticipated) reactions	42
Victim–target differentiation	38
Purposive, planned, systematic, organized action	32
Method of combat, strategy, tactic	31
"Extranormality," in breach of accepted rules, without humanitarian constraints	30
Coercion, extortion, induction of compliance	28
Publicity aspect	22
Arbitrariness; impersonal, random character; indiscrimination	21
Civilians, noncombatants, neutrals, outsiders as victims	18
Intimidation	17
Innocence of victims emphasized	16
Group, movement, organization as perpetrator	14
Symbolic aspect, demonstration to others	14
Incalculability, unpredictability, unexpectedness of occurrence of violence	9
Clandestine, covert nature	9
Repetitiveness; serial or campaign character of violence	7
Criminal	6
Demands made on third parties	4

(Alex P. Schmid, Albert J. Jongman, et al. *Political Terrorism: A New Guide to Actors, Authors, Concepts, Data Bases, Theories, and Literature.* New Brunswick, Transaction Books, 1988, pp. 5–6.)

The terrorist bombings of the World Trade Center in 1993, the Alfred P. Murrah Federal Building in Oklahoma City in 1995, and U.S. military and diplomatic facilities abroad in the late 1990s awakened people in the United States to the reality of terrorism directed at U.S. targets at home and abroad. Before the 1990s, public concern about terrorism focused on the use of small arms and light weapons, explosives, and incendiaries (Chapter 9). Public concern about the use of biological, chemical, and nuclear weapons was then largely limited to their use by *nation-states* that had the capability to produce and deploy such weapons. During the 1990s, public concern broadened when the potential for terrorist attacks by *individuals and nongovernmental groups*, using a range of weapons, was widely publicized in the United States. This potential was based, in part, on evidence of the weaponization of biological and chemical agents by Iraq, allegations of weaponization of smallpox and

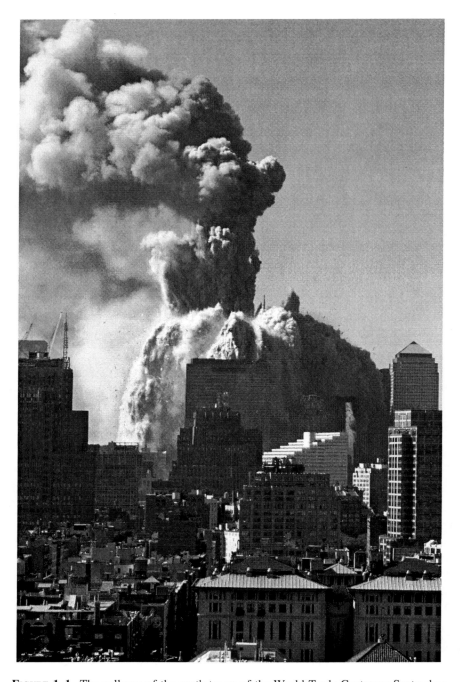

FIGURE 1–1. The collapse of the north tower of the World Trade Center on September 11, 2001 (Copyright Steve McCurry/Magnum Photos).

other biological agents by the Soviet Union and Russia, an intentional outbreak of salmonellosis in Oregon, and the use of the chemical nerve agent sarin in attacks in Japan (Chapters 10 and 11).

In the late 1990s, the U.S. government began developing and funding new programs for preparedness against terrorism, mainly in major U.S. metropolitan areas. These new initiatives involved health, safety, and other professionals in these metropolitan areas, and the Centers for Disease Control and Prevention (CDC), the National Institutes of Health (NIH), and other federal agencies; academic institutions; and some nongovernmental organizations.

THE TERRORIST EVENTS IN THE UNITED STATES IN 2001

The general public's and health professionals' concerns about terrorism on U.S. soil were tragically confirmed by the September 11 attacks on the World Trade Center (Figure 1–1) and the Pentagon (Figure 1–2), followed soon after by letters contaminated with anthrax spores that were mailed to two U.S. senators and several news-media organizations (Figure 1–3). These events highlighted the importance of public health professionals and their organizations, both in responding to these events and in helping to prepare for and

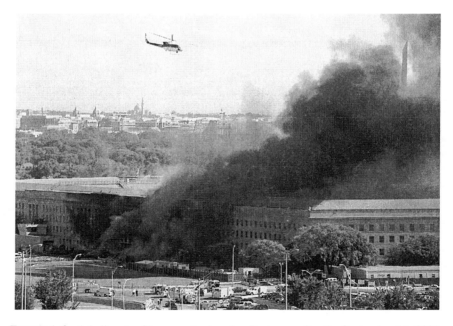

FIGURE 1–2. A helicopter flies over the burning Pentagon after the September 11, 2001, attack (AP/Wide World Photos).

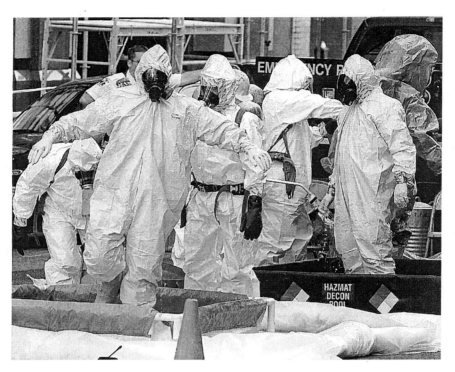

FIGURE 1–3. Hazardous materials' specialists are decontaminated after inspecting a suspicious letter in Trenton, N.J., in October 2001. The envelope contained an unknown white, powdery substance, but tests indicated it was harmless. Many suspicious letters were inspected after envelopes containing anthrax spores were sent to two U.S. senators and several news-media organizations (AP/Wide World Photos).

prevent future terrorist acts and threats. The involvement in this response, not only of public health professionals but also of others throughout society, underscored the fact that public health is what we, *as a society*, do collectively.

In response to the September 11 attacks, a range of public health and medical services were provided (Chapter 2). Emergency medical care was provided to injured survivors. Mental health services were provided to survivors of the attacks, victims' families, residents in nearby communities, and rescue and recovery workers (Chapter 3). Epidemiological surveillance was quickly established to help recognize adverse health effects of possible terrorist attacks with biological or chemical weapons. Environmental sampling was performed in lower Manhattan to assess the levels of contamination of asbestos and other hazardous substances that had resulted from the attacks and subsequent fires and collapse of buildings (Chapter 4). Occupational health and safety programs were established to help protect rescue and recovery workers (Chapter 5). Local, state, and federal public health agencies provided the public and health care providers with necessary information (Chapter 7). Governmental agencies, health care institutions, and nongovernmental organizations worked to coordinate the responses of government workers, health and safety professionals, and volunteers.

In response to the dissemination of anthrax, epidemiologists, environmental scientists, and others performed extensive investigations (Chapter 6). Health care providers diagnosed and treated those directly affected and provided prophylaxis and advice to thousands of others. Public health agencies provided information to the public and health professionals (Chapter 7 and Box 13–1 in Chapter 13). Specialists decontaminated postal service facilities, government buildings, and news-media offices.

These terrorist attacks led to much discussion of how health professionals can help minimize the health consequences of future terrorist acts and threats and help prevent them from occurring.

PREVENTION OF TERRORISM AND ITS CONSEQUENCES

The extent to which terrorist attacks or threats will occur in the future in the United States or elsewhere is not known. Based on past experience, terrorist attacks with small arms, explosives, and incendiaries are more likely than attacks with biological, chemical, or nuclear or radioactive weapons. The United States and other countries need to heighten their preparedness to meet these threats. (See Box 1–1.)

Public health professionals distinguish among primary, secondary, and tertiary levels of prevention, and use this framework in developing and implementing policies and programs. *Primary prevention* attempts to prevent disease or injury from occurring. Examples of primary prevention of terrorism include national laws and regulations to control the purchase and possession of small arms; international treaties to control the production, distribution, storage, and use of chemical weapons; and strategies to control, and ultimately eliminate, nuclear weapons.

Secondary prevention attempts to identify and control disease at an early, treatable stage. With regard to terrorism, examples of secondary prevention include physicians' and other health care providers' recognizing and treating the signs and symptoms of diseases that might be caused by terrorist use of biological or chemical agents, and screening asymptomatic individuals for evidence of exposure or subclinical infection with anthrax or other potential bioterrorist diseases, as deemed appropriate in specific bioterrorist events. Immunization against smallpox, anthrax, or other potential bioterrorist agents may be used for either primary or secondary prevention.

Box 1–1. Guiding Principles for a Public Health Response to Terrorism.

In order to prevent future acts of terrorism and their adverse public health consequences, the public health community should support policies and programs that:

1. Address poverty, social injustice, and health disparities that may contribute to the development of terrorism;
2. Provide humanitarian assistance to, and protect the human rights of, the civilian populations that are directly or indirectly affected by terrorism;
3. Advocate the speedy end of the armed conflict in Afghanistan and promote nonviolent means of conflict resolution;
4. Strengthen the public health infrastructure (which includes workforce, laboratory, and information systems) and other components of the public health system (including education, research, and the faith community) to increase the ability to identify, respond to, and prevent problems of public health importance, including the health aspects of terrorist attacks;
5. Ensure availability of, and accessibility to, health care, including medications and vaccines, for individuals exposed, infected, made ill, or injured in terrorist attacks;
6. Educate and inform health professionals and the public to better identify, respond to, and prevent the health consequences of terrorism, and promote the visibility and availability of health professionals in the communities that they serve;
7. Address mental health needs of populations that are directly or indirectly affected by terrorism;
8. Assure the protection of the environment, the food and water supply, and the health and safety of rescue and recovery professionals;
9. Assure clarification of the roles, relationships, and responsibilities among public health agencies, law enforcement, and first responders;
10. Prevent hate crimes and ethnic, racial, and religious discrimination, including profiling; promote cultural competence, diversity training, and dialogue among people; and protect human rights and civil liberties;
11. Advocate the immediate control and ultimate elimination of biological, chemical, and nuclear weapons; and
12. Build and sustain the public health capacity to develop systems to collect data about the health and mental health consequences of terrorism and other disasters on victims, responders, and communities, and develop uniform definitions and standardized data-classification systems of death and injury resulting from terrorism and other disasters.

(Statement adopted by the Governing Council of the American Public Health Association, October 2001.)

Tertiary prevention attempts to prevent disabling consequences of disease or injury by helping individuals regain their optimal level of function after a disease or injury and accompanying damage has already occurred. With regard to terrorism, examples of tertiary prevention include treatment and rehabilitation of individuals who have been seriously burned or otherwise injured by a terrorist bomb, and treatment and supportive care of persons affected by chemicals during a terrorist attack.

Of these three levels of prevention, primary prevention has the greatest human appeal and is the most effective from a cost-benefit perspective. For example, effective immunizations against a potential bioterrorist agent before the attack occurs may be more cost-effective than immunizing or treating people after they have been exposed or become ill. The efficacy and safety of specific immunizations and immunization programs need to be carefully evaluated, however; for some programs, adverse reactions and other costs may outweigh the potential benefits.

MAJOR CHALLENGES OF TERRORISM FOR PUBLIC HEALTH

Improving Public Health System Capabilities to Respond to Health Consequences of Terrorist Acts

The possibility of future threats or acts of terrorism requires strengthening of the public health system in the United States. Although the system functioned reasonably well in 2001 (Chapters 2–6), public health agencies, especially state and local health departments, have suffered from decades of underfunding—perhaps as a result of the success of public health in reducing the occurrence of many illnesses and injuries and in helping to increase life expectancy. These agencies need to be more adequately supported, and improved in many areas (Chapter 13). Epidemiology, surveillance, and laboratory capabilities need to be improved by increasing the number and improving the competencies of epidemiologists and laboratory scientists and by more adequately funding laboratory facilities (Chapter 14). The surge capacity of medical care facilities needs to be increased. The effectiveness, safety, and availability of vaccines, antimicrobials, and antitoxins for bioterrorist agents need to be upgraded through more intensive research (Chapter 15) and improved supply systems. Mental health capabilities also need to be improved (Chapter 3), and the general public, health professionals, and policymakers need to be made more aware of their importance. Environmental and occupational health capabilities (Chapters 4 and 5) need to be strengthened with planning for better coordination of responses after terrorist attacks. Better protection of food and water supplies and the ambient air is needed (Chapter 16). We also need better ways of communicating with the public as well as of mobilizing and coordinating the vast resources of public volunteers and civil-society organizations (Chapter 7).

Strengthening the public health system's capacity to respond to terrorism will strengthen some of its capabilities in dealing with other problems of public health importance. For example, improving the surveillance, epidemiology, and laboratory capabilities of state and local health departments to address terrorism will have beneficial effects on their abilities to address other problems of public health importance.

Yet, public health professionals should be aware that responding to and developing preparedness for terrorism may

- Shift attention and divert critically needed human, financial, and other resources away from other important public health needs, adversely affecting the health and well-being of individuals and communities. There is already evidence of this, with major new funding being made available for bioterrorism preparedness while substantial funds are being cut from budgets for necessary public health programs and services.
- Require public health professionals and their organizations to work with the military, police, and other law enforcement and investigatory agencies in ways that may compromise their trust with the communities they serve and their freedom to communicate important public health information.
- Compromise the civil rights and human rights of individuals and organizations (Chapters 17 and 19).[6]

Controlling Terrorist Weapons

Terrorist weapons include small arms, explosives, and incendiaries (Chapter 9); biological weapons (Chapter 10); chemical weapons (Chapter 11); and nuclear, radiological, and related weapons (Chapter 12). Approaches to controlling these weapons include development and implementation of (a) national, state, and local laws and regulations to control the trade, sale, possession, and use of small arms as well as access to materials that can be used in bombs and incendiaries; and (b) international treaties and regulations to control biological, chemical, and nuclear weapons. Health professionals can help document the adverse health impact of these weapons and advocate their control.

Addressing Factors That May Breed Terrorism

Many different factors can lead to the development of terrorism and the recruitment of would-be terrorists, including historical, political, economic, social, philosophical, ideological, religious, and psychological factors (Chapter 18). Health professionals can help contribute to a better understanding of these factors and help address them and their underlying causes, which include gross disparities in health status and access to health services within the United States and among the countries of the world.

ROLES OF HEALTH PROFESSIONALS

Health professionals have a variety of roles with regard to terrorism, including:

Responding to Health Consequences of Terrorist Acts and Threats

Diagnosing and reporting

Diagnose illnesses and injuries caused by biological or chemical agents and to report these cases immediately to their state and local health departments. Many of the diseases and injuries caused by these agents are rare and may cause nonspecific signs and symptoms. Health care providers need to educate themselves about these diseases and injuries, their clinical presentation, and methods of confirming (or ruling out) diagnoses. They also need to have a low threshold for requesting clinical and public-health consultation when they encounter patients with suspicious illnesses or injuries.

Providing primary preventive measures

Educate their patients and the communities they serve about primary preventive measures—including use of appropriate vaccines, prophylactic antimicrobials, and antitoxins, and avoidance of certain high-risk activities or contacts. Recommending and administering these measures when appropriate should specifically be part of public health and medical care responsibilities.

Preventing secondary spread of disease

Educate people about specific measures to prevent secondary spread of disease among household and other close contacts of an affected person, and recommend and administer these measures when appropriate.

Assisting in the investigation of outbreaks of disease

Assist epidemiologists and others in their investigations of bioterrorist outbreaks when they occur.

Discouraging inappropriate responses

Discourage people from taking actions that may be unsafe or counterproductive, such as hoarding antibiotics or purchasing gas masks.

Developing Improved Preparedness for Future Terrorist Acts or Threats

Educating the public and other health professionals

Educate their patients, the general public, and other health professionals about the health consequences of terrorism and about prudent measures that can be undertaken to prevent or mitigate these consequences. It is challenging to inform and warn the public without creating undue alarm (Figure 1–4).

Participating in preparedness planning

Help improve preparedness for terrorist attacks by participating in the development or improvement of local, state, or national preparedness training. Effective preparedness has the potential to improve the treatment of injured individuals and to save lives, and to provide improved support for victims and their families. Effective preparedness can also assure communities and the nation as a whole that emergency and longer-term services will be provided in response to terrorist acts or threats. Some preparedness planning can improve the overall infrastructure for public health and medical care and the ability to respond to other emergency and long-term problems.

Evaluating preparedness policies and programs

Critically evaluate preparedness policies and programs and previous responses to the health consequences of terrorism, so that these policies and programs can be made more appropriate in the future.

Taking Actions to Help Prevent Terrorism

Helping reduce access to biological agents that can be used as bioterrorist weapons

Health professionals, especially those working in clinical or research laboratory settings, may be able to help restrict access to potential bioterrorist weapons and to equipment that could be used in refining these weapons or producing them in large quantities for possible bioterrorist use.

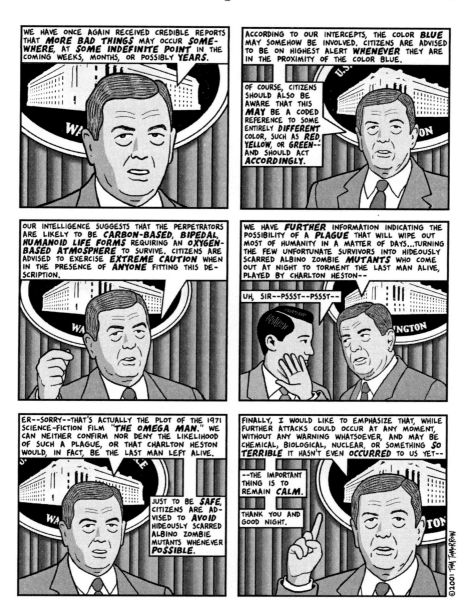

FIGURE 1–4. Informing and warning the public (Copyright 2001 by Tom Tomorrow).

Advocating the control, reduction, and elimination of weapons of mass destruction

A serious attempt to prevent terrorism must include measures to control weapons of mass destruction and ultimately eliminate them. For example, health professionals should advocate the reversal by the United States of its unilateral rejection of the international community's recent attempts to strengthen the Biological Weapons Convention with strong inspection and verification protocols. As with nuclear weapons, the best civil defense can never really offer protection from truly catastrophic scenarios. Real biological security can only come from merging the best global controls over weapons technologies with the commitment to eradication of specific diseases worldwide. Similarly, health professionals can advocate strengthening international treaties to control, and ultimately eliminate, chemical and nuclear weapons. (See Chapters 10–12.)

Promoting a Balance Between Response to Terrorism and to Other Public Health Concerns

Maintaining support for other public health priorities

Health professionals must maintain and strengthen support for other public health priorities. For example, more than 400,000 people in the United States die each year of tobacco-related disease, and another 100,000 die of alcohol-related disease. Hundreds of thousands suffer from HIV/AIDS. There are approximately 30,000 gun-related deaths in the United States each year. Attention to these urgent problems by public health professionals, policymakers, and the general public should not be diverted.

Promoting the Protection of Civil Rights and Human Rights

Health professionals can help promote the protection of civil rights and other human rights of individuals in the United States and in other countries (Chapters 17 and 19). They can also promote the prevention of military measures in the "war on terrorism" that may cause hundreds of casualties among civilians, as have already occurred among many civilians in Afghanistan as a result of U.S. airstrikes.[7]

CONCLUSION

Terrorism is a threat to public health and to society as a whole. Health professionals can do much to mitigate the health consequences of terrorist threats or acts, and to help prevent them. Preventing terrorism and its health consequences should be in the curricula of schools of public health, medicine, nursing, and other health fields and disciplines. Health professionals of all types need to learn more about terrorism and their roles in addressing it. At the same time, health professionals must maintain and promote a balanced perspective that gives terrorism preparedness an appropriate priority amidst the many other health problems people suffer from as well as the underlying societal factors that contribute to the development of these health problems. While public health departments in the United States are receiving large amounts of categorical funding for bioterrorism preparedness, these same departments are losing money for programs that address current public health problems because of the economic crises of state and local governments.[8]

How public health professionals respond to the current terrorist crisis could have a profound impact on the future of public health. Precedents that are set now will probably influence many aspects of public health in the years to come, including the availability and distribution of human, financial, and other resources for public health; the organization of public health and its relationships to the military, police, and other enforcement and regulatory agencies; the roles of communities and nongovernmental organizations in influencing governmental decisions concerning terrorism and the response to it; policies and programs to control weapons of mass destruction; and even the future occurrence of terrorist acts and threats. The Governing Council of the American Public Health Association, in October 2001, approved guiding principles for a public health response to terrorism (see Box 1–1). Public health values, such as promotion of health; prevention of disease, injury, disability, and premature death; support of human rights and social justice; and visionary and leadership by public health professionals will continue to be critically important as we address the dangers of terrorism.

REFERENCES

1. Institute of Medicine. *The Future of Public Health.* Washington, DC: National Academy of Sciences, 1988.
2. Hoffman B. *Inside Terrorism.* New York: Columbia University Press, 1998.
3. Jenkins BM. *The Study of Terrorism: Definitional Problems.* Santa Monica, CA: RAND Corporation, P-6563, December 1980.
4. Schmid AP, Jongman AJ, et al. *Political Terrorism: A New Guide to Actors, Authors, Concepts, Data Bases, Theories, and Literature.* New Brunswick, NJ: Transaction Books, 1998, pp. 5–6.
5. Geiger HJ. "The Impact of War on Human Rights." In: Levy BS, Sidel VW (eds). *War and Public Health.* New York: Oxford University Press, 1997, pp. 39–50.
6. Annas GJ. Bioterrorism, public health, and civil liberties. N Engl J Med 2002;346: 1337–1342.
7. Filkins D. Flaws in U.S. air war left hundreds of civilians dead. *New York Times,* July 21, 2002.
8. Elliott vs. Public health funding: Feds giveth but the states taketh away. *AMA News,* October 28, 2002. Available at: http://www.ama-assn.org/sci-pubs/amnews/pick_02/hll21028.htm.

BACKGROUND READINGS

Terrorism

Bodansky Y. *Bin Laden: The Man Who Declared War on America.* Roseville, CA: Prima Publishing, 1999.

Carr C. *Lessons of Terror: A History of Warfare Against Civilians: Why It Has Always Failed, and Why It Will Fail Again.* New York: Random House, 2002.

Chomsky N. *The Culture of Terrorism.* Boston: South End Press, 1988.

Chomsky N. *9-11.* New York: Seven Stories Press, 2001.

Cooley JK. *Unholy Wars: Afghanistan, America and International Terrorism.* London: Pluto Press, 1999.

Heymann PB. *Terrorism and America: A Commonsense Strategy for a Democratic Society.* Cambridge, Mass.: MIT Press, 1998.

Hoge JF Jr, Rose G. (Editors). *How Did This Happen? Terrorism and the New War.* New York: Public Affairs, 2001.

Kushner HW. (Editor). *The Future of Terrorism: Violence in the New Millennium.* Thousand Oaks, CA: Sage Publications, 1998.

Laqueur W. *A History of Terrorism.* New Brunswick, NJ: Transaction Publishers, 2001

Lifton RJ. *Destroying the World to Save It: Aum Shinrikyo, Apocalyptic Violence, and the New Global Terrorism.* New York: Henry Holt and Company, 1999.

Miller J, Engelberg S, Broad W. *Germs: Biological Weapons and America's Secret War.* New York: Simon & Schuster, 2001.

Reich W (Editor). *The Origins of Terrorism: Psychologies, Ideologies, Theologies, States of Mind.* Washington, DC: Woodrow Wilson Center Press, 1990.

Zinn H. *Terrorism and War.* New York: Seven Stories Press, 2002.

The Response of Health and Safety Professionals to Terrorism

Henderson DA, Inglesby TV, O'Toole T. *Bioterrorism: Guidelines for Medical and Public Health Management.* Chicago: AMA Press, 2002.

The Second National Symposium on Medical and Public Health Response to Bioterrorism: Public Health Emergency and National Security Threat. *Public Health Reports* 2001; 116(Suppl 2):1–118.

Bevelacqua A, Stilp R. *Terrorism Handbook for Operational Responders.* Albany, NY: Delmar Publishers, 1998.

Maniscalco PM, Christen HT. *Understanding Terrorism and Managing the Consequences.* Upper Saddle River, NJ: Prentice Hall, 2002.

Landesman LY. *Public Health Management of Disasters: The Practice Guide (with an Epilogue on the September 11, 2001, Tragedy).* Washington, DC: APHA, 2001.

Institute of Medicine, National Research Council. *Chemical and Biological Terrorism: Research and Development to Improve Civilian Medical Response.* Washington, DC: National Academy Press, 1999.

Sifton DW (Editor). *PDR Guide to Biological and Chemical Warfare Response.* Montvale, NJ: Thomson/Physicians' Desk Reference, 2002.

2

The public health response to the World Trade Center disaster

TIMOTHY H. HOLTZ, JESSICA LEIGHTON, SHARON BALTER, DON WEISS, SUSAN BLANK, AND ISAAC WEISFUSE

The attack on the World Trade Center (WTC) complex on September 11, 2001, caused the single largest loss of civilian life from an act of terrorism on American soil. It was also one of the largest human-generated technological disasters faced by a local, state, or federal public health system.[1] The sudden, unexpected loss of 2,617 lives, including first responders, sent the New York City (NYC) Department of Health (DOH) into an emergency response phase that lasted for more than one month. The presence of an emergency preparedness plan, with predetermined committees and team leaders, enabled the DOH to respond to both the immediate and the longer-term impacts of the disaster.[2]

The DOH response to the WTC disaster shifted with time. Initially, it consisted of providing care and triage for injured persons, providing shelter to displaced persons, assessing the threat to routine health services, assessing hospital staffing and resource needs for responding to substantial numbers of casualties, commencing environmental health sampling and coordination, and performing a rapid epidemiological assessment of injuries. Within days after the attack, priorities shifted to worker-injury surveillance and injury prevention; surveillance for bioterrorism; environmental health concerns due to building collapse and fires; ensuring food and water safety; rodent and vector control; and educating the public regarding the health implications of decomposing human remains and building collapse.

In this chapter, we outline the process of emergency preparedness by the NYC DOH, the initial response to the disaster, the challenges posed to those addressing environmental health concerns, and the four distinct surveillance activities implemented despite logistical challenges. We also review key issues in the response that stemmed from a preliminary evaluation performed by senior DOH staff one month after the terrorist attacks. We believe that the NYC DOH response to the WTC disaster provides guidance to improve our preparedness for future public health disasters, whether natural or intentional.

PREPAREDNESS OF THE NYC DOH

Emergency response capabilities of the NYC DOH evolved in the late 1990s. Historically, the Department did not see itself as a front-line emergency response agency. This changed with the growing understanding of the role of public health in emergency situations. The creation of the Mayor's Office of Emergency Management (OEM) in 1996, charged with coordinating emergency response in NYC, accelerated the change process. From the outset, OEM leaders recognized the significance of minimizing morbidity and mortality during any emergency and saw the critical role of the DOH in emergency preparedness. The NYC DOH was a core participant in citywide emergency preparedness activities, including staffing the OEM incident command center located at 7 WTC during heat waves, snow storms, and other extreme climatic events; actively participating in citywide emergency planning; and participating in simulated exercises and drills.

Two other events influenced the NYC DOH approach to emergencies. The 1999 West Nile virus outbreak made the NYC DOH, for the first time, the lead agency in responding to an emergency.[3] Emergency activities included starting active citywide surveillance for a new pathogen, enhancing communication with providers, setting up telephone hotlines for providers and concerned citizens, applying larvicides to control mosquito populations, monitoring the health effects of larvicide use, and creating a speakers' bureau to discuss the outbreak with community groups. The second event was planning the Year 2000 celebration, which started soon after the first West Nile virus outbreak concluded in the fall of 1999. DOH leaders realized that a larger organizational structure dedicated to emergency preparedness and response was required to respond to potential public health concerns in the event of a terrorist attack or disruption of electrical power. The position of Emergency Preparedness Coordinator and standing committees comprising senior agency personnel were created to plan for emergencies. Year 2000 planning also allowed the Department to practice with backup communication systems, such as 800-megahertz radios, which became critical in the aftermath of the WTC disaster.

As of 2000, seven emergency preparedness committees existed in the NYC DOH: surveillance, medical/clinical, sheltering, environmental, laboratories, operations, and management information systems (MIS). In addition, an emergency operations center, with an incident command system (ICS) structure, was created, with roles and responsibilities for all senior management and committees during an emergency. Committee leaders met monthly as a group, and quarterly update meetings were held for all group members as well as others involved in emergencies.

The NYC DOH needed to communicate its new emergency roles and responsibilities to its employees. In the spring of 2001, a letter was sent to all DOH staff by the Commissioner of Health explaining the DOH's role in emergencies. The DOH also established a relationship with the Center for Public Health Preparedness at the Mailman School of Public Health at Columbia University. This center provided technical advice to the Emergency Preparedness Coordinator, and trained 745 school health nurses in August 2001 regarding emergency concerns.

EVENTS OF SEPTEMBER 11, 2001

September 11 was a clear, late-summer day in New York. At 8:46 a.m., at the height of the morning rush hour, a hijacked Boeing 767, with 92 passengers and crew members aboard, crashed into floors 93 through 98 of 1 World Trade Center (WTC). For minutes, a stunned city attempted to determine whether it was an accident or a malicious act. Occupants of 1 WTC rushed to the emergency exits, while hundreds of persons above the crash site were trapped by the ensuing fire. Occupants of 2 WTC began to evacuate their building as well. When a second Boeing 767 airliner, with 65 passengers and crew members aboard, crashed into floors 78 through 84 of 2 WTC at 9:02 a.m., the purpose and magnitude of the attack on the 110-story buildings were apparent.

Hundreds of NYC fire, police, and rescue teams rushed to the scene from throughout the city's five boroughs and entered the burning buildings to organize the evacuation. Thousands of building occupants were guided to plaza exits by these first responders. As the evacuation continued, the fires, ignited by burning jet fuel, heated the interior of the steel-frame buildings, causing the floor support joints to weaken. At 9:59 a.m., 2 WTC collapsed in an imploding column of smoke, dust, and debris as the weight of the floors above the fires produced an accordion effect below. Thirty minutes later, as the evacuations continued, 1 WTC collapsed (Figure 1–1).

Injured and noninjured survivors from the WTC evacuation and building collapse fled in all directions from lower Manhattan Island (Figure 2–1). Thousands of people escaped the island to Brooklyn and New Jersey across bridges and on boats, while most others made their way northward in Manhattan on foot. Injured persons were evaluated in hospitals throughout the city, although a limited number of major casualties were treated. No major health-care facility was destroyed in the attack; thus, the therapeutic capacity of local medical care services was not interrupted or overwhelmed. Hundreds of volunteer medical personnel from throughout the city flocked to the neighborhoods near the disaster site to search for survivors; fewer than 10 survivors were found.

In total, 343 New York City firefighters, 23 police, and three emergency rescue crewmen were killed, as well as 37 security guards and Port Authority of New York and New Jersey personnel and one New Jersey firefighter who stayed behind to assist them. The fires continued to burn the entire WTC complex. Eventually, all seven buildings were destroyed or damaged beyond repair (Figure 2–2).

As of April 2002, there were 2,617 people listed as dead as a result of the WTC attack. An independent investigation determined that at the floor of the crash site and above in 1 WTC, approximately 1,360 people died and none

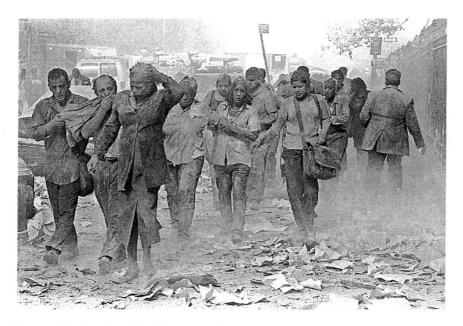

FIGURE 2–1. People make their way amid debris near the World Trade Center approximately 1 hour and 40 minutes after the first attack (AP/Wide World Photos).

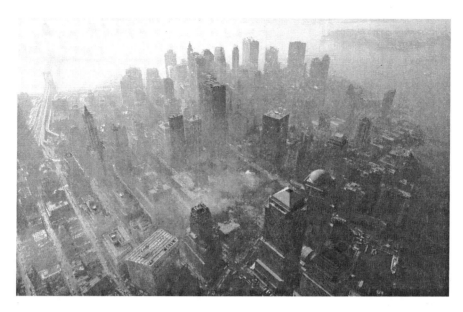

FIGURE 2–2. Aerial view of devastation at the World Trade Center site as it appeared on October 4, 2001 (Photograph by Andrea Booher/FEMA News Photo).

survived. Below the crash site, 72 people died and more than 4,000 survived. In 2 WTC, only four of the 600 who died there worked below the floors of the crash site.[4] Credited with making the evacuation successful were widened stairwells, back-up power, and having an emergency evacuation plan that was frequently rehearsed.

Data based on 2,617 death certificates filed with the DOH Office of Vital Records through January 25, 2002, describe the demographics of the victims.[5] A plurality of victims were young men between the ages of 35 to 39 years. Sixty percent of victims were listed as non-Hispanic white males, with another 15 percent non-Hispanic white females. Nine percent of victims were Hispanic, 8 percent were black, and 6 percent were Asian. Forty-three percent of victims were residents of New York City, another 21 percent were residents elsewhere in New York State, and 25 percent were residents of New Jersey. While only 1 percent were residents of foreign countries, 20 percent were born in one of 115 countries other than the United States (Table 2–1). All but 65 were at work when they were killed. Only nine deaths occurred after September 11.

INITIAL PUBLIC HEALTH RESPONSE

The NYC DOH activated the Emergency Operations Center (EOC) within 30 minutes after the attacks. The EOC Coordinator activated the emergency response protocol, mobilizing the seven emergency committees that would

TABLE 2–1. WTC Disaster Deaths, by Birthplace (Preliminary Data, Reported by January 25, 2002).

COUNTRY OF BIRTH	NUMBER
United States	2,106
United Kingdom	53
India	34
Dominican Republic	25
Jamaica	21
Japan	20
China	18
Colombia	18
Canada	16
Germany	16
Philippines	16
Trinidad and Tobago	15
Guyana	14
Ecuador	13
Italy	13
Ukraine	11
Korea	9
Poland	8
Russia	8
Haiti	7
Ireland	7
Pakistan	7
Taiwan	7
Cuba	6
Yugoslavia	6
Other	143
Total	2,617

(Office of Vital Statistics.[5])

function within the ICS structure for the next month. The Commissioner of Health and the liaison to the NYC OEM, after being briefly caught up in the evacuation from 7 WTC (which burned down and collapsed at 5:00 p.m. on September 11), relocated to the new OEM command center to coordinate the response with other city agencies. Because of the proximity of DOH central offices to the WTC (5 to 10 blocks away), DOH staff members evacuated their offices; fortunately, none was injured.

The EOC responded to immediate needs on September 11. Although the main DOH building is not a clinical care facility, casualties began arriving before 10:00 a.m. DOH physicians, nurses, and other personnel created and staffed a makeshift triage center and acute-care clinic. Within the first 6 hours of operations, approximately 45 persons were triaged, with problems ranging from chest pain, corneal abrasions, and anxiety; to more serious injuries, such as limb fractures, respiratory distress from smoke and dust inhalation, and severe anxiety. Persons were transported to acute-care facilities as needed, although no one was critically ill.

The sheltering plan was activated on September 11, in conjunction with the American Red Cross. Twelve sites were initially opened, all in school buildings. School health nurses were called in to staff each site, provide basic medical care, and provide referral services for those requiring medical attention. The school health program master-staff list was used to assure that staff members were available for continued coverage of the shelters and other emergency needs, such as picking up schoolchildren stranded by the disaster. Persons made homeless by the disaster, including tourists and those in residential areas adjacent to the WTC site, were housed in 11 shelters in schools and buildings in Manhattan and Staten Island. At the peak level of service, 140 persons were staying in DOH shelters nightly. Approximately 130 DOH public health nurses were involved in staffing the shelters 24 hours per day in 12-hour shifts for the next 12 days. In addition, hotels throughout the city opened their doors to displaced families and recovery workers in the weeks after the disaster.

EOC leaders recognized the need for essential public health services to continue uninterrupted. During the evening of September 11, the vital records department moved to an upper Manhattan DOH site, where it communicated daily with the Office of the Chief Medical Examiner to issue death certificates and burial permits for recovered bodies. Funeral directors were notified of the relocation that night by telephone. Later, for bodies that were not recovered, a court decision was necessary to determine death rather than mandating that families wait 3 years for missing-persons' death certificates.

On September 12, lost telephone service in lower Manhattan (crucial telephone cables were destroyed in the fire) disrupted electronic mail capability, and difficult transportation problems in lower Manhattan forced the EOC to evacuate the lower Manhattan DOH buildings and relocate to the NYC Public Health Laboratory building, where temporary quarters were created for all seven emergency response committees. This was the first time in history the DOH had to to leave its 10-floor, 1935-era building.

Persons affected by the disaster needed to receive reliable information regarding health concerns related to the disaster and where to go to access medical and mental health services (see Chapter 7). An emergency public health hotline number was distributed to media outlets, with DOH staff members answering the phones 24 hours a day. The LifeNet Hotline for mental health counseling was also established on September 12, in English, Spanish, and Chinese.

Distributing accurate information to health-care providers, the general public, and rescue and recovery workers was an early priority for the DOH. The surveillance committee sent regular broadcast fax and electronic mail alerts to emergency department personnel, infection control nurses, and staff members of infectious disease laboratories regarding health concerns related to the disaster, bioterrorism surveillance, and vaccine availability (Table 2–2).[6] The CDC's Health Alert Network augmented these activities by distributing information to local health officials regarding incident response and technical problems. The DOH sent public health advisories and press releases concerning the low risk for disease from decomposing human remains, exposure to bloodborne pathogens among workers at the site, and air quality, to address concerns raised by recovery workers and residents of lower Manhattan (Table 2–2). Later advisories discussed the need to use wet methods, such as wet mopping, or high-efficiency particulate air (HEPA) vacuuming to clean homes and businesses, how to commence reoccupation, and air-quality issues (Box 2–1).

Soon after the disaster, reports were received that special-needs populations, such as the elderly and persons with acquired immunodeficiency syndrome (AIDS), living south of 14th Street were having problems accessing services. This interruption was caused by blocked streets, closed pharmacies, and lack of transportation. The New York State (NYS) AIDS Institute performed a needs assessment with DOH assistance, which resulted in local agencies' becoming involved in ensuring that necessary services were delivered.

The surveillance committee initiated multiple surveillance systems on September 11. The initial system generated data regarding emergency department visits for acute injuries sustained from the attack. The DOH sent staff members to four lower-Manhattan hospitals to conduct chart review and perform emergency-department log abstraction. A citywide hospital needs assessment was initiated in conjunction with the Greater New York Hospital Association (GNYHA). It eventually encompassed 62 acute-care hospitals to ensure the continuation of bed availability, supplies, vaccine stock, and the collection of information on the number of deaths, WTC-related emergency-department visits, and morgue capacity. Prospective surveillance for unusual disease clusters and bioterrorism-related events, and injury surveillance for recovery workers were begun 2 days after the attack.

Risks posed by asbestos to volunteers and workers at the WTC site were immediate concerns (see Chapter 4). Asbestos had been used for fireproofing in the construction of 1 WTC (North Tower) through the 40th floor, and also in the elevator shafts.[7] Sampling for asbestos, dioxin, benzene, and other substances commenced within 2 days after the attack. The DOH worked with the U.S. Environmental Protection Agency (EPA), the NYC Department of

Environmental Protection (DEP), and the NYS Department of Environmental Conservation (DEC) to position air monitors throughout the WTC site. On September 11 and September 13, the DOH evaluated ash samples from locations in and around the WTC site for radiological activity. Radiation was not detected above background levels. In addition, the DOH confirmed the existence of radiological material licenses for two companies that had used industrial nickel-63 for gas chromatograph machines that had been located in the WTC. The U.S. Department of Energy (DOE) began testing debris around the site on September 15 and performed aerial assessments on September 19 and 24, checking for sources of radiation in the debris. None was found at the WTC site, nor at the Fresh Kills landfill on Staten Island, where WTC debris was taken.

On the federal level, the Federal Response Plan (Figure 2–3) was immediately activated, allowing the U.S. Department of Health and Human Services (DHHS) to release federal resources under Emergency Support Function 8 (Health and Medical). Despite an air travel ban, an air shipment of intravenous supplies, bandages, dressings, respiratory support supplies, and medications arrived on the night of September 11, including the first emergency mobilization of the National Pharmaceutical Stockpile (NPS).

In addition, the U.S. government activated the National Disaster Medical System, a federally coordinated system of emergency medical teams that can be deployed immediately to provide medical attention to victims and rescue workers. Four Disaster Medical Assistance Teams (DMATs), consisting of 35 persons each, arrived in New York on September 11 from as far away as Long Beach, California. These DMATs set up in four quadrants around the disaster site and maintained a 24-hour presence there for two months after the disaster. They became crucial for collecting information regarding rescue and recovery worker safety and health (see Chapter 5). DHHS also dispatched seven Disaster Mortuary Operational Response Teams, with morticians, anthropologists, and forensic scientists who are trained to identify bodies in mass-casualty situations.

The Centers for Disease Control and Prevention (CDC) sent five epidemiologists with the NPS, who were soon followed by additional epidemiologists, occupational health specialists, and industrial hygienists to assist with the recovery effort.[8] In total, more than 100 CDC staff members and Epidemic Intelligence Service (EIS) officers worked in New York during the next two months. Other federally coordinated responses established after the attacks included counseling through the Substance Abuse and Mental Health Services Administration; Veterinary Medical Assistance Teams to care for search-and-rescue dogs; and Medicare and Medicaid personnel to assist residents of lower Manhattan having difficulty accessing services.

TABLE 2–2. Public Health Advisories (PHAs), Broadcast Fax Alerts, and Press Releases Issued by the New York City (NYC) Department of Health (DOH) and Department of Mental Health (DMH) after the World Trade Center (WTC) Disaster, 2001.

DATE	TYPE	SUBJECT/TITLE
Sept. 12	Broadcast fax alert #1 to hospitals and emergency departments	Bioterrorism surveillance, acute hospital needs, reporting fatal cases, handling corpses, smoke and dust advisory, tetanus/diphtheria (Td) vaccine availability
	PHA	Air quality, dust, asbestos and health concerns in the affected area of the WTC disaster
	Press release	Mental Health Hotline (LifeNet) established to assist those experiencing emotional crisis or distress in the aftermath of the WTC disaster
Sept. 13	Broadcast fax alert #2 to hospitals and emergency departments	DOH relocation, asbestos and dust advisory, bioterrorism surveillance, reporting fatal cases, mental health needs, rescue worker exposures to body fluids, West Nile virus testing, Td vaccine availability
Sept. 14	Press releases	NYC DOH headquarters temporarily relocates, DOH operations continue
		U.S. Department of Health and Human Services sends 35 members of the CDC Epidemic Intelligence Service to NYC
	Work alert	DOH employee instructions on work, pay, activities
Sept. 16	PHA and press release	Health of rescue personnel, public safety and decomposing human remains, what to do for possible exposure to bloodborne pathogens
Sept. 17	Broadcast fax alert #3 to hospitals and emergency departments	Health risk from decomposing human remains, air quality and environmental risks, infectious disease surveillance, reporting fatal cases, West Nile virus testing, Td vaccine availability
	PHA and press release	Recommendations for people re-occupying commercial buildings and residents re-entering their homes

Date	Communication	Content
Sept. 18	Press releases and PHA	DOH asks restauranteurs of closed restaurants below Chambers St. in Manhattan to allow health officials access to conduct inspections Following the WTC disaster, the NYC DMH provides services to those in need
Sept. 21	Press release	West Nile virus update
Sept. 22	Press releases	Vital records update: How to obtain birth and death certificates during the WTC disaster response DOH distributes health recommendations for residential and commercial re-occupation
Sept. 24	Broadcast fax alert #4 to hospitals and emergency departments	Bioterrorism and infectious disease surveillance, health risk from decomposing human remains, acute stress disorders, asbestos and dust advisory, reporting fatal cases, West Nile virus testing, Td vaccine availability, immunization registry
Sept. 25	Press releases and PHA	Operators of closed restaurants near the collapsed towers are asked to allow health officials access for inspections DOH, Office of the Chief Medical Examiner, and Office of the Criminal Justice Coordinator expedite death certificates for families who request them
Oct. 5	Broadcast fax alert #6 to hospitals and emergency departments	Anthrax case in Florida, recommendations for antibiotic prophylaxis and anthrax vaccination in NYC, disease surveillance, acute stress disorders

Box 2–1. Recommendations for People Re-occupying Commercial Buildings and Residents Re-entering Their Homes.

What steps should I take upon returning to my workplace or home? If you were evacuated from a residence or workplace south of Warren Street, west of Broadway, and north of Exchange Street, and have been approved to resume tenancy by your building manager, you are advised to wear a dust mask upon entering this area to decrease the possibility of dust inhalation and throat irritation. Outside these boundaries, masks are not necessary, but may be worn for your own comfort. If there is dust present indoors, it should not be necessary to wear this mask if you following the cleaning procedures detailed below.

In a workplace, speak to your supervisor to see if there are special startup and cleaning procedures. In very dusty places, clean-up may be necessary before equipment can be restarted. Follow the cleaning procedures discussed below.

In your home, you should first make sure that conditions are safe. You should enter your home dressed in a long sleeve shirt and pants, and with closed shoes. Upon entry:

- Check for the smell of gas. If the apartment smells of gas, leave immediately and report it to your building manager and to Con Edison.
- Check for broken glass and fixtures. Wrap any broken glass in paper and mark it "broken glass." If large pieces of glass are broken, ask your building superintendent for instructions on disposal.
- Run hot and cold water from each of the taps for at least two minutes, or until water runs complete clean.
- Flush toilets until bowls are refilled. For air pressure systems, you may need to flush several times. If there are any problems with the toilet or plumbing system, call a plumber—do not try to fix the problem yourself.
- Follow the cleaning procedures discussed below.

I have heard that asbestos was released from the collapse of the World Trade Center. What are the health effects of asbestos? Because some asbestos was used in the building of the World Trade Center, City, State, and Federal agencies have been collecting dust, debris, and air samples since the World Trade Center collapse. As expected, some asbestos was found in a few of the dust and debris samples taken from the blast site and individuals working in this area have been advised to take precautions. However, most of the air samples taken have been below levels of concern. Based on the asbestos test results received thus far, there are no significant health risks to occupants in the affected area or to the general public.

In general, asbestos-related lung disease results only from intense asbestos exposure experienced over a period of many years, primarily as a consequence of occupational exposures. The risk of developing an asbestos-related illness following an exposure of short duration, even to high level, is extremely low.

(continued)

(continued)

What should I do with food left in my apartment? The power outage in much of lower Manhattan may have caused refrigerated and frozen food to spoil. Raw or cooked meat, poultry and seafood, milk and milk-containing products, eggs, mayonnaise and creamy dressings, and cooked foods should be thrown out if power was out for two or more hours. Frozen foods that have thawed should be thrown away. Do not re-freeze thawed food.

Throw away any food that may have been contaminated with dust, except for food in cans, jars, or containers with tight-fitting lids. Wash cans and jars with water and wipe clean. When it comes to food left in your building, *if in doubt, throw it out.*

How should I clean the dust in my apartment when I move back in? The best way to remove dust is to use a wet rag or wet mop. Sweeping with a dry broom is not recommended because it can make dust airborne again. Where dust is thick, you can directly wet the dust with water, and remove it with wet rags and mops. Dirty rags can be rinsed under running water, being careful to not leave dust in the sink to dry. When done, used rags and mops should be put in plastic bags while they are still wet and bags should be sealed and discarded. Cloth rags should be washed separately from other laundry. Wash heavily soiled or dusty clothing or linens twice. Remove lint from washing machines and filters in the dryers with each laundry load. Rags should not be allowed to dry out before bagging and disposal or washing.

To reduce dust recirculation, the Health Department recommends using HEPA (high efficiency particulate air) filtration vacuums when cleaning up apartments, if possible. If a HEPA vacuum is not available, it is recommended that either HEPA bags or dust allergen bags be used with your regular vacuum. If these options are not available, wetting down the dust and removing it as described above is recommended.

Carpets and upholstery can be shampooed and then vacuumed.

- If your apartment is very dusty, you should wash or HEPA vacuum your curtains. If curtains need to be taken down, take them down slowly to keep dust from circulating in the air.
- To clean plants, rinse leaves with water. Pets can be washed with running water from a hose or faucet; their paws should be wiped to avoid tracking dust inside the home.

How can I remove dust from the air? Air purifiers may help reduce indoor dust levels. HEPA air purifiers are superior to other models in filtering the smallest particles. Air purifiers are only useful for removing dust from the air. They will not remove dust already deposited on floors, shelves, upholstery or rugs. Keep windows closed when using an air purifier.

Additional recommendations include:

- Keep outdoor dust from entering the home;
- Keep windows closed;
- Set the air conditioner to re-circulate air (closed vents), and clean or change the filter frequently;

(continued)

Box 2–1. *(continued)*
- Remove shoes before entering the home for several days (once you first make sure there is no broken glass)
- Avoid sweeping or other outdoor maintenance

(For more information, visit the Health Department website at www.nyc.gov/health.)

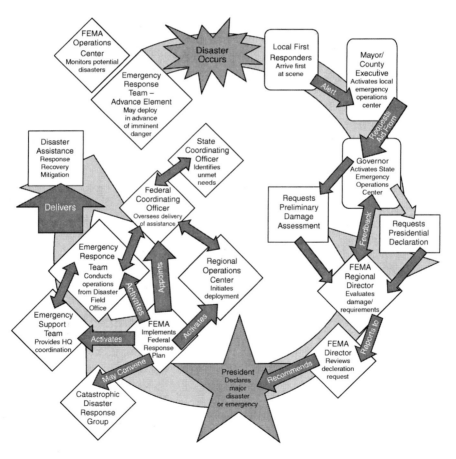

Figure 2–3. Federal Response Plan actions after a disaster occurs (Federal Response Plan).

ENVIRONMENTAL HEALTH ASSESSMENT
AND RISK COMMUNICATION

The WTC attack highlighted the need for further recognition and under-standing of terrorism-related environmental health effects on the public and on rescue and recovery workers (see Chapter 4). The collapse and prolonged burning of the Twin Towers and five other WTC buildings created exposures to substantial amounts of dust, debris, and products of combustion (see Fig-ure 4–1). As a result, persons who were near the disaster site during the col-lapse or who assisted in the rescue and recovery, as well as residents and workers in the surrounding community, were potentially exposed to contam-inants. During the first days after the attack, the degree and range of conta-mination were unclear. The smell of the burning debris extended to many parts of the city, and the smoke was apparent for miles. Assessment of po-tential exposures required the immediate coordination of federal, state, and local agencies responsible for the environment, health, and worker protection.

Beginning September 11, Hazardous Materials Units of different city, state, and federal agencies were at the WTC site to assess the existence of poten-tial contaminants. Because of the multiple agencies conducting or planning environmental sampling, to ensure the development of an efficient, techni-cally sound, and comprehensive plan to monitor environmental hazards, co-ordination among the agencies was necessary. Although communication was difficult because of unavailable telephone service, the NYC DOH, NYC DEP, the U.S. EPA, the NYS DOH, the NYS Department of Environmental Con-servation, the Consolidated Edison power company, the Port Authority of New York and New Jersey, and researchers from Mount Sinai Medical Cen-ter met on September 12 to determine how to coordinate both worker-protection concerns and environmental sampling efforts. These interagency meetings, which became conference calls, grew to include representatives of other agencies and organizations: the Occupational Safety and Health Admin-istration (OSHA), the National Institute for Occupational Safety and Health (NIOSH), the National Institute of Environmental Health Sciences (NIEHS), the NYS Department of Laboratories, Bechtel Corporation, the NYC Coali-tion for Safety and Health, and Public Employee Safety and Health.

Health and Safety of Rescue Workers

Immediately after the September 11 attack, residences and worksites sur-rounding the WTC site were evacuated because of building damage, lack of electricity, potential exposure to hazardous conditions, and the need to keep the area clear for emergency or clean-up vehicles. While rescue and recov-ery efforts were underway, protection of workers and volunteers near the site from physical and chemical environmental hazards became a primary concern (see Chapter 5). Within one day, NYC DOH and NIOSH staff members identified the types of personal protective equipment (PPE) needed and coordinated ordering thousands of each item. The NYC DOH provided the initial 24-hour staffing for 14 days for the distribution of equipment and fit-checking of respirators. Thousands of workers and volunteers received instructions on how to wear, clean, and maintain respirators, and were checked at least once by DOH staff. DOH staff also placed toilet facilities and hand-washing stations for volunteers and workers at the WTC site.

Stressing the need for PPE was a priority. Workers at the site were required to wear hard hats to protect themselves from falling debris; goggles to protect their eyes from dust and debris; and respirators to protect against exposure to dust and noxious substances emanating from the fires. Guidelines were developed, and signs, flyers, and posters were printed to advise workers about why PPE was necessary. However, recommended PPE, such as respirators, was often not worn (see Chapter 5). The 24-hour staffing by DOH personnel continued until OSHA formally began oversight of equipment distribution on September 24. Personal air monitoring was conducted, starting September 15, by organizations and agencies, including Consolidated Edison, the Port Authority, NIOSH, OSHA, and academic institutions.

Environmental Exposures

Environmental monitoring for exposure assessment is a complex technical task. Daily interagency environmental and worker protection conference calls were used to develop a coordinated and integrated effort to ensure that environmental risks were adequately assessed. Through these calls, agencies discussed what substances should be sampled on the basis of expected risk, where monitors should be located, methodologies for sample collection, standards to be used for risk assessment, analytical techniques for laboratory analyses, sampling results, and plans for analyzing the data.

The initial approach to the sampling was to locate the monitors at the perimeter of the site, at locations where emergency and debris-carrying vehicles were leaving the site, on the debris pile, and at locations in the surrounding community. If levels of the contaminants were acceptable in the highest-risk locations, they would probably be acceptable in other areas. To ensure a safe environment for the workers, residents, and students reoccupying workplaces, homes, and schools after the initial weeks, additional monitors were set up in the community.

To compile the environmental data in one place and to begin the analysis of daily and long-term trends, the NYC DOH initiated the development of a database for data from multiple sources. As a result of daily environmental and worker protection conference calls as well as data from NYS DEC sent by electronic mail, the NYC DOH was able to receive and input environmental sampling data from several agencies. This database, and the criteria set for data submission by all agencies, served as the basis for a database that is now managed by the EPA. Approximately 66,000 results were entered in a database for samples collected from September 11 to November 13.

Substances monitored included asbestos, particulate matter (both $PM_{2.5}$ and PM_{10}), dioxins, polychlorinated biphenyls (PCBs), carbon monoxide, heavy metals, volatile organic compounds (VOCs) such as benzene, and others. Samples were taken from media including air, bulk dust, and water. Samples were collected at the WTC site, in the nearby community, in other NYC boroughs, at the Fresh Kills landfill on Staten Island, and in New Jersey. Results for these samples are available on the EPA website at <www.epa.gov>.

Asbestos was a known building component in the WTC and thus became an immediate contaminant of concern. Asbestos was found in approximately one-fourth of bulk samples on the site, usually in small concentrations (0.5 percent to 3 percent). The highest concentration of asbestos found in a bulk sample was 40 percent (during the first month). From September 11 to December 31, 2001, the EPA collected and analyzed 4,229 samples for airborne asbestos in lower Manhattan. Twenty-seven of these samples exceeded the Asbestos Hazard Emergency Response Act (AHERA) standard. (Because no standards for asbestos in outdoor air exist, city, state, and federal agencies decided to use the most protective indoor air standard to test for asbestos in the outdoor air. This standard is the AHERA standard of 70 structures per square millimeter [s/mm^2]. The AHERA standard is normally used to decide when children can safely re-enter school buildings after asbestos-removal activities.) Of these 27 samples that exceeded the AHERA standard, 13 were collected before October 1, indicating that almost half of the elevated levels occurred within the first three weeks after the attack.

Communication regarding environmental sampling and health risks was a great challenge, yet was a key component in helping the community understand the environmental risk posed by this disaster. An increased level of concern has existed regarding air quality. Within the first weeks, the NYC DOH developed fact sheets that were hand-delivered by DOH staff to homes in the community to specify what needed to be done to re-occupy homes (Box 2–1). These fact sheets were also posted on the NYC DOH website with links to the DEP website describing obligations of building owners.

A key message that the agencies and scientists tried to communicate to people living and working in the community was the difference in health risks associated with asbestos compared with those associated with the smoldering fires that were finally extinguished 100 days after the disaster. With asbestos, most health effects are associated with long-term exposures and take a substantial period of time to develop. Brief spikes in outdoor asbestos levels, such as those located around the WTC site, have generally not been associated with long-term health effects. Workers and residents near the WTC site reported experiencing such symptoms as a scratchy throat, eye irritation, and cough. These symptoms, caused by smoke and odors from the persistent fires, were thought unlikely to result in long-term health conditions.

Food and Water Safety

Ensuring food and water safety proved to be a time-intensive activity for the DOH. Restaurant inspections began on September 13 using DOH and NYS sanitarian staff members. Because of the rapid evacuation from lower Manhattan, patrons and owners left restaurants with food sitting on counters and tables. The Commissioner of Health ordered the NYC Department of Sanitation to begin disposing of all food waste and garbage near the WTC on September 15. The famous Fulton Fish Market was moved uptown to Hunts Point on September 17 because of the inability to provide routine sanitation pick-up at its former location. Public health advisories were released on September 18 and 25, asking owners to allow DOH inspectors inside their establishments. Certain restaurants were forcibly entered. In total, these efforts included inspection of approximately 1,100 restaurants in lower Manhattan, removal of tons of spoiled food from food establishments and supermarkets, and placement and monitoring of 1,000 rodent bait stations near the WTC site. Sanitarians performed more than 400 sanitary inspections at 226 food-service establishments in the 10-block secure zone near the WTC during the three weeks after the attack, totaling 10,320 staff hours.

Impromptu food distribution sites were erected by volunteer organizations to serve the thousands of volunteers sifting through WTC rubble and debris. DOH inspectors attempted to limit the number of rogue feeding centers and individuals roaming the area around Ground Zero distributing prepared food. This proved difficult, but, in meetings with the American Red Cross, the Salvation Army, and City Harvest, the number consolidated to 33 sites by September 19. Inspectors visited these three times a day to monitor food safety and instruct volunteers on safe food-handling practices. Handwashing and toilet facilities were provided early for volunteers at the WTC site, and later maintained by the EPA and serviced daily by a portable-toilet company.

The DOH sampled the water supply at selected sites near the WTC site for three weeks after the disaster. Coliform counts never exceeded threshold values. Residents and building owners were advised to flush out all water reservoir tanks and fill them with fresh water before DOH inspections took place. No outbreak of waterborne illness was reported.

SURVEILLANCE

Surveillance of disaster-related health effects is a key component of an appropriate and effective public health response by a local health department.[9] The NYC DOH initiated four distinct surveillance systems immediately after the WTC attack.

Rapid Assessment of the Physical Injuries Related to the Attack

To rapidly assess injuries and health service use, the NYC DOH sent field investigation teams to review emergency department and inpatient medical records at the four Manhattan hospitals closest to the WTC site and a fifth Manhattan hospital serving as a burn referral center. Assessments began within six hours of the attack. Trained medical-record reviewers obtained demographic and clinical data regarding all patients who were seen at these hospitals between 8:00 a.m. on September 11 and 8:00 a.m. on September 13. A uniform record was used to collect data. Information collected included age, sex, mode of arrival, date and time of initial treatment, type of injury or illness, whether the injury was related to the WTC disaster, and disposition.

A total of 1,688 patients received emergency care during the assessment interval.[10] Sixty-five percent (1,103) were survivors treated for incident-related injuries or illness. The relationship between injury or illness and the attack could not be determined for 6 percent (96) of patients because of incomplete documentation. Arrival of injured survivors at nearby hospitals began within minutes of the attack and peaked 2 to 3 hours later. A total of 810 (73 percent) were treated and released, 181 (16 percent) were hospitalized for additional treatment, and four (0.4 percent) died during emergency care. Within the first 48 hours after the attack, 790 survivors were treated for injuries at these hospitals; half received care within 7 hours (Table 2–3). Individuals with the most serious injuries, such as burns, fractures, and head injuries, were admitted to hospitals. Most patients were treated for inhalational injuries (49 percent) or ocular injuries (26 percent). Of those treated, 29 percent were identified as rescue workers. Rescue workers had a higher rate of ocular injuries (39 percent) compared with others treated (19 percent) ($p < 0.0001$), and a lower rate of burns (2 percent, compared with 6 percent, $p < 0.01$). Surveillance data indicated a single large wave of survivors, followed by a second group on the next day that largely comprised rescue workers.

Because of time constraints, the assessment was not population-based and did not attempt to assess the total number of incident-related injuries. Many people were seen in other NYC hospitals, in other areas of New York, New

TABLE 2–3. Physical Injuries Sustained by WTC Attack Survivors: Five New York City Hospitals, 8:45 a.m. September 11 to 8:00 a.m. September 13, 2001.

TYPE OF INJURY*	Hospitalized (n = 139)§		Treated and Released (n = 606)		Undocumented Disposition (n = 45)		Total (n = 790)	
	NUMBER[†]	PERCENT[‡]	NUMBER[†]	PERCENT[‡]	NUMBER[†]	PERCENT[‡]	NUMBER[†]	PERCENT[‡]
Inhalation	52	37	300	50	34	76	386	49
Ocular	10	7	185	31	9	20	204	26
Laceration	25	18	80	13	5	11	110	14
Sprain or strain	17	12	85	14	6	13	108	14
Contusion	29	21	66	11	3	7	98	12
Fracture	27	19	19	3	0	0	46	6
Burn	27	19	12	2	0	0	39	5
Closed head	8	6	6	1	0	0	14	2
Crush	6	4	2	0.3	0	0	8	1

*Excludes unspecified injuries or illnesses.

§Includes 2 survivors who died during emergency care.

[†]Totals might exceed total number of survivors because certain survivors might have sustained multiple injuries.

[‡]Totals might exceed 100 percent because certain survivors might have sustained multiple injuries.

(Source: Centers for Disease Control and Prevention. Rapid assessment of physical injuries related to the attack on the World Trade Center—New York City, September 11, 2001. *Mor Mortal Wkly Rep* 2002; 51:30–35.)

Jersey, and Connecticut, and at emergency triage stations outside hospitals, where no documentation took place. The population assessed was probably representative of the immediate survivors and rescuers.

Hospital Needs Assessment

In collaboration with the Greater New York Hospital Association (GNYHA) and the NYS DOH, the NYC DOH rapidly set up a daily hospital-assessment system focused on three areas: (1) surveillance of incident-related and all-cause emergency department visits and hospital admissions, as well as mortality; (2) daily hospital census, including numbers of occupied and empty hospital beds, numbers of acute-care and intensive-care inpatient beds, as well as emergency department beds; and (3) staffing and supply needs.

To obtain this information, all NYC hospitals were asked to complete and fax a daily data report form. The 13 facilities near the WTC site were telephoned daily to ensure full reporting. Because hospitals that are not close to the WTC site in lower Manhattan did not experience major increases in admissions and emergency department visits, data on census and staffing and supply needs were no longer collected from these hospitals after the first week. Disaster-related hospital surveillance continued for 14 days.

Sixty-two hospitals from all areas of New York City reported incident-related visits and admissions (unpublished DOH/GNYHA data). In total, 14 percent (range: 4 to 52 percent) of 5,523 emergency department visits and 4 percent (range: 1 to 15 percent) of 441 hospital admissions were incident-related. The median number of total incident-related emergency department visits per hospital was 58 (range: 0 to 648), and the median number of total incident-related inpatient admissions per hospital was 2 (range: 0 to 111). Fifteen incident-related deaths were reported. Sixteen hospitals in Manhattan were most heavily affected, defined as having more than 100 incident-related visits. Four hospitals with the highest number of incident-related emergency department visits also had the highest proportion of incident-related emergency department visits and hospital admissions. One-third of 1,745 emergency department visits during the surveillance period at these four hospitals were incident-related. One-fourth of 111 incident-related admissions were to one hospital near the WTC site.

Significant numbers of patients were treated outside of New York City and in New Jersey. No data were available on the number of individuals in and around the WTC site at the time of the attacks. Therefore, calculating a rate of emergency department visits and hospital admissions among the "exposed" population was not possible.

Syndromic Surveillance

Timely detection of an intentional biological-agent release is both essential and problematic for public health agencies (see Chapter 10). Reliable technology does not exist to detect a biological agent at the moment and point of a mass release. Because some potential bioterrorist agents cause illnesses that begin with nonspecific influenza-like symptoms such as malaise and fever, syndromic surveillance has been proposed as a potential early warning system. The NYC DOH and the CDC established a syndromic surveillance system in New York City in the days after the WTC attack because of increased concern of a parallel bioterrorist attack.

EIS officers were stationed at 15 sentinel emergency departments throughout the five boroughs of New York beginning on September 13. A one-page abstraction form, completed by either a hospital staff member or an EIS officer, was used to code emergency department discharge diagnoses into one of 12 syndrome categories. Seven of these categories—respiratory illness with fever, sepsis, rash with fever, meningitis/encephalitis, gastrointestinal illness, botulism-like illness, and unexplained death with fever—were designed to identify and collect data on illnesses potentially caused by an infectious agent. EIS officers facilitated form completion, performed data entry, did chart reviews, investigated clusters, and communicated findings to hospital staff.

Data were analyzed each morning covering the preceding 24-hour period. Spatial and temporal clusters were detected by using SaTScan.[11] Supplemental temporal analyses were performed by using a modification of the cumulative sum feature of SAS.[12] A total of 49 alarms occurred from September 13 to October 10. (SaTScan compares the proportion of cases of the syndrome of interest [number of syndrome cases to number of nonsyndrome emergency department visits] to its baseline value within a geographic circle to the same proportions outside the circle. The circle drawn is arbitrary but it reruns this analysis 999 times, changing the size and location of the circle, homing in on the most significant cluster. It reports the clusters (circles) with the smallest p values. We varied the p values from the SaTScan analyses that were used to determine significance for an alarm, and examined such parameters as age distribution, overlapping syndromes, alarms of several days in a row, and the combination of a cumulative sum alarm and a SaTScan alarm.)

Response to alarms began by reviewing the paper forms and then the age distribution of cases in the cluster. (In two instances, alarms were determined to be caused by form miscoding.) Next, chart reviews were performed when (1) a cluster involved multiple hospitals, or (2) the proportion of children under 13 years of age comprised less than half of the total number of cases. Table 2–4 presents statistical alarms by syndrome and analytical method. Gastrointestinal illness was the most frequent syndrome to generate an alarm,

TABLE 2–4. Statistical Alarms by Syndrome and Analytical Method

SYNDROME	CITYWIDE CUSUM ALARMS (n)	LOCALIZED ALARMS (n)	LOCALIZED ALARM TYPE* (n)			CASES TO TRIGGER SATSCAN ALARM (RANGE)
			S	C	B	
Respiratory illness with fever	2	11	5	2	2	8–19
Sepsis	1	13	4	7	1	2–7
Rash with fever	0	8	2	2	2	2–9
Meningitis/ encephalitis	1	4	2	2	0	2–4
Gastrointestinal illness	3	13	2	7	2	12–28
Total	7	49	15	20	7	2–28

*C—cumulative sum (CUSUM), S—SaTScan, B—both

followed by sepsis, respiratory illness with fever, and rash with fever. No alarm occurred for a botulism-like syndrome. One unexplained death was detected. No alarm was determined to represent the release of a biological agent. The system was labor-intensive and was replaced on October 18 by an electronic system based on emergency department chief-complaint logs that is now (April 2002) in place in 30 hospitals.

Injuries Among Rescue and Recovery Personnel

Immediately after the disaster, the DOH began an assessment of the number and types of injuries suffered by people who were involved in the rescue, recovery, and excavation efforts. For the purpose of this surveillance project, a *rescue worker* was defined as any person working or volunteering at the disaster site. The four medical centers in closest proximity to the WTC site, and five DMAT sites that provided most of the urgent medical care to rescue workers, were enrolled in the surveillance system. Variables included age, worker type, injury type, worker activity at the time of injury, PPE worn, and medical encounter disposition. A retrospective component for the initial 72 hours after the disaster, using hospital chart reviews, was conducted by DOH and CDC staff. Prospective surveillance was initiated on September 14 and was conducted by onsite medical personnel at the four medical centers and five DMAT sites treating the injured.

Approximately 7,000 visits were recorded during the 2 months after the WTC attack (unpublished DOH/CDC data). These include rescue and recovery workers as well as other workers evaluated for injuries, other medical conditions, and nonmedical conditions (such as requests for PPE and other supplies). Construction workers accounted for the greatest proportion of prospective surveillance visits (35 percent), followed by police (21 percent) and firefighters (15 percent). Twenty-four percent of visits were among workers not involved in rescue and recovery; for 5 percent of visits, worker type was unknown. Denominator data were unavailable to compute rates. Visits for musculoskeletal complaints were common (13 percent), followed by eye complaints (11 percent), respiratory complaints (9 percent), headaches (9 percent), and blisters (6 percent). Forty percent of visits were for other medical and nonmedical reasons (such as requests for medications, supplies, and PPE), and for 12 percent the visit type was missing. No death was reported during the prospective surveillance period.

A daily summary report was made available to various federal, state, and local agencies and participating medical providers. This prospective system provided prompt descriptions of injury patterns as well as the first real-time summary of DMAT activities in the field, while responding to evolving requests for information. The DOH EOC used results from this system to alert rescue leaders about what injuries were occurring and what they should be doing to prevent them. For example, Woods' lamps (for diagnostic purposes) were provided to the DMAT teams because a substantial proportion of eye injuries were corneal abrasions.

SUPPORT SYSTEMS: OPERATIONS AND MANAGEMENT INFORMATION SYSTEMS

The MIS and operations committees faced difficult challenges in the first month after the attack. Because of the relocation of the DOH, setting up temporary phone, fax, and internet lines became necessary. Staff relied on two-way radio and cellular telephone communication. The broadcast fax and electronic mail health-alert system was moved to a temporary location to keep local health-care providers up-to-date concerning DOH activities. Because of preparation for the year 2000, offsite data storage enabled the recovery of all necessary information for DOH work; thus, no data were lost. For 24 hours each day, DOH drivers transported staff members, including physicians, epidemiologists, and environmental investigators, as well as patient specimens, suspicious packages, and hazardous waste for disposal. Operations also provided security, escorts through police lines, safety and health monitoring, and support for onsite clean-up and inspections.

MENTAL HEALTH

A key component of the public health response to the WTC disaster was to address the short- and long-term mental health needs of city residents (see

Chapter 3). Both the NYS Office of Mental Health (OMH) and the NYC Department of Mental Health (DMH) deployed staff members into the field to provide clinical support to the relief operations for the families receiving services at the American Red Cross Family Assistance Center for injured survivors and evacuees. They also provided counseling support for rescue and recovery workers as well as volunteers. To assist in service coordination and planning, DMH also identified residents with home damage, those displaced from jobs, and WTC workers who were absent during the attacks as being in need of services. OMH and DMH met specifically with the New York Fire Department's counseling services representative soon after the disaster, and assisted with services for fire and police department personnel. The mental health of DOH personnel was addressed through crisis counseling sessions and debriefing sessions through the Employee Assistance Program.

Funding for mental health services was provided by the Federal Emergency Management Agency (FEMA) through a $22.7 million grant for the Crisis Counseling Assistance and Training Program's Immediate Services Program. This grant program, entitled "Project Liberty," covered immediate crisis outreach and counseling, public education, and referral services for affected persons for 60 days after the disaster.

The impact of the WTC disaster on the mental health of survivors, families of the deceased, and other city residents could potentially be substantial. Two months after the attack, 7.5 percent of Manhattan residents reported symptoms consistent with a diagnosis of current post-traumatic stress disorder (PTSD) related to the attacks, and 9.7 percent reported symptoms consistent with current depression.[13] Residents living nearest to the WTC had a prevalence of PTSD of 20 percent. The degree of elevated mental health symptoms among other population groups around the city are unknown. A national telephone survey immediately after the attacks determined that 44 percent of adults reported one or more symptoms of stress.[14] Community-based health-care providers, city psychiatric hospitals, and academic research centers will be conducting studies to assess the level of acute and long-term mental health symptomatology among selected population groups.

KEY ISSUES IN THE PUBLIC HEALTH RESPONSE
TO THE WTC DISASTER

There were several critical characteristics of New York City's public health response to the WTC disaster. The DOH was able to respond well to the emergency, despite the loss of use of the main building and land-line phone systems. Emergency response teams mobilized successfully for 24-hour-a-day coverage. As part of this response, DOH staff members became knowledgeable about public health concerns that were not a part of daily routine, such as worker safety and health and the technical aspects of environmental air monitoring. DOH staff members also demonstrated flexibility by responding to situations for which they had not yet planned, but for which they had resources needed at the time, including: providing acute medical care to victims of the disaster, working at an alternative worksite for several weeks without adequate telephone and computer support, and contributing expertise in addressing the occupational health and safety needs of rescue and recovery workers.

The DOH realized that several operational problems required attention. To identify these problems, senior managers involved in the emergency preparedness committees met one month after the response. This meeting helped identify acute problems in the response, including communication problems among emergency committees and agencies, personnel concerns, technical and infrastructure problems raised by the event, and training and assessment concerns.

Communication between emergency committees was identified as a key problem. During the EOC activation from September 11 to 28, twice-daily update meetings were held. Because of competing demands, however, committee-leader participation was not uniform. Because of telephone difficulties, we were unable to include the NYC DOH liaison to the OEM in the DOH EOC meetings, leading to duplication of effort and inefficiencies. Incident command center liaisons changed every workshift, and new persons rotating into the shift schedule were not well oriented to recent citywide conditions and problems. This situation might have led to decreased coordination between the NYC DOH and OEM efforts.

As a result of the evacuation from the NYC DOH headquarters building, access to personnel data and other information was not readily available. Access to employees was further hampered by the inconsistent availability of telephones to reach employees or DOH worksites.

Other than the school health program, a master list of DOH employee home phone numbers did not exist on September 11. It became difficult to ensure the continuous availability of DOH staff members to respond to the emergency so that essential DOH functions could continue. This difficulty led to overuse of the same staff members and a feeling of neglect and frustration among underutilized staff members.

Emergency committees did not feel adequately prepared for the different concerns that they faced during the response. Identified gaps in their knowledge included occupational safety and health, environmental health impacts of explosions and building collapse, and mental health needs of DOH employees involved in the response. For example, reports came from DOH staff members working at the WTC site of observing body parts recovered from the debris, resulting in emotional stress to employees. Critical-incident sessions were held one month after the disaster to allow DOH staff members to psychologically process what they had seen, and to refer those in need for further mental health services.

New initiatives targeted gaps in preparedness that were identified. Certain senior managers were not oriented to the emergency ICS. Therefore, training sessions on ICS were held for 40 senior staff members in December 2001 with the assistance of the Columbia University's Center for Public Health Preparedness. The human resources department of the DOH now has a master list of home telephone numbers of all employees so that staff can be contacted at any time during an emergency activation. We now recognize the importance of redundancy in resources, including communication, and are seeking to create redundant network and telecommunications connectivity for critical DOH locations, including offsite data storage for existing registries and surveillance systems. In addition, the DOH is presenting seminars for all staff members on key environmental health concerns related to the WTC disaster.

SIMILARITIES TO THE GENERAL SLOCUM DISASTER

The WTC attack resulted in the largest number of fatalities in New York City as a result of a single event since the beginning of the collection of vital statistics data in 1866 (Table 2–5). Yet the similarities are striking between the WTC disaster and the *General Slocum* passenger ship disaster, the second largest disaster in New York City, nearly one century earlier. The *General Slocum* was carrying picnic-goers, predominantly women and children, from one neighborhood to another through New York harbor. The ship caught fire and sank, killing 1,030 people. Many died when they jumped off the ship

TABLE 2–5(A). Worst Disasters in New York City, 1849–2001.

YEAR	DISASTER	NUMBER OF DEATHS
2001	World Trade Center attack, September 11	2,800 (estimated)
1904	*General Slocum* passenger ship fire	1,030
2001	American Airlines Flight 587 plane crash, Queens	265
1911	Triangle Shirtwaist Factory fire (all women)	146
1960	United DC-8 and TWA Super Constellation midair collision, Brooklyn	135
1975	Eastern Airlines 727 plane crash, JFK airport	113
1990	Happy Land Social Club fire, The Bronx	87
1945	US Army B-25/Empire State Building plane crash	14

(*Source:* Famighetti R, ed.[18])

TABLE 2–5(B). Selected Epidemics for Comparison, New York City.

YEAR	EPIDEMIC	NUMBER OF DEATHS
1918	Influenza	12,562
1994	Human Immunodeficiency Virus	8,039
1849	Cholera	5,071
1904	Meningitis	2,219
1901–1902	Smallpox	720
For comparison:		
2000	Average number of deaths per day in September	152

Data confirmed by the Vital Statistics Unit, NYC Department of Health.

and drowned. The response to the disaster included an unfruitful rescue operation, difficulty in the recovery of bodies, the creation of a special morgue in the city, concern regarding the mental health impact of the disaster, and the creation of a special relief fund. The public response mirrored that of the response to the WTC disaster, including relatives of victims going to hospitals to check for their loved ones, crowds lining up to view the hulk of the ship, and mass funerals.

CONCLUSION

The WTC disaster presented unique public health challenges to the NYC DOH. The sudden loss of thousands of lives, coupled with an environmental disaster of unequal proportions, thrust the DOH into the front line of the emergency response. The presence of an emergency response plan reflected the amount of forethought that went into disaster preparedness years before September 11, 2001. Unfortunately, the WTC disaster was followed two months later by another disaster, the crash of American Airlines flight 587 (bound from New York to the Dominican Republic), and the intentional dissemination of anthrax in New York City and elsewhere (see Chapter 6), requiring the DOH to further increase its efforts and to continue its emergency response through the end of 2001.[15]

The DOH responded to each public health problem in comprehensive and methodical fashion, with assistance from other local, state, and federal agencies. This response included providing shelter to displaced residents, assessing the risk from environmental contaminants, maintaining surveillance systems for illnesses and injuries caused by the WTC attack and subsequent recovery effort and by the dissemination of anthrax, and communicating essential health messages to health-care providers and an anxious public. Simultaneously, the DOH dealt with tremendous logistical challenges in carrying out its work, and managed to maintain essential core DOH services, such as vital event registration, sexually transmitted disease control, tuberculosis control, and West Nile virus surveillance and control.

The long-term impact of the WTC attack on the health of the population of New York City has yet to be determined. Disaster-related effects can range from environmental disease, to mental illness, to the long-term impact of the loss of primary wage-earner income.[16] Creation and maintenance of a registry by the DOH and the CDC of all surviving WTC occupants, first-responders, and lower-Manhattan schoolchildren will attempt to measure this long-term impact. Although each disaster has it own unique epidemiological profile, the ongoing analysis and evaluation of this database will assist the DOH in future planning for disasters and in emergency preparedness.[17]

Many parallels exist between New York City's experience of September 11 and previous disasters in the city. These parallels serve as a reminder that, despite stark differences between life across many decades, the core public-health response remains remarkably similar in times of disaster. Undoubtedly, responders to disasters, including public health departments, will have to address these needs again in the future. The lessons learned from the NYC DOH response to the WTC disaster will provide guidance for our responses to future terrorist events in New York City and elsewhere.

Acknowledgment

We would like to thank Dr. Neal Cohen and Dr. Benjamin Mojica for their tremendous dedication, insight, and leadership at the New York City Department of Health during the response to the attack on the World Trade Center. We would also like to thank all of our colleagues at the Department of Health, who are too numerous to mention, for their hard work toward safeguarding the health of the residents of New York City.

REFERENCES

1. Lillibridge SR. Industrial disasters. In: Noji EK, ed. *The Public Health Consequences of Disasters.* New York, NY: Oxford University Press, 1997.
2. Landesman LY. *Public Health Management of Disasters: The Practice Guide.* Washington, D.C.: American Public Health Association, 2001.
3. Nash D, Mostashari F, Fine A, et al. The outbreak of West Nile virus infection in the New York City area in 1999. *N Engl J Med* 2001; 344:1807–1814.
4. Cauchon D. For many on September 11, survival was no accident. *USA Today*, December 19, 2001:1A, 3A.
5. Office of Vital Statistics. *The City of New York Summary of Vital Statistics 2000.* New York: New York City Department of Health, 2002.
6. Layton M, Ackelsberg J. *Alert #4—Terrorist Attack at the World Trade Center in New York City: Medical and Public Health Issues.* New York: New York City Deparment of Health, 2001:1–9.
7. Landrigan PJ. Health consequences of the 11 September 2001 attacks. *Environ Health Perspect* 2001; 109:A514–A515.

8. Centers for Disease Control and Prevention. New York City Department of Health response to terrorist attack, September 11, 2001. *Mor Mortal Wkly Rep* 2001; 50:821–822.
9. Wetterhall SF, Noji EK. Surveillance and epidemiology. In: Noji EK, ed. *The Public Health Consequences of Disasters.* New York: Oxford University Press, 1997.
10. Centers for Disease Control and Prevention. Rapid assessment of physical injuries related to the attack on the World Trade Center—New York City, September 11, 2001. *Mor Mortal Wkly Rep* 2002; 51:30–35.
11. Kulldorff M. A spatial scan statistic. *Communications in Statistics: Theory and Methods* 1997; 26:1481–1496.
12. SAS/STAT software: Changes and enhancements through release 6.12. Cary, NC: SAS Institute, Inc., 1997.
13. Galea S, Ahern J, Resnick H, et al. Psychological sequelae of the September 11 terrorist attacks in New York City. *N Engl J Med* 2002; 346:982–987.
14. Schuster MA, Stein BD, Jaycox LH, et al. A national survey of stress reactions after the September 11, 2001, terrorist attacks. *N Engl J Med* 2001; 345:1507–1512.
15. Centers for Disease Control and Prevention. Investigation of bioterrorism-related anthrax and interim guidelines for clinical evaluation of persons with possible anthrax. *Mor Mortal Wkly Rep* 2001; 50:941–948.
16. Sidel VW, Onel E, Geiger HJ, et al. Public health responses to natural and human-made disasters. In: Last JM, Wallace RB, eds. *Public Health & Preventive Medicine,* 13th ed. Norwalk, CT: Appleton & Lange, 1992.
17. Nicoll A, Wilson D, Calvert N, Borriello P. Managing major public health crises. *Br Med J* 2001; 323:1321–1322.
18. Famighetti R, ed. *The World Almanac and Book of Facts* 1999. Mahwah, NJ: Primedia Reference, Inc., 1998.

3

Addressing mental health needs

ZEBULON TAINTOR

The terrorist attacks on the World Trade Center (WTC) and the Pentagon and the dissemination of anthrax in 2001 led to several different types of mental health problems, including anxiety, depression, and post-traumatic stress disorder (PTSD). Anxiety was further increased by perceived threats of additional terrorist attacks—a goal of psychological warfare.

Studies of the mental health effects of earthquakes may be relevant to the September 11 terrorist acts.[1-3] Earthquakes bear similarity to the WTC attack because they have an epicenter of destruction, and those in the area are traumatized by their experience and have realistic concerns about recurring events. Depression tends to persist because losses are permanent, while anxiety wanes as life returns to normal and disasters do not recur.

The first part of this chapter considers the challenges that terrorism poses to mental health, as well as the deficiencies and strengths in the mental health system that were highlighted by the terrorist acts of 2001. The second part of this chapter offers a preliminary list of recommendations for possible future terrorist acts and threats.

CHALLENGES THAT TERRORISM POSES TO MENTAL HEALTH

Terrorism is a mental health term. A *terrorist* is one who seeks to terrify victims. Terror involves sheer fear of specific, awful things that can happen; and

49

anxiety, which is fear without a conscious object. Mental health workers recognize the real possibilities of awful outcomes, including death, sickness, injury, and disfigurement affecting oneself, loved ones, and others in one's community or nation. Possible future terrorist attack scenarios cannot involve much realistic reassurance about prevention, and thus may take therapists into uncharted territories. Psychological approaches to primary prevention of severe emotional reactions to trauma, such as prolonged anxiety, depression, or other symptoms, involve considering which defense and coping mechanisms are reinforced by particular strategies. For example, repression and denial are defenses that may work for some people, while others may need to explore their feelings in detail and practice suppression and altruism.

Strengths of the System

The terrorist acts of 2001 shed light on certain strengths of the mental health system. In terms of strengths, the WTC disaster was perhaps the first one in which mental health concerns were highlighted from the start. Experts appeared in the mass media to warn about what might happen and what should be expected. Free and open discussions probably served to help people detect their own symptoms and to reduce the stigma of asking for help. The mass media stimulated discussion that kept mental health needs on the public agenda. Mental health professional organizations generated cogent statements and recruited volunteers. Ten thousand physicians volunteered their services through the Medical Society of the State of New York. Psychiatrists, psychologists, social workers, and other types of counselors were all mobilized as volunteers within hours of the WTC disaster (see Box 3–1). Disaster Psychiatry Outreach, which had previously helped victims of the Swissair, EgyptAir, and TWA airplane crashes in the late 1990s, was officially designated by New York City[4] to staff the crisis center, which was established in the Armory at 29th Street and Lexington Avenue (and subsequently at Pier 94).[5]

All major hospitals, clinics, and institutions mobilized to support their staff members and their families and to provide services beyond their walls. Within hours of the disaster, the main problem was an oversupply of everything that had been mentioned publicly as being in short supply, from water to dry clothing. These communications fostered a sense of community—of being in it all together, of being able to *do* something. Since one of the objects of terror is to create a sense of impotent paralysis, these and other joint efforts were conducive to positive mental health.

Health care in the United States often is thought to lack a system. It is diverse and fragmented, duplicative in some areas and lacking in others. The United States is notorious for lacking mandates for coverage of mental ill-

Box 3–1. The Experiences of Two Mental Health Professionals.

The mental health community in New York City seemed to struggle in responding to the World Trade Center (WTC) attack. The response was initially not very orderly, but may have been as effective as humanly possible under the circumstances. The major factor that worked in making the response effective was the existence of many mental health workers in New York City who were skilled and concerned professionals ready to provide counseling for those in need. The chaos of the early days of the response evolved into a working structure that gave psychological help to many thousands of individuals and families.

Mental health professionals responding to the WTC disaster had a variety of experiences in providing services. The following are summary accounts of two of their experiences.

Cindy Ness, a therapist and a resident of lower Manhattan, was in Philadelphia when the disaster occurred. She performed work for a behavioral health company with which she had previously done trauma counseling. Two days after the disaster, she began debriefing groups of employees who had worked at the WTC. Many of them seemed unsure about what they should be doing—staying at home with their children or coming to work where they might be of some help, though none was really clear about how they could help. The two most common needs that emerged were their need to reestablish a sense of safety and their need to make meaning out of the incident by doing something active.

Ms. Ness also met with employees of an insurance company that had offices in the Twin Towers and elsewhere in New York. Many of their employees had worked on eight floors in the North Tower at the level where the first plane attacked. All were presumed dead. She spoke with company employees who worked at its midtown-Manhattan office. These employees seemed more at a distance from their emotions and were deeply concerned about their co-workers in the North Tower. The image of their fellow employees trapped at the WTC was quite real for them.

Ms. Ness also worked at a family center that another company had established for its employees. She spoke with many family members, assisting them in dealing with their grief and, at times, self-recrimination—many family members stated that they wished they had died instead.

Another psychologist, Dr. Katie Gentile, who teaches counseling courses on trauma and related subjects at John Jay College in New York and directs the Women's Center there, worked in a number of settings. Starting in October, she co-led a weekly psychotherapy group of engineers who had worked in the WTC. Each session lasted three and a half hours. The number of engineers who met ranged from seven to ten, with some participants attending regularly and others more erratically. Several of them had survived the 1993 bombing at the WTC, which took place down the hall from their offices. Many of them were wounded in that earlier attack, and most suffered severe

(continued)

Box 3–1. *(continued)*

symptoms of post-traumatic stress disorder afterward—one had not slept more than three hours at a stretch since the 1993 bombing. They all said that they knew that a second attack was coming. They were already hypervigilant: each time there was a bomb threat (and there were many) or a loud noise they jumped with fear.

As Ms. Gentile worked with this group, humiliation was a central theme. It was humiliating for them to need help, especially as their work involved fixing things. It was humiliating for them to be handicapped in functioning and not to be employed. It was humiliating for them not to be asked to help in the recovery effort, especially since their unique expertise about the WTC buildings was not recognized, appreciated, or utilized. It was humiliating that "their" buildings disappeared in smoke and ashes. Three months after the WTC attack, their nightmares worsened. They had difficulty facing the prospect of Christmas. They felt humiliated at their lack of income and, therefore, their means to buy good gifts. Some feared the sight in public spaces of Christmas packages, which they thought might contain bombs.

The stories of their experiences did not come out all at once, nor was their narrative coherent. At first, only a few dominated the discussions and told stories, while others stared blankly or in shock. Over time, the others joined in and all of the participants began telling their stories with more affect. Most of them related horrific accounts of being temporarily trapped in the WTC as people jumping from the upper floors were falling outside. All of them related accounts of seeing people injured, burned, and killed.

—Charles B. Strozier and Katie Gentile

ness equivalent to coverage for physical illness. Yet, the diversity of its health care allows several systems to come into play in a disaster. (See Box 13–2.)

After September 11, the New York State Office of Mental Health, acting as part of the State Emergency Management Agency (SEMA), moved quickly, as it had in previous emergencies, to establish a command center, which was operating within 45 minutes. It emptied space and opened buildings at the ten psychiatric centers in the New York metropolitan area to receive stable medical patients transferred from city hospitals. It moved in 60 tractor-trailer loads of food and supplies, prepared to serve 20,000 meals a day, and dispatched 350 professional staff members to provide services. With federal government designation of the area as a disaster area, it received, as the designated agency for mental health training, $22.7 million from the Federal Emergency Management Agency (FEMA) and $8 million from the Substances Abuse and Mental Health Services Administration (SAMHSA).[6,7]

Key officials in the city, state, and federal governments worked together well and made it clear who was designated to do what. A broad outreach program, called Project Liberty, was created.[8]

Immediate concerns included incidents of anger and violence directed at Muslims and people wearing turbans (see Box 3–2). Rumors abounded. Public figures addressed the expectation of additional attacks, a challenge since warnings had to be conveyed and reassurance was of limited value. The emphasis in these communications was on how the community could respond in caring for community members, and how it could demonstrate strength and resiliency (see Chapter 7).

The dissemination of anthrax (Chapter 6) in 2001 also had impacts on mental health. Moods rose and fell according to the ease with which diagnoses were made, treatment instituted, and lives saved. Despite some missteps due to inexperience with and inadequate scientific information on, the diagnosis and treatment of anthrax, anxiety rapidly subsided, except for concerns about the deaths of two women in New York and Connecticut who had no obvious anthrax contact.[9] Still, anxiety about anthrax led to widespread use of antibiotics like ciprofloxacin (Cipro), for which adverse psychiatric reactions have been reported.[10]

Deficiencies of the System

Well-laid contingency plans depended on means of communication and transportation that suddenly were not available. Cell-phone towers had been destroyed. Air traffic was grounded. A massive telephone switching station was destroyed, interrupting both local telephone service and e-mail transmission. The methods of personal communication that still worked were jammed as people tried to contact loved ones. This situation left the mass media as the primary method of communication. Initially, the media reflected the confusion of officialdom, but Mayor Rudolph Giuliani and the municipal government increasingly used the media effectively.

The massive outpouring of aid and volunteers was itself somewhat of a problem in that resources had to be diverted to deal with well-wishers. Bad feelings resulted when some of the people who wanted to help were turned away. The ambiguity about whether the WTC site was a crime site or a disaster site and the ongoing concern about personal injuries among rescue and recovery workers (Chapter 5) limited access so that many volunteers and supplies that had been contributed did not penetrate the perimeter. Dr. Antonio Abad, a forensic psychiatrist who was the first to arrive at the WTC disaster site from the nearby court clinic, stayed there two weeks as a member of what became the "ad hoc" team. He has provided the following summary:

Box 3–2. Anger, Racism, and Hate Crimes.

The events of September 11 have caused Americans to experience horror, fear, anxiety, panic, sadness, and mistrust. Anger and hatred directed towards terrorists are also very common feelings to experience after such a disaster.[1] In a study of ethnic Albanians after the 1998–1999 war in Kosovo, almost 90 percent of people reported having strong feelings of hatred toward Serbs; almost half reported feelings of revenge; and, of these, about one-third claimed they would act on their feelings.[2] Similar feelings may have occurred in Americans after September 11.

Soon after the September 11 attacks, repeated television images of Osama bin Laden were displayed, representing a target for hatred and anger. Since he was not accessible to the American public, hatred was directed towards groups he resembled in some people's minds, such as Muslims, Arab-Americans, Sikhs, and other Middle Easterners and Southeast Asians. Some people acted on these intense feelings of hatred and committed hate crimes.

Hate crimes are violent acts against people, property, or organizations that represent a particular group or belief.[3] This representation may be false; clearly not all Muslims are terrorists, and not all terrorists are Muslim. This false representation is due to a distortion of facts that the perpetrator of the hate crime has developed or learned. The perpetrators of these crimes are often trying to send a message to these groups that they are not liked, accepted, or wanted. In some cases, the perpetrator belongs to an organized hate group, but, in many cases, he or she is acting alone.[3] The perpetrator often has a previous history of antisocial behavior, and may be under the influence of drugs or alcohol. While hate crimes can be committed against any group, racial bias is the most frequent cause of a hate crime.[3]

The events of September 11 led to many bias-related hate crimes. Less than one week after the attacks, the Federal Bureau of Investigation (FBI) was investigating 40 potential hate crimes against Arab-Americans and others mistaken for belonging to terrorist groups.[4] By the end of November, the American-Arab Anti-Discrimination Committee (ADC) had confirmed 520 violent acts or threats directed against Muslims, Arab-Americans, Sikhs, and other people perceived to be Arab.[5] Hate crimes nearly quadrupled in the months following September 11. These offenses ranged from murder, to arson, to assault and battery. Specific hate-based murders included:

• A Sikh owner of a gas station was killed in Mesa, Arizona;
• A Pakistani Muslim owner of a grocery store was killed in Dallas;
• Two Sikh store-owners were killed in Fresno and Tulare County, California; and
• An Egyptian owner of a grocery store was killed in San Gabriel, California.[6–8]

In addition, in Northridge, California, a Sikh man was beaten with a metal pole. A Middle Eastern taxi driver was severely beaten by two passengers. Two Afghan-

(continued)

(continued)

American teenagers were attacked by a mob of people. In Upstate New York, three teenagers committed arson at a Sikh temple. There were many other reports of beatings and vandalism in other mosques and temples throughout the country.

Besides these grotesque acts of hate and racism, many other subtle acts of discrimination were also reported, including 27 cases of airline racism, employment discrimination, and law enforcement profiling.[5]

The victims of these heinous hate crimes are likely to suffer severe emotional consequences. Due to fear or possibly even embarrassment, many victims do not report hate crimes, possibly leading to ineffective coping—perhaps a reason why these victims experience crime-related psychological problems for several years more than victims of non-bias crimes.[3] These problems may manifest as fear, anger, depression, physical ailments, and social consequences.

Post-traumatic stress disorder (PTSD) can also develop in these victims. In addition, race-related stressors increase the risk of PTSD and psychological distress symptoms.[9]

Many approaches were used to curtail these hate crimes and racist attitudes. Numerous rallies, marches, and candlelight vigils representing anti-hate, anti-racism sentiments took place throughout the United States in the fall of 2001. One of the largest of these occurred on September 29, when over 20,000 people marched in an "anti-war, anti-racist" rally in Washington, D.C. President George W. Bush and other government officials have repeatedly condemned hate crimes and other racially motivated acts of terror.[4] The U.S. Commission on Civil Rights made a hotline available soon after September 11 for people wishing to report hate crimes committed against Arabs, Muslims, and other South Asian victims. In addition, Human Rights Watch issued a Universal Declaration of Human Rights, signed by several organizations.[6] This document called for condemning the terrorist attacks, as well as rejecting scapegoating that might lead to hate crimes and racially driven harassment towards Arab-Americans and others perceived to be Arab.

Although there was limited media exposure and condemnation of racism and hate crimes after September 11, the public needed to be even better informed about them to help prevent them. If teachers, physicians, and other professionals help educate the public about tolerance and patience during threats of terror, then perhaps fewer crimes may be committed.

—Nimmi Kapoor

BOX REFERENCES
1. Holloway H, Norwood A, Fullerton C, et al. The threat of biological weapons. *JAMA* 1997; 278:425–7.
2. Cardozo B, Vergara A, Agani F, et al. Mental health, social functioning, and attitudes of Kosovar Albanians following war in Kosovo. *JAMA* 2000; 284:569–77.
3. Hate crimes today: An age-old foe in modern dress. *American Psychological Association*, 1998. (Accessed March 10th, 2002, at http://www.apa.org/pubinfo/hate/)
4. *Copley News Service*, September 17, 2001. Bush demands respect for Muslims in America; FBI probing hate crimes. Finlay Lewis, Copley News Service.

(continued)

Box 3–2. *(continued)*

5. ADC Fact Sheet: The Condition of Arab Americans Post-9/11. Washington, D.C., Nov. 20, 2001. (Accessed February 20th, 2002.)
6. *HRW World Report 2001: Racism and Human Rights.* Human Rights Watch Press release, New York, 2001. (Accessed February 20th, 2002, at http://www.hrw.org/press/2001/09/us-reprisal0921.htm.)
7. *Washington Post,* January 20, 2002, "Sept. 11 Backlash Murders and the State of 'Hate'; Between Families And Police, a Gulf on Victim Count," Alan Cooperman, Washington Post staff writer.
8. *Washington Post,* November 04, 2001, "Beating of Pakistani Cab Driver Called a Hate Crime; Two Passengers Charged With Assault," Josh White, Washington Post staff writer.
9. Loo CM, Fairbank JA, Scurfield RM, et al. Measuring exposure to racism: development and validation of a Race-Related Stressor Scale (RRSS) for Asian American Vietnam veterans. *Psychol Assess* 2001; 13:503–20.
10. Schuster MA, Stein B, Jaycox L, et al. A national survey of stress reactions after the September 11, 2001, terrorist attacks. *N Engl J Med* 2001; 345:1507–12.
11. Ursano R. Post-traumatic stress disorder. *N Engl J Med* 2002; 346:130–2.

During the first 2 weeks immediately after September 11, the mental health *ad hoc* team performed many clinical interventions involving most rescue, security, and support personnel working at Ground Zero. These activities included distributing more than 10,000 "psychoeducational" documents. The team also directly provided supportive interventions or debriefed more than 1,500 individuals, facilitated the evacuation of hundreds of workers who urgently needed treatment and rest, and referred many more workers to mental health facilities throughout the city. In addition, for clinical and research purposes, they performed long-term follow-up of a cohort of 500 individuals involved during the first week after September 11 in rescue, support, and medical services at Ground Zero. From my perspective, the following systems problems occurred:

- Civilian volunteers provided most of the mental health services at the Ground Zero area during the first two weeks after the disaster.
- Limited access of civilians to the disaster site, because of security reasons and delayed credentialing processes, caused a serious shortage of staff members, and contributed to high levels of distress and exhaustion among civilian volunteers, including clinicians.
- Problems were caused by delayed and limited deployment of mental health teams provided by federal agencies and nongovernmental disaster relief organizations.
- No organized official psychiatric personnel were available until September 18, except for those from the New York Police Department and the Health and Hospitals Corporation teams.
- Official mental health services were unable to meet the demands at the site, as evidenced by consistent requests to the *ad hoc* team to continue providing services after they had been deployed.
- The civilian *ad hoc* team was required to provide coordination among governmental agencies and civilian volunteers.
- Civilian volunteers who were at high risk of mental health problems left the area without registration, psychoeducation, and follow-up referrals, as compared with government personnel, who received these services.

• Nongovernmental disaster-assistance agencies did not provide significant mental health services at Ground Zero during the first 2 weeks after the catastrophe.[11]

Although the ad hoc team grew eventually to more than 100 clinicians, it still needed many more workers. It was not totally clear why more workers were not there. The mass media did not specify what kind of workers were needed. In addition, it was not clear who needed assistance. For example, rescue and recovery workers acknowledged their physical needs and sought treatment for them; most of them, however, denied having needs for emotional support or treatment of mental health problems.

In general, there was no private way of recruiting those able to meet relevant needs. On September 11, a call was made for physicians and nurses to go to hospitals, but this was cancelled within hours when an overwhelming number of volunteers appeared. There was no call for medical volunteers to go to the triage sites that were rapidly established near Ground Zero (Figure 3–1). There was no request for mental health professionals—except through their professional associations, which reached them by e-mail messages, faxes, and some telephone calls. But, as James Stone, New York State Commissioner of Mental Health, observed, there was no way to be sure which volunteers had been trained to do what.

IMPROVING MENTAL HEALTH SYSTEM RESPONSES TO TERRORISM

Future threats of terrorism could involve hijackings; truck bombs; nuclear power plants; "dirty nukes"; contamination of water supplies; and biological, chemical, and nuclear weapons. While it is reassuring to read about plans to

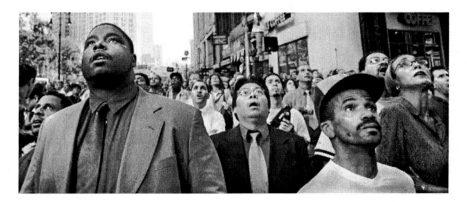

FIGURE 3–1. Onlookers behold the collapse of the south tower of the World Trade Center at 9:59 a.m. on September 11, 2001 (Photograph by Patrick Witty).

cope with each of these threats, no plans include any consideration of mental health. Yet each of these threats has its own form of accompanying terror. While there are other, presently unimagined possibilities, one must start somewhere. Some threat-specific special considerations are noted for the following needs.

Assisting Affected Individuals

What can be learned from the WTC disaster? Calculations for Project Liberty, the main public effort aimed specifically at mental health, determined that there were 2.5 million people at risk of being affected by mental health problems, with widening circles of decreasing severity—like ripples spreading out from the impact of a stone landing in a pond. These calculations will be reviewed as data accumulate from actual experiences. In the rush to provide physical aid, comfort, and triage, only partial records were kept of who was served, and there is no way of knowing, apart from records of those employed at the WTC and nearby businesses, who was in the area at the time of the attack. Thousands of people streamed from Ground Zero to what became makeshift triage areas at New York University Downtown Hospital (several blocks away), open spaces immediately north of the WTC site, and on the Liberty Island trade center in the adjacent Hudson River. Mental health professionals were not called to these places, although there was no safety risk or perimeter control. Instead, many health professionals wasted their time waiting at hospitals in uptown Manhattan to which victims never came. Many people with immediate mental health problems were therefore overlooked. Subsequent outreach efforts were not effective in targeting populations at high risk, such as recent or undocumented immigrants whose native language is not English. Up until seven months after the WTC attack, there was no generally accepted list of those killed—another source of anxiety.[12-16] There was additional anxiety about the possible mistaken identification of victims.[17,18]

Despite the presence of all the relevant disaster relief agencies, the deployment of organized mental health services at Ground Zero by federal agencies and nongovernmental disaster-relief organizations was delayed and limited. For the future, all large cities should create contingency plans capable of dealing with the types and numbers of mental health needs generated by the WTC attacks. These plans should ensure the effective integration of all available mental health resources, and the appointment of official mental health teams that are ready to deploy immediately after a catastrophe.

Training of authorized mental health team members before a catastrophe occurs and development of clinical and psychoeducational protocols are urgently needed within governmental agencies and nongovernmental organizations. Each possible terrorist attack in the future will pose its own challenges. For example, attacks with biological, chemical, and nuclear or radiological weapons are likely to cause restricted access to the disaster site. If physical isolation of affected individuals occurs, methods will be needed overcome that isolation.

Records of WTC workers who survived the attack are fragmentary. As of March 2002, there was no consensus on whether to try to contact all survivors and, if so, how. Most businesses and other organizations that had been based at the WTC, in order to address the mental health needs of their employees, either used their employee assistance programs or contracted with private firms. Follow-up has been limited. The New York Fire Department has allowed statements of general findings (but not about specific patients) from clinicians at St. Vincent's Hospital, which has been successful in getting mental health workers into firehouses;[19] in contrast, the New York Police Department, which contracted with Columbia University for mental health services, has not released[19] any observations.[20]

Ideally, in the future, everyone at risk of mental health problems should be contacted, with their privacy respected. A contact would be limited to assessing the degree of trauma ("What happened?") and defense and coping mechanisms ("How are you dealing with it?").

Work with survivors of other disasters has found that the large numbers initially reporting distress decrease to 5 to 15 percent in about six months.[1–3] In the first four weeks, everyone in the area is likely to feel some distress, which should be seen as a normal reaction to a disaster. During this time, it is best to provide brief counseling, support, and assistance through self-help groups, and ensure involvement in activities. After six months, the 5 to 15 percent who still are distressed may include some people who need referral for mental health treatment.

While there is a consensus on the helpfulness of cognitive behavioral therapy, medication, group and individual psychotherapy, and self-help and support groups, there is controversy concerning debriefing and eye movement desensitization. *Debriefing* involves getting a patient to review the traumatic event in detail and bring out all of her or his memories—virtually reliving it. The rationale for debriefing is that incompletely repressed memories cause continuing symptoms. Debriefing is seen by its proponents as a way of dealing better with memories by bringing them out into the open. Others see it as stripping defenses, such as repression and denial, without providing alternative defense or coping mechanisms. Reliving the experience may make it harder to move on. In this view, debriefing is unnecessary for many and potentially harmful for some disaster survivors.[2] Eye movement desensitization assumes that images of the trauma are lodged in the brain somewhat like a frozen frame of a motion picture. It further assumes that guiding the eyes to different parts of the image, and then entirely out of the frame of the image, such as to objects in the room where the person is now located, may be effective. A potential problem with eye movement desensitization is that it may further ingrain an image that would otherwise fade slowly. In addition, there are other approaches to desensitization that do not involve eye movements at all.[2]

The September 11 attacks have been compared to the London Blitz. Although PTSD was not recognized then, the high degree of organization involved in being part of the British war effort probably kept people from feeling isolated or impotent, thus minimizing anxiety and depression—and PTSD. After September 11, a high percentage of Americans were affected emotionally, as evidenced by rises in sales of antidepressants[21] and antianxiety[22] medications—a 30 percent increase in the first four weeks.[23] The perceived physical threat also sparked increased gun sales nationally,[24] raising concern about a possible future increase in gun-related fatalities.

There have been reports of survivor guilt—that is, people entering therapy to deal with the fact that they lived while loved ones they thought should have lived (rather than themselves) were killed.[25] Helping children deal with the attacks has posed special problems based on their incomplete knowledge of the world and different ways of showing distress.[26] On the other hand, the schools have been venues for outreach, with each teacher and administrator provided with manuals developed by, and available from, the NYU Child Study Center.[27]

Much PTSD occurred in New York after the WTC attack. Thirty-minute telephone interviews of 1,008 adults living in Manhattan below 110th Street, conducted five to eight weeks after September 11, found 9.7 percent reporting symptoms consistent with current depression (within the past 30 days) and 7.5 percent reporting symptoms consistent with current PTSD. Overall, 13.6 percent of the respondents reported symptoms consistent with either of these diagnoses, and 3.7 percent reported symptoms consistent with both. Projected onto Manhattan's population, the study suggests that about 87,000 people needed mental health services for depression and about 67,000 for PTSD.[28] The study found a higher incidence of symptoms among Hispanics, a finding for which there is no easy explanation. It also found that those experiencing panic attacks on or shortly after September 11 were more likely to experience symptoms subsequently, which may be a useful prognostic indicator.

Experience in other disasters has demonstrated that it is difficult to predict who will still have symptoms after the initial 6-month period, during which a wide range of emotional reactions are regarded as normal. After 6 months, it is usual for some people who have been coping well to experience difficulties. In response to these and other mental health needs, the mass media in the New York area have encouraged people to seek service through advertisements for Project Liberty and published articles.[29]

Helping Families Cope and Grieve

Dr. Martin Gittelman, a New York psychologist who cared for families of WTC attack victims, observed that: (a) Families of native-born, employed Americans are doing as well as could be expected. (b) Undocumented workers' families dropped out of follow-up activities and did not want to be detected or deported. (Among those affected, they had the greatest economic needs.) (c) Members of the families of Muslim victims were especially reluctant to come forward. (d) Language barriers reduced access to assistance—especially needed were Spanish-language materials.[30]

Affected families needed outreach services, but efforts were complicated by the absence of a list of their names and addresses. Families have been organizing among themselves, but, as of March 2002, did not receive a newsletter or periodic e-mail information. Contacts of families affected by the WTC disaster by families affected by the 1995 Oklahoma City bombing were helpful. In the future, families affected by the WTC disaster might serve as resources for families affected by other terrorist acts or disasters.

As with affected individuals, families who lost loved ones in the WTC disaster until 6 months afterward have been distressed, but experiencing a normal grieving process (Figure 3–2). However, the 6-to-8–month period is

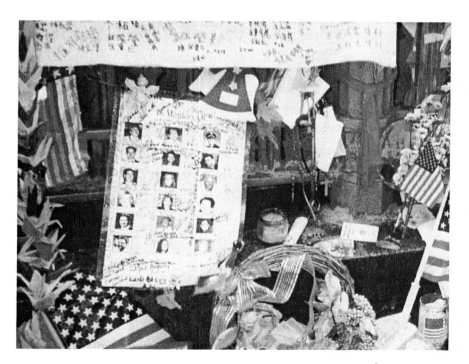

FIGURE 3–2. A makeshift memorial near the World Trade Center site (Photograph by Barry S. Levy).

stressful, and four suicides are known to have occurred in families who lost a loved one in the WTC disaster, despite all the awareness of this risk and massive outreach efforts.[30] A book in memory of firefighters who died has been published.[31] The families that have been involved with one another and have had other supports are presumably at less risk than those who are not. It can be expected that the 5 to 15 percent of those affected who are still experiencing distress six months afterward will include family members who received such support, as described above. Some families may elect to be seen as a group in family therapy. Future terrorist-attack sites may differ, with more or less area, physical damage, and risk to rescue and recovery workers and the general population, but the effects on families are unlikely to differ much because they most likely will be remote from the site of the attack. For individuals they may differ, however, since some affected individuals may be isolated (requiring that families be given means to communicate with them) or chronically ill or disfigured (requiring continued support and treatment for the family as a whole).

Since one-third of working adults in New York City have no health insurance, it is not surprising that families affected by the WTC attacks have been concerned about ongoing care (see Box 13–2 in Chapter 13). At present, an attempt is being made to arrange lifetime health insurance coverage for them. If successful, a major source of anxiety and possible economic hardship will be removed and an important precedent set.

Preparing and Supporting First-Responders and Counselors

Dr. Abad has noted that during the first two weeks after September 11, the mental health *ad hoc* team performed many clinical interventions for most rescue, security, and support personnel working at Ground Zero.[11] All of the activities described thus far in this chapter were performed by a group that gradually increased in number from 12 to 100, who patrolled the site, engaging rescue and recovery workers in conversations about how they were doing.

I provided treatment to first-responders at Bellevue Hospital, who were distinguished from victims in that they felt challenged to work beyond reasonable limits and to deny any emotional anguish. For example, a firefighter who was being treated for a moderately severe eye injury that should have been painful instead said he felt nothing. He told me he was so happy about saving some of his fellow firefighters that his eye injury did not matter. "Situational mania" described him best.

Over time, however, energy levels decreased and the euphoria of providing help did not persist after repeatedly dealing with serious injury and death, so stoicism developed.[32] The defense mechanisms involved in stoicism include repression (unconscious mechanisms that prevent some feelings from being perceived), denial (denying feelings), and suppression (consciously willing unwanted feelings out of one's mind)—defenses that may give way abruptly. Since first-responders and counselors cannot be trusted to monitor themselves well, every team should include someone who is monitoring the care of these carers.

Regular relief and rest are essential for these first-responders and counselors, necessitating access to disaster sites for the first-responders and counselors who relieve them. A designated team of trained personnel is not enough. There must be multiple teams to handle large numbers of victims and to relieve each other.

Treatment for first-responders and counselors is similar to that for others with similar diagnoses, except that there is likely to be more peer support and more obvious reward for having served others. Treatment must also consider that first-responders and counselors are likely to have been at the disaster site longer than the victims, with risk of exposure to toxins needing to be considered (Chapter 5). Follow-up of New York firefighters, performed by St. Vincent's Hospital, found (a) effective use of therapists if they were deployed at fire department locations, and (b) persistence of the following problems: increased alcohol use, strained relationships, irritability, difficulty concentrating, insomnia, and avoidant responses, such as firefighters being determined to avoid appearing weak.

Workers at Ground Zero frequently refused to wear hard hats and masks, and often refused to wear gloves (Chapter 5). Denial of potential vulnerability seemed to be an important part of the professional armor for working at Ground Zero. At least one member of each team of first-responders and counselors should ensure that safety regulations and guidelines are followed and hazardous occupational exposures thereby limited. This approach might be easiest in radiation situations, where threats are most easily measured and there is long experience in calculating exposure risks.

Diagnosing and Treating PTSD and Other Disorders and Dysfunctional Responses

Even six months after a disaster is too soon to make definite diagnoses of PTSD and other chronic mental health disorders because premature diagnoses are harmful and should be discouraged. The prevailing philosophy is that adverse mental or emotional reactions to awful events are to be expected, should be talked out or somehow dealt with, and can be overcome. Issues that might be encountered in treatment may vary according to specific terrorist acts or threats. For example, attacks involving nuclear power plants or "dirty nukes" may lead to a fear of cancer or birth defects in offspring (Chapter 12). Hijackings may lead to survivor guilt or concern that one should have done more to prevent the outcome. Water supply threats may lead to phobic responses to drinking tap water or obsessive-compulsive concerns and practices. Terrorist acts or threats involving chemical agents may lead to fear of residual or long-term damage. Acts or threats involving biological agents may lead to fear of infecting others.

Strengthening the Fabric of Communities through Collective Responses

Government agencies at the federal, state, and local levels need to rethink their roles vis-à-vis terrorism. Public anxiety in New York on and after September 11 was enhanced by public uncertainty about who was in charge and whether Ground Zero was a crime scene or a disaster site. Access guidelines developed in advance of various possibilities can help facilitate assistance from nongovernmental organizations (NGOs) to government agencies, as was done after September 11. For example, the New York City list of mental health resources, which was issued within days of the tragedy, was useful. NGOs, however, were not allowed access to first-responders, and NGO staff members were not trained or credentialed for dealing with the aftereffects of terrorist attacks or disasters.

Charity problems, which abounded after September 11,[33] created a sense of inequity[34] that threatened to divide communities.[35] The amount of funding available from charities, in addition to government agencies, very much affected the affordability of ongoing care. By September 28, at least $482 million had been pledged to charitable funds.[36] Generous compensation payments loomed.[37] The American Red Cross raised so much money that it suggested keeping some to help with subsequent disasters; it later had to backtrack, as contributors protested that they wanted their donations used for September 11 victims and their families.[38] The amount raised far exceeded, on a per-recipient basis, amounts raised after any other tragedy.[39] A precedent was established: those who lost homes or jobs received $2,500 each—the single largest disbursement of charity aimed specifically at those who were newly unemployed and homeless.[40] The job market has been followed closely as a barometer of loss and need,[41] with revival not necessarily resulting in the rehiring of the people who lost their jobs.[42]

Concern that some people would receive too much or too little led to the suggestion—fortunately not followed—to list recipients publicly.[43] At the same time, relief agencies had trouble gaining access to a database that would enable them to do their work.[44] For future disasters, a confidential pooling of recipient data should be planned. The charity problem was exacerbated by public arguments on whether the fund would be controlled by the mayor[45] or the New York State attorney general.[46] After this debate was resolved,[47] there was the additional problem of distributing the money—another issue that can be anticipated and planned for future disasters.[48] Unanticipated large financial losses occurred for hospitals,[49] a problem that also needs to be addressed in future disaster planning by government agencies and charitable organizations.

Community planning for future disasters must consider potentially divisive effects of charitable contributions. Broad-based groups should develop formulas for disbursing funds in the future, gaining consensus on who gets assistance and how much—such as by using the scale paid to airplane disaster victims. The plan of the American Red Cross for setting aside some of the funds for future disasters would have been sensible, had its solicitations explicitly stated this plan.

Commissioner Stone noted that future planning must address the need that communities feel for some constructive personal connection to the event, the importance of having roles for volunteers, and the need for more contingency planning. The family center at Pier 94 in New York provided "one-stop shopping" for medical, psychological, financial, housing, and other needs; however, the space provided was insufficient for those in need to talk and associate freely.

Adding to the Knowledge Base for Effective Prevention

The terrorist attacks of September 11 have led to several research projects on the efficacy of mental health and other interventions. There is a need to draw lessons from what was done well and where problems occurred. People and organizations that have been involved in responding to the mental health consequences of the WTC attack understandably want to preserve the privacy of those affected and are reluctant to open lists of victims and survivors to any researcher,[50] but a balance probably will be struck to ensure that long-term findings are derived and conclusions are disseminated. Little new information has been reported from service systems research on the WTC disaster, as agencies are still in the debriefing stage.

Questions remain, such as: Who should be trained to do what? What responsibilities should everyone have? What should be the roles of primary health care and of the specialty mental health sector? New York Governor George Pataki has noted that a lesson learned from September 11 is that all health care workers need to have first-responder training at the same level as police and firefighters and should be among the first people to arrive at the scene of any terrorist attack. Research is needed to define these roles. Research is also needed on communication technology and content that will effectively and promptly alert health professionals but not unduly alarm the general public. Since diagnoses by health professionals depend on an appropriate index of suspicion and since terrorism depends on making people anxious, we must find ways to inform health professionals without unduly alarming others.

CONCLUSION

The mental health of the population is a prime target of terrorists. The September 11 attacks inflicted great damage and posed challenges that were met well, despite problems of access to Ground Zero. The course of emotional problems resembled that after earthquakes, with expectations that distress during the first few months after the event will be regarded as normal, even while requiring attention to crisis work, counseling, and support groups for survivors, family members of victims, first-responders, and others. The six-month mark is when some previously well individuals can be expected to need help, even while the bulk of the people who were distressed initially are recovering. Although government agencies and the health care system coped well in response to the WTC attack, future planning for disasters should more clearly define responsibilities for various personnel at disaster sites, including how to provide optimal access for prequalified response teams. Support issues that involve charitable organizations and government agencies should be resolved in advance. Plans to respond to terrorist attacks in the future must adequately include mental health.

REFERENCES

1. Shinfuku N. To be a victim and a survivor of the Great Hanshin-Awaji Earthquake. *J Psychosom Res* 1999; 46:541–548.
2. Katz C, Pandya A, DeLisi L. Psychiatric interventions in disasters. *Psychiatric Research* (in press). Available from ckatz@aol.com.
3. Desai NG, Gupta DK, et al. *Mental Health Service Needs and Service Delivery Models in the Earthquake Disaster Affected Population in Gujerat: A Pilot Phase Study.* New Delhi, India: Institute of Human Behavior & Allied Sciences (IHBAS), 2002.
4. Lagnado L. Disaster psychiatry volunteers minister to the distraught. *Wall Street Journal*, September 17, 2001, A20.
5. Perez-Pena R. Service center offers help to the victims of terrorism. *New York Times*, September 24, 2001, B10.
6. Lagnado L. New York rushes to spend grants for counseling. *Wall Street Journal*, October 5, 2001, B1.
7. Donovan A. Grants to help post-traumatic stress. *New York Times*, November 27, 2001, B8.
8. Project Liberty. *Office of Mental Health Quarterly*, December 2001.

9. Chen D, Greenhouse S. As anthrax cases mount, the tranquil rhythms of suburban havens are disrupted. *New York Times*, November 1, 2001, B9.

10. Parker-Pope T. Antibiotics like Cipro are linked to tendon, psychiatric problems. *Wall Street Journal*, October 26, 2001, B1.

11. Abad A. Report from Ground Zero. *Bulletin of the World Association for Psychosocial Rehabilitation* 14(1): 2–9, 2002.

12. Ellison M. Number of New York dead may be 2,000 less than official tally. *The Guardian*, October 20, 2001, p. 17.

13. Lipton E. Toll from attack at Trade Center is down sharply. *New York Times*, November 11, 2001, A1.

14. Lipton E. Tally of Twin Towers deaths is down sharply. *New York Times*, November 30, 2001, A1.

15. Cardwell D. City refines its counting of the dead. *New York Times*, November 25, 2001, A43.

16. Trade Center count of missing and dead falls below 3,000. *New York Times*, December 20, 2001, B7.

17. LeDuff C. After error, a funeral under the right name. *New York Times*, December 2, 2001, B7.

18. Worth R. DNA matches surge, aiding identification of victims. *New York Times*, December 21, 2001, B6.

19. Lagnado L. FDNY tries to rescue its own. *Wall Street Journal*, March 2, 2002, B1.

20. Kupersann E. Stoic firefighters wrestle with post-disaster emotions. *Psychiatric News*, March 1, 2002, pp. 7, 37.

21. Parker-Pope T. Anxious Americans seek antidepressants to cope with terror. *Wall Street Journal*, October 12, 2001, B1.

22. Lewin T. Bioterrorism and anxiety are swelling prescriptions. *New York Times*, November 1, 2001, B10.

23. Rosach J. Drug makers find Sept. 11 a marketing opportunity. *Psych News*, March 1, 2002, p.9.

24. Butterfield F. Steep rise in gun sales. *New York Times*, December 16, 2001 A1.

25. Goode E. Therapists hear survivors' refrain: if only. *New York Times*, September 25, 2001, F1.

26. Lagnada L. Kids confront Trade Center trauma. *Wall Street Journal*, November 2, 2001, B1.

27. Manual for Administrators and Mental Health Professionals (71pp) and Manual for Parents and Teachers (44pp) can be downloaded from www.aboutourkids.org.

28. Galea S, Ahern J, Resnick H, et al. Psychological sequelae of the September 11 terrorist attacks in NYC. *N Engl J Med*, 2002; 346:982–987.

29. Lagnado L. Bracing for trauma's second wave. *Wall Street Journal*, March 2, 2002, B1.

30. Gittelman M. Presentations at American Association for Psychosocial Rehabilitation, February 26 and April 22, 2002.

31. Barron J. Book of photos serves as a glossy homage to lost firefighters. *New York Times*, December 2, 2001, B7.

32. Amid dig, emotions are buried. *New York Times*, November 18, 2001, B1.

33. Donovan A. $17 million given since attack in donations large and small. *New York Times*, September 28, 2001, B10.

34. Barstow D. Survivors say plan for fund is stingy. *New York Times*, December 21, 2001, B6.

35. Henriques D. Gifts for the rescuers are dividing the victims' survivors. *New York Times*, December 2, 2001, A1.
36. Henriques D, Barstow D. Fund for victims' families already proves sore point. *New York Times*, October 1, 2001, A1.
37. Henriques D. Victims' fund is likely to pay average of $1.6 million each. *New York Times*, December 21, 2001, A1.
38. Barstow D. In Congress, harsh words for Red Cross. *New York Times*, November 7, 2001, B1.
39. Ingrassia R. Charity giving raises hard questions. *Daily News*, September 25, 2001, p. 29.
40. Barstow D. Those who lost homes or jobs are to get $2500 grants. *New York Times*, December 12, 2001, B11.
41. Eaton L. The mystery of the disappearing jobs. *New York Times*, March 10, 2001, X-1.
42. Dunham K. New York's job market is reviving. *Wall Street Journal*, March 12, 2002, B10.
43. Henriques D, Barstow D. Plan to list who receives disaster aid stirs concern. *New York Times*, September 27, 2001, B1.
44. Bank D. Relief agencies gain control of database for Sept. 11 aid. *Wall Street Journal*, November 2, 2001, B2.
45. Barstow D, Henriques D. Mayor asserts he, not state, will oversee charity efforts. *New York Times*, October 2, 2001, A1.
46. Barstow D. Spitzer plans to coordinate charity efforts for victims. *New York Times*, September 26, 2001, B10.
47. An accord on charities. *New York Times*, October 3, 2001, B10.
48. Charity and red tape. Editorial, *New York Times*, October 30, 2001, A16.
49. Steinhauer J. Sept 11 exacts economic toll from hospitals in New York. *New York Times*, October 30, 2001, D1.
50. Lagnado L. It's trying time for health chief in New York City. *Wall Street Journal*, October 12, 2001, B1.

4

Addressing environmental health issues

LUZ CLAUDIO, ANJALI GARG, AND PHILIP J. LANDRIGAN

The environmental aspects of the World Trade Center (WTC) disaster were extraordinary. Over a million tons of steel, dust, cement, asbestos, and other debris fell to the ground. The enormous heat (up to 2000° F) from the fires and explosions transformed many materials, such as computers, carpeting, furniture, and air conditioning fluid, in the WTC into a gaseous cloud of potentially toxic dust, which took weeks to dissipate[1] (Figure 4–1).

The six-story-high pile of compacted rubble that resulted from the fires and collapse of the WTC towers became known as the Pile, or Ground Zero. During the first days after September 11, immediate physical dangers were everywhere. Buildings adjacent to the towers collapsed or suffered major damage. Intense fires continued to burn, and a massive cloud of dust and smoke spread with the prevailing winds for miles from the site. For several months after the attack, nearby communities experienced the smell of acrid smoke from the long-burning fires. All of this devastation occurred in the middle of an intensely populated urban center.

Lower Manhattan encompasses not only a vibrant working community, but also a significant residential neighborhood. Nearly 20,000 people live within one-half-mile of Ground Zero; almost 3,000 of them are children.[2] When the WTC was destroyed, the communities of lower Manhattan were enveloped in smoke and soot. All residents were placed at risk of exposure to poten-

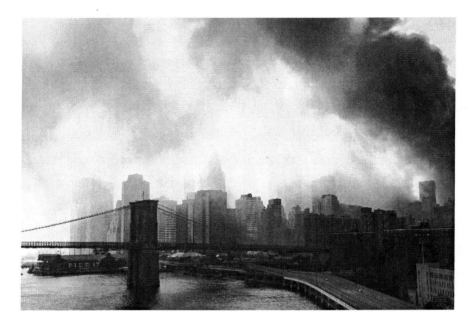

FIGURE 4-1. On September 11, 2001, lower Manhattan disappeared behind a black veil of smoke (© Thomas Hoepker/Magnum Photos).

tially toxic compounds, with particular concern expressed for women and children. Many offices and apartments were coated with dust that entered those structures through shattered windows or inadequately protected air-handling systems. Following the initial shock of the largest death toll ever from terrorism on U.S. soil, federal, state, and local government officials, along with scientists from across the nation, began the enormous process of recovering human remains, removing and disposing of debris, and evaluating the potential continued health threats to rescue and recovery workers and residents of the surrounding community from environmental health exposures related to the attacks.

ENVIRONMENTAL HEALTH THREATS

A number of contaminants, such as asbestos, particulate matter, lead, and polychlorinated biphenyls (PCBs) were released into the environment after the WTC attack (see Table 4–1). The levels of contamination and the adverse health effects on rescue and recovery workers (see Chapter 5) and residents of the surrounding community are being assessed by regulatory agencies and environmental health scientists.

TABLE 4-1. Contaminants Potentially Present* at the World Trade Center Site.

CONTAMINANT	EXAMPLES OF HEALTH EFFECTS	SOURCE
Asbestos	Carcinogenic. Causes tissue scarring in the lungs when inhaled over long periods and can lead to asbestosis, mesothelioma, and lung cancer.	Used as an insulator and fire retardant, applied to steel beams.
Benzene	Flammable and carcinogenic. Short-term effects include dizziness, headaches, and tremors. Long-term exposure can lead to leukemia.	Combustion of plastics.
Biohazards	Exposure to blood and body parts can transmit infectious diseases such as hepatitis and AIDS. After long periods, they may pose little hazard to health, although finding human remains can cause psychological trauma.	Human remains of the victims trapped in the rubble.
Chromium	Carcinogenic when inhaled at high concentrations. Dermal contact can cause skin ulcers.	Video and computer monitors.
Copper	In large amounts can cause dizziness, headaches, vomiting, and damage to the kidneys and liver.	Electrical wiring and cables.
Diesel fumes	Asthma trigger. Can aggravate symptoms in asthmatics.	Truck traffic and heavy machinery from the cleanup effort.
Dioxins	Chloracne is a short-term effect of exposure. Strong evidence for carcinogenic, teratogenic, reproductive, and immunosuppressive effects. Persist and bioaccumulate in the environment and and food chain.	Combustion of polyvinyl chloride found in electrical cables and others insulating materials and some plastics.
Freon	Damages the ozone layer. When burned, can produce phosgene, a potent cause of severe and life-threatening pulmonary edema.	Refrigeration and air-conditioning equipment.
Lead	Neurotoxic. Damages the central nervous system, especially in children. Can also cause kidney and reproductive damage in adults.	Video and computer monitors, rust-proofing paint used on steel beams.

(continued)

TABLE 4–1. (*continued*)

CONTAMINANT	EXAMPLES OF HEALTH EFFECTS	SOURCE
Mercury	Neurotoxic. Damages the peripheral nervous system, especially in children.	Thermometers and other precision instruments.
Particulate matter	Asthma trigger. Can aggravate symptoms in asthmatics. Can also aggravate cardiovascular disease. Smaller particles ($PM_{2.5}$) may be more potent than larger particles (PM_{10}).	Pulverized concrete and other materials (large particles); smoke, dust, and soot from combustion (small particles).
Polychlorinated biphenyls	Carcinogenic. May also cause hormonal problems and reproductive and developmental abnormalities. Persist in the human body and the environment.	Transformers and other electrical equipment.
Sulfur dioxide	Pulmonary toxicant. Can cause severe airway obstruction when inhaled at high concentrations. Can burn the nose and throat.	Combustion of many materials.

*Not all of the pollutants listed were tested for at the World Trade Center site.

Asbestos

The release of asbestos fibers from the WTC site into the neighboring community was a major environmental concern. Asbestos is a known carcinogen, particularly in workers who are exposed to high doses over long periods of time.[3,4] Long-term health risks of exposure to asbestos include lung cancer and mesothelioma, a malignancy virtually specific to asbestos exposure. During the construction of the lower 40 floors of the North Tower, asbestos was sprayed onto steel beams for fireproofing. This spray contained between 5 percent and 30 percent chrysotile asbestos.[5]

The collapse of the Twin Towers caused the asbestos fibers that had been tucked into the walls of the buildings to disperse in a huge dust cloud. After September 11, the U.S. Environmental Protection Agency (EPA) obtained samples of the air, dust, water, river sediments, and drinking water, and analyzed them for the presence of asbestos and other contaminants that might pose a health risk to the public and to rescue and recovery workers (Figure 4–2). All of the 70 samples taken at and around Ground Zero between February 27 and March 1, 2002, demonstrated asbestos levels of fewer than 70 fibers (structures) per square millimeter, the standard under the Asbestos Hazard Emergency Response Act (AHERA) for allowing children to re-enter school buildings after asbestos abatement.[6] At least 17 samples obtained earlier, however, had demonstrated levels that were above this standard; of these 17 samples, six had been collected after September 30, 2001. (See Chapter 2.)

Although air levels of asbestos may have been below the range that would require regulatory action, dust that had accumulated outside, on window sills and sidewalks, and inside homes of residents throughout the area needed to be treated as if it contained asbestos and lead. Due to uneven release of asbestos, only some samples may have contained it, but all dust exposures had to be considered potentially hazardous. The New York City Department of Health (DOH) issued guidelines for residents returning to their homes.[7] In order to reduce dust recirculation, the DOH recommended using high-efficiency particulate air (HEPA) filtration vacuums for cleaning up apartments wherever possible. Wetting down the dust and removing it was also recommended in order to reduce the dispersion of the asbestos particles. Unfortunately, recommendations for proper clean-up did not reach all residents before they returned to their homes. Some researchers believe that the probability of developing mesothelioma or other asbestos-related disease is small for residents because exposures would have to have occurred for much longer periods for these diseases to occur. Other researchers, however, believe that certain susceptible individuals, such as cigarette smokers, may be at higher risk of asbestos-related lung cancer as a result of this exposure, given the synergistic relationship between asbestos and cigarette smoking in causing lung

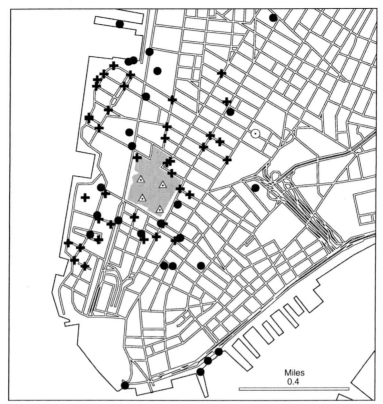

● EPA Asbestos Air Monitoring Site with other Parameters (PCBs, Dioxins, PAHs, Metals, Silicates, Direct Reading Acid Gases and VOCs, Freon at Sites Close to Work Zone)

● EPA/NYSDEC Particulate and Organic Monitoring Sites (PM 2.5, PM10, PM Speciation, Asbestos, VOCs, Reactive VOCs, Dioxins/Furans)

⊙ EPA/Office of Research and Development Network Site (Network also included eight of the EPA and EPA.NYSDEC air sites)

△ EPA Work Zone Sites (Direct reading acid gases and VOCs, Freon)

✚ NYCDEP Asbestos Sampling Site

FIGURE 4–2. U.S. Environmental Protection Agency (EPA), New York State Department of Environmental Conservation, and New York City Department of Environmental Protection air monitoring sites in lower Manhattan implemented in response to attack on World Trade Center. (U.S. Environmental Protection Agency, Region 2, World Trade Center Disaster Response. Basemap data included in the map [roads, building footprints, and parks] were provided by the New York City Department of Information Technology and Telecommunications.)

cancer—cigarette smokers who have been occupationally exposed to asbestos have a 55-fold risk of lung cancer compared with the general population.[8]

Particulate Matter

The force of the airplane explosions and collapse of the WTC buildings shattered cement structures, sending plumes of dust and smoke far into the air.

The resulting particles, of varying size and composition, had the potential to aggravate illnesses, such as asthma, bronchitis, chronic heart disease, and cardiac failure, in people who breathed air emanating from Ground Zero.[1,9,10]

The EPA regulates particulate matter according to size. Particles measuring 10 microns or less (PM_{10}) are considered inhalable because they can penetrate the airways below the larynx. Smaller, fine particles of 2.5 microns or less ($PM_{2.5}$) are considered in the respirable range because they can penetrate deeper into the unciliated regions of the lungs, and thereby cause more toxicity.[11]

The level of concern to protect sensitive populations, including children, the elderly, and people with chronic heart or lung disease, is 40 $\mu g/m^3$ for $PM_{2.5}$ measured over a 24-hour period.[6] Above this level, the EPA recommends that sensitive groups reduce their exposure. Air monitoring conducted by EPA at sites near the WTC showed that daily average measurements for $PM_{2.5}$ were below the standard (Figure 4–3). When hourly measurements were considered, however, occasional peaks of fine particulates were recorded above 40 $\mu g/m^3$, mainly at night, when winds were calm and thermal inversions reduced dispersion of particles.[12]

Lead

Lead may have been released from several sources during the destruction of the WTC. Small quantities of lead are present in the solder used for circuit

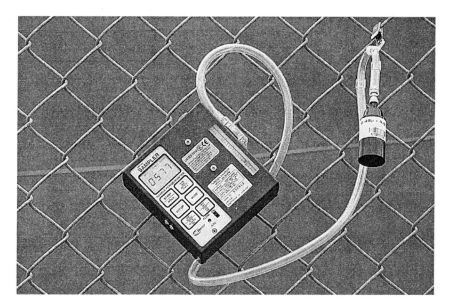

FIGURE 4–3. Air monitor positioned on fence at World Trade Center site perimeter (Photograph by Earl Dotter).

boards of computers and in the components of computer monitors.[13] Because there were possibly tens of thousands of computers in WTC offices, the levels of lead from this source may have been significant.

In addition, it was common practice at the time of the construction of the buildings during the late 1960s and early 1970s to use lead-containing paint to rustproof steel beams. Investigations have demonstrated lead particles from paint chips and dust originating from the site to have been at moderately high levels, ranging from 38 to 635 μg/gr of dust.[14]

Some investigators of the WTC disaster have suggested that dust samples in homes and parks should have been carefully monitored for lead content. Many nearby residents, who may not have been able to properly decontaminate their homes of lead, contracted with professional cleaning services to assist them. The Federal Emergency Management Agency (FEMA) assisted families with this expense. But the widespread use of clean-up companies that were not certified could have created other problems, because clean-up workers did not have the proper training and equipment to handle hazardous materials.

Polychlorinated Biphenyls

Polychlorinated biphenyls (PCBs), used as lubricants and coolants in capacitors, transformers, and other equipment because they are good insulators, were present in electrical equipment at the WTC. PCBs are toxic to the developing brain.[15,16] They accumulate in the food chain and are persistent in the environment and biological tissues.

PCBs were detected occasionally during the recovery process. All air samples analyzed by the EPA for PCBs near Ground Zero were below the EPA screening level, and no PCBs were detected in the vast majority of samples.

Hazards to Workers

Immediately after the WTC attack, the main goal of operations at Ground Zero was to find and rescue any survivors who may have been trapped in the rubble. Thousands of volunteers from throughout the United States came to New York to offer their assistance. Emergency responders from New York, in spite of their own losses, returned immediately to search for survivors. Early on, officials of the Port Authority of New York and New Jersey, who were concerned about the safety of rescue and recovery workers digging through the rubble without appropriate personal protective equipment, such as respirators, requested recommendations from academic occupational health and safety programs in the New York metropolitan area.

The occupational health and safety team that was formed found that the most serious immediate problems were traffic hazards, and safety hazards that were causing falls, cuts, and crush injuries. As the site was stabilized, other occupational hazards became apparent, such as workers' being given respirators without adequate instruction in their use. As the operation changed from rescue to recovery, an appropriate respirator program was implemented by the Occupational Safety and Health Administration (OSHA), in collaboration with the Irving Selikoff Occupational Health Center at the Mount Sinai School of Medicine, including medical screening, fit-testing, and training of workers. Because these measures were not implemented immediately after the attack, workers may have been adversely affected by toxic substances in smoke and dust. Several workers developed asthma, and one worker was treated for carbon monoxide poisoning. (See also Chapter 5.)

Hazards to Children

Children are particularly vulnerable to environmental toxins because (a) they are closer to the ground than adults and thus are more likely to inhale materials stirred up from dust; (b) they breathe more air per kilogram of body weight; (c) their organ systems are more sensitive than those of adults; and (d) they have more years of future life in which to develop exposure-related cancer and other diseases with delayed onset.

The public schools in lower Manhattan underwent extensive environmental testing. Levels of fine particulates, PCBs, dioxin, lead and other metals, asbestos, and volatile organic compounds were almost always well below applicable standards. Potential long-term consequences of exposure to contaminants such as asbestos still need to be monitored, however.

Asthma is a special concern for children. Asthmatics are more susceptible to many air pollutants that can trigger wheezing, shortness of breath, chest discomfort, and other symptoms.[17] Some air pollutants that were liberated into the air during the collapse of the WTC, such as fine particulates, are known to be potent triggers of asthma symptoms. Children were also at risk of exposure to toxic products of combustion that may have been generated during the explosions and fires, including benzene, dioxins, furans, and polycyclic aromatic hydrocarbons (PAHs).

FUTURE NEEDS

Follow-up Assessment

While federal regulatory and research agencies have continued to evaluate levels of contamination and adverse health effects among workers and nearby residents, additional follow-up was initiated of vulnerable individuals who were in lower Manhattan on September 11, and the next few weeks, including:

- *Then-pregnant women and their subsequently-born children*: The possible physical and psychological consequences that the terrorist events may have had on pregnant women and their children are not known and needed to be studied. Researchers at the Mailman School of Public Health of Columbia University and the Mount Sinai School of Medicine in New York have jointly been studying women who were acutely or chronically exposed, as well as their infants. Samples of blood and other bodily fluids have been obtained from these women to assess their exposures. Their children were evaluated at birth and will be periodically evaluated over the first several years of their lives to discover any adverse health effects of toxic substances and also their levels of stress and anxiety.
- *Children residing and attending schools in lower Manhattan*: Small numbers of children in lower Manhattan are being studied for one year by the Centers for Disease Control and Prevention (CDC), the Agency for Toxic Substances and Disease Registry, and the New York City and New York State departments of health, focusing on asthma and other respiratory problems (but not psychological effects).
- *Workers*: Five academic centers, funded by the National Institute of Environmental Health Sciences (NIEHS) in collaboration with the CDC (including the National Institute for Occupational Safety and Health), the EPA, the New York State and New York City departments of health, contractors, and major labor unions, are assessing long-term consequences of occupational exposure at Ground Zero with questionnaires, activity logs, blood samples, pulmonary function tests, and other examinations. Among these five academic centers, the Irving J. Selikoff Occupational Clinical Center at the Mount Sinai School of Medicine has been conducting clinical examinations of firefighters and other exposed workers. Other NIEHS-funded academic centers have been involved with exposure assessment and study design. Preliminary results from a pilot study on ironworkers who were present at Ground Zero, which utilized questionnaires, physical examinations, and pulmonary function tests, found that they sustained clinically significant exposures to airborne irritants, which resulted in upper and lower airway inflammation and an increase in reactive airways disease/asthma. In addition, a very high prevalence of psychiatric sequelae was found among these workers.

REFERENCES

1. Claudio L. Environmental aftermath. *Environ Health Perspect* 2001; 109:A528–A536.
2. New York Department of City Planning. Population 2000 Census Community Districts. Available at www.ci.nyc.ny.us/html/dcp/html/popcd.html.

3. Manning CB, Vallyathan V, Mossman BT. Diseases caused by asbestos: mechanisms of injury and disease development. *Int Immunopharmacol* 2002; 2:191–200.

4. Nishimura SL, Broaddus VC. Asbestos-induced pleural disease. *Clin Chest Med* 1998; 19:311–329.

5. Reitze W, Nicholson W, Holiday D. Application of sprayed inorganic fiber containing asbestos: occupational health hazards. *Am Ind Hyg Assoc J* 1972; 33:178–191.

6. U.S. Environmental Protection Agency. EPA Response to September 11. Available: www.epa.gov/epahome/wtc. [cited: March 11, 2002].

7. New York City Department of Health. New York City Department of Health Continues to Respond to the World Trade Center Disaster: Information for Residents of Lower Manhattan. Available: http://www.ci.nyc.ny.us/html/doh/html/alerts/911res.html [cited: March 11, 2002]

8. Selikoff IJ, Hammond EC, Churg J. Asbestos exposure, smoking, and neoplasia. *JAMA* 1968; 204:106–112.

9. Samet JM, Dominici F, Curriero FC, et al. Fine particulate air pollution and mortality in 20 U.S. cities, 1987–1994. *N Engl J Med* 2000; 343:1742–1749.

10. Pope CA 3rd, Burnett RT, Thun MJ, et al. Lung cancer, cardiopulmonary mortality, and long-term exposure to fine particulate air pollution. *JAMA* 2002; 287:1132–1141.

11. Schwela D. Air pollution and health in urban areas. *Rev Environ Health* 2000; 15:13–42.

12. Dr. George Thurston, Associate Professor of Environmental Medicine at New York University. Presentation at the "Environmental Health Issues Related to the World Trade Center Disaster" symposium, held at New York University on Oct 18, 2001.

13. Lee CH, Chang SL, Wang KM, Wen LC. Management of scrap computer recycling in Taiwan. *J Hazard Mater* 2000; 73:209–220.

14. Dr. Paul Lioy, Professor of Environmental and Community Medicine, The University of Medicine and Dentistry of New Jersey. Presentation at "Environmental Health Issues Related to the World Trade Center Disaster" symposium held at New York University on Oct 18, 2001.

15. Schantz SL. Developmental neurotoxicity of PCBs in humans: What do we know and where do we go from here? *Neurotoxicol Teratol* 1996; 18:217–227.

16. Jacobson JL, Jacobson SW. Intellectual impairment in children exposed to polychlorinated biphenyls in utero. *N Engl J Med* 1996; 335:783–789.

17. Pope CA, 3rd. Epidemiology of fine particulate air pollution and human health: biological mechanisms and who's at risk? *Environ Health Perspect* 2000; 108(Suppl 4):713–723.

5

Protecting the health and safety of rescue and recovery workers

BRUCE LIPPY

The full extent of the injury and illnesses suffered by rescue and recovery workers after the World Trade Center (WTC) disaster is not known, but clearly thousands of incidents occurred. Unfortunately, protection for workers at Ground Zero was given a relatively low priority.[1] This chapter examines the events at the WTC disaster site and, to a lesser degree, at the Pentagon, and provides recommendations for protecting rescue and recovery workers after terrorist attacks.

Hazards Faced by Rescue Workers

The destruction of the WTC, then the world's largest office complex, and the extensive damage to the Pentagon, the largest office complex under one roof, created extraordinarily dangerous environments for rescue and recovery workers and required them to face an exceptional array of hazards. The force of the collapse of the WTC's Twin Towers pulverized 425,000 cubic yards of concrete, and the collapse and fire twisted 200,000 tons of steel beams, intertwining them with the cables from the 104 elevators in each tower and miles of rebar from the concrete. The resulting six-story, shifting pile of debris was potentially life-threatening to any rescue or recovery worker attempting to move over, under, or around it. When combined with the open fires, smoke, caustic dust, jet fuel, and extreme heat, the situations at the WTC and the Pentagon represented unique "multi-threat events."[1]

The magnitude of the disaster created enormous difficulties for the rescue and recovery workers (Figure 5–1). The collapse of the Twin Towers destroyed much of the land-line communication and cell-phone service in lower Manhattan. The temporary grounding of airlines stranded many urban search-and-rescue team members from elsewhere who had intended to participate in rescue and recovery efforts. Much equipment was also stranded. Bucket brigades were organized to move debris so that rescue could proceed, but this practice was very inefficient and exceptionally wearying for the long lines of participants who passed debris in buckets to one another. Shoes and boots melted from working on the hot surfaces. The psychological stress of finding so many human remains affected rescue and recovery workers.

The rescue phase of the operation was characterized by the phrase "Risk a life to save a life." Not everyone recognized that those taking the greatest risks should have the training and expertise to recognize the magnitude of these risks. The 20 Federal Emergency Management Agency (FEMA) urban search-and-rescue teams from many parts of the United States who partici-

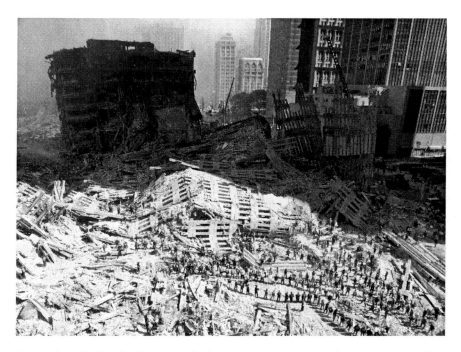

FIGURE 5–1. Police, firefighters, and other emergency rescue workers confront a bedlam of steel and stone at Ground Zero (Photograph by Mario Tama/Getty Images).

pated comprised well-trained experts (Figure 5–2); many others at the site, however, including numerous volunteers, did not have sufficient training and were therefore at considerably increased risk.

Hazards Faced by Recovery Workers

At the WTC site, unlike the Pentagon or the site of the 1995 Oklahoma City bombing, there was never any formal declaration of the end of the rescue phase and the start of the recovery phase.[2] Because 343 firefighters had died at the WTC and the feelings of the New York Fire Department (NYFD) firefighters for their fallen comrades were so intense, no official in the incident command structure was willing to declare that the search for survivors was over. This extended the "Risk a life to save a life" mentality and complicated the protection of thousands of workers—ironworkers, laborers, carpenters, heavy-equipment operators, and others—who were not trained to deal with emergencies. These workers were exposed to the same hazards as rescue workers: smoke, dust, organic vapors, asbestos, acid mists, chlorofluorocarbons, fibrous glass, broken glass, infectious disease risks from human remains, live electric lines, and boxes of ammunition (Figure 5–3).

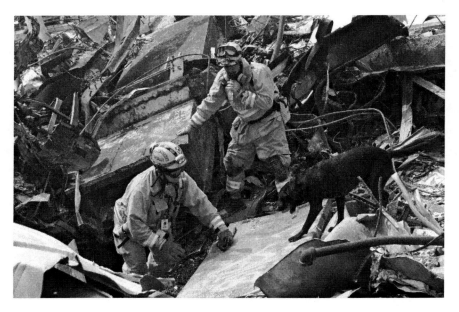

FIGURE 5–2. Two rescue workers and a search dog amidst the World Trade Center ruins (Photograph by Andrea Booher/FEMA News Photo).

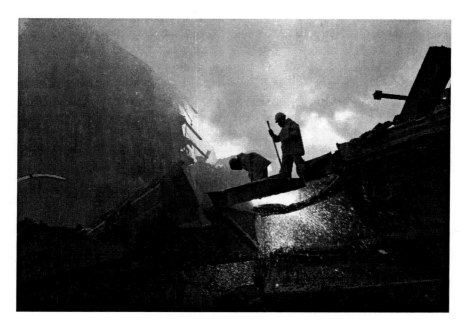

FIGURE 5–3. Ironworkers balance precariously as they cut through the rubble of the World Trade Center (Courtesy of the American Red Cross).

DEFICIENCIES IN SYSTEMS

Delayed Health and Safety Plan

It took far too long to produce a viable health and safety plan to protect workers at Ground Zero. Attempts to create a plan began shortly after the attack. Early drafts were too focused on chemical hazards and not sufficiently focused on the construction safety issues, which were the largest risks. The final plan was not issued until October 29—48 days after the attack—adversely affecting the timely creation and approval of a safety awareness program for the site. Consequently, formal training onsite did not occur until November 29. By January 29, 2002, there were 1,467 recovery workers who had attended the mandatory 3-hour safety and health awareness program, but the delay had already doomed the chances of changing the safety culture at the site.

   The health and safety plan was delayed, in part, because of the difficulty of getting all of the key signatories to approve it. There were nine different agencies that had to agree before it could be issued. While several New York City and federal government decision-makers delayed approving the document, the drafters excluded key stakeholders, especially unions, from the review process, believing that including them would further extend the process. As a safety and health representative for the International Union of Operating Engineers, I was twice denied access to the drafts, even though union members were operating all of the cranes, grapplers, bulldozers, and backhoes on the site.

John Moran, a construction safety and health expert representing the National Institute of Environmental Health Sciences (NIEHS), reported that the Revision A draft of the plan had "many serious potential deficiencies." He added, "The primary deficiencies relate to a complete lack of overall S&H [safety and health] site coordination on this multi-employer site, lack of a clear S&H [safety and health] organizational structure to facilitate attention to concerns that workers or their representatives might have, and a complete lack of participation by workers or their representatives."[3]

After labor representatives were given the opportunity to review the plan, their suggestions were carefully reviewed by New York City Department of Design and Construction (DDC) and Bechtel and incorporated into later drafts. The final version was greatly improved over earlier drafts and, once approved, became the basis for managing safety and health at the site.

Inappropriate Gaps and Overlaps in Responsibilities of Federal, State, and Municipal Government Agencies

Health and safety officials participating in a conference in December 2001 that was sponsored by the National Institute for Occupational Safety and Health (NIOSH) agreed that "the lack of a clear command structure at the World Trade Center [site] thwarted efforts to enforce PPE (personal protective equipment) use and risk-reduction behaviors." They repeatedly expressed the "need to rapidly establish a single controlling authority or unified command."[4] New York City's Office of Emergency Management was responsible for the city's overall handling of the disaster. The NYFD controlled Ground Zero rescue and recovery while the DDC oversaw the four prime contractors and many subcontractors at the site. Nine government agencies had significant involvement with environmental health issues at the site.[1]

One of the most significant factors that prevented a unified structure at the WTC site was the death of 85 percent of the members of the Special Operations Command of the NYFD at the site. Those killed included the hazardous materials ("hazmat") experts for New York—the individuals most needed to guide this type of complex response. Including firefighters, more than 400 emergency responders died at the site. (See Chapter 2.)

Compliance with safety and health requirements was a much more significant problem at Ground Zero than at the Pentagon or at the Fresh Kills site in Staten Island, where debris from the WTC was disposed. The DDC had overall responsibility for enforcing safety requirements at the WTC site, but the scope of the disaster and the number of organizations involved greatly complicated consistent enforcement. The DDC had no contractual mechanism to enforce safety requirements with the four prime "contractors" at the site (who worked without contracts). The primary guidance concerning occupational health and safety at Ground Zero was the site health and safety plan, which did not become effective until almost seven weeks after the attack.

When the final plan was approved, it included a clause giving each worker the right and responsibility to stop work any time unsafe conditions arose. Yet even Occupational Safety and Health Administration (OSHA) inspectors appeared reluctant to use this enforcement hammer.[5] (OSHA can stop work that is considered an imminent danger.) DDC sought police assistance on several occasions to deal with construction workers arguing with Bechtel safety inspectors, who were trying to enforce site rules. Compliance was much better for PPE items that were part of the safety culture of construction work, such as hardhats, than for items like respirators, which were not.

There are important differences in the planned enforcement of occupational safety and health standards during a crisis. The Williams-Steiger Occupational Safety and Health Act (1970), which created OSHA, gave the agency the power to ensure that all employers covered by the Act provide their employees places of employment free from recognized hazards through the enforcement of standards promulgated under the Act.[6] OSHA, however, is one of 27 departments and agencies participating in the Federal Response Plan (FRP), which is designed to coordinate and apply the resources of the federal government to any disaster that is beyond the capabilities of an individual state to handle. Under the Stafford Act, FEMA serves as the primary coordinating agency for disaster response and recovery activities and is specifically directed to establish disaster-specific safety and health guidance and policies for deployed personnel, in cooperation with the U.S. Department of Health and Human Services, OSHA, and other agencies. FEMA is also required to establish a Federal Interagency Occupational Safety and Health Committee comprising safety staff members of deploying agencies in order to monitor and coordinate disaster safety and health operations. The OSHA standards are referenced in the FRP as being applicable even during an emergency.[7] (See Figure 2–3 in Chapter 2.)

OSHA's role under the FRP is to "make available safety and health specialists to provide safety-specific assistance to affected disaster response agencies as required by the Federal Coordinating Officer. Requirements may include safety consultation and training programs, air contaminant sampling and analysis, and other safety services preparatory to, during, and/or following disaster operations under the FRP."[7]

OSHA received considerable criticism during the WTC clean-up for working in a consulting, rather than an enforcement, mode. A strong argument can be made, however, that OSHA was following its prescribed role under the FRP. Whether this was the correct role for the agency was often discussed. OSHA, however, did keep with the plan. For example, on October

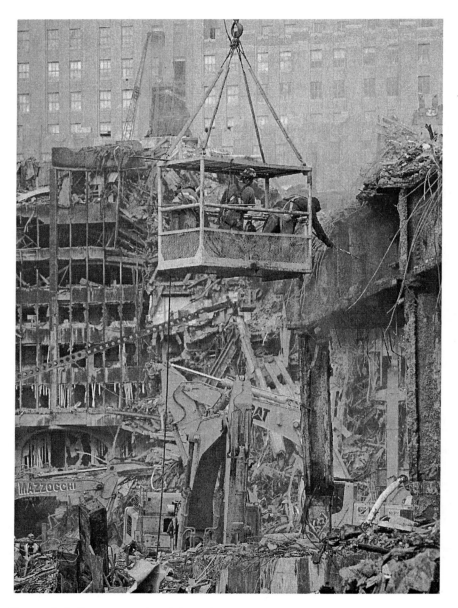

FIGURE 5–4. Recovery workers being hoisted in a personnel basket at World Trade Center site (Photograph by Earl Dotter).

12, it fielded a team of specialists to perform crane inspections and to check slings and rigging used by the cranes, earning praise from the safety officer for one of the prime contractors.[8] The team inspected 17 cranes over 3 days, and found that 10 cranes had a total of 38 serious safety deficiencies—the most serious of which was the practice of lifting workers in personnel baskets (Figure 5–4). New York City does not allow these elevated working platforms on normal construction jobs because of the risk of fatalities from falls if a cable or basket fails. The proper protection for workers is to attach a safety lanyard from their body harness to the cable above the point of connection to the personnel basket. This was not properly done at the WTC site. Early in the recovery phase, workers were not even tied off to the side of the basket.[9]

OSHA had at least six officers assigned to each shift—an unprecedented manpower commitment. An associate director of the Center to Protect Workers' Rights stated that OSHA "made a big difference" by providing "outstanding manpower," and imagined how much improved incident and injury rates would be for any large construction project where there were six OSHA inspectors on site at all times.[10]

By September 25, 2001, safety representatives from the four prime contractors were advised that OSHA would eventually be switching from a consultative to a compliance role at Ground Zero. But that never happened. Instead, on November 20, OSHA entered into a cooperative partnership with the DDC, the NYFD, the Building and Construction Trades Council of Greater New York, and the four prime contractors at the site. The voluntary agreement, called the WTC Emergency Project Partnership Agreement, included a joint labor-management safety committee for the entire site; daily environmental, safety, and health meetings among prime contractors and subcontractors; assignment of a full-time environmental-safety-and-health manager by each prime contractor; weekly environmental, safety, and health reports that tracked OSHA-recordable injuries and illnesses, restricted-work cases, and sampling reports; logs maintained at the site for all first-aid rendered; enhanced personal and environmental monitoring for hazardous substances; and safety orientation training for all new workers at the site.[11]

Difficulties with Communication

Communication about worker safety and health issues began shortly after the WTC attack. The New York City official responsible for site safety was brought into the planning process on September 13. During the second week after the disaster, daily safety meetings began to be held, coordinated by the DDC and involving all of the contractors, OSHA, Bechtel, and union safety personnel. Another regular meeting was held by the NYC DOH at Pier 92

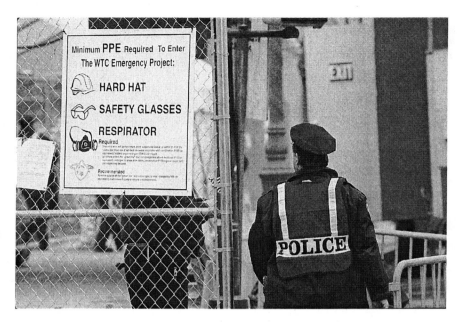

FIGURE 5–5. Sign warning workers to wear personal protective equipment at World Trade Center site (Photograph by Earl Dotter).

and involved broader participation of stakeholders responsible for safety issues. These meetings provided a regular source of current and critical information and a chance for each organization to update the others. The problem came in disseminating this information to the workers at the site. Initially, the concern was just getting information out in any format. Hand-painted signs showed up. (See Figure 5–5.)

Risk communication could have been handled much better at the site. Handout materials were produced by many organizations, but most flyers were too wordy, not focused on the key issues at Ground Zero, and not crafted for worker populations. More successfully, the Operating Engineers National Hazmat Program produced small plastic cards for inside cabs of heavy equipment that contained on their front side a message from the union's general president, urging the members to follow the site safety rules, which were then listed. On their other side was a list of PPE available from the union at the "hazmat trailer." The Operating Engineers published all of their materials in Spanish, which should have been done more widely at the site.

A major problem with communication was the difficulty posed by respirators. Given the loud noise at the site, wearing a half-face respirator made it nearly impossible to communicate. Consequently, workers were constantly tugging respirators down to pass along important information or just to talk to someone to relieve the great stress and sadness of working at Ground Zero.

This difficulty was undoubtedly one of the reasons so many workers chose not to wear the respirators provided.[12]

Inadequate Respiratory Protection

Almost immediately after the attack, agencies scrambled to provide respirators to rescue and recovery workers who were working in the smoking rubble. Hardware stores in Manhattan were emptied of respirators by organizations like FEMA that were trying to provide respirators to those at the site. Large suppliers of industrial masks were initially swamped with orders. Organizations at the WTC site sometimes competed with each other to fill orders intended for the same workers. The OSHA requirement that employers are fully responsible for ensuring adequate respiratory protection for their employees appeared to have been waived as agencies and unions took the lead in obtaining respirators and other PPE.

Little or no training, however, accompanied the provision of the respirators. Workers interviewed on September 19 had no idea which organization had provided their respirators. One could find every conceivable type of half-face and disposable respirator on site. The quantity of half-face respirators handed out was far greater than the number of workers at the site: OSHA provided 130,000; the EPA, 22,000; and the International Union of Operating Engineers 11,000; among others. Without training, workers were throwing away the respirators, instead of disposing of only the used cartridges.

Experts from the NIOSH Respiratory Protection Branch in Morgantown, West Virginia, following agency selection criteria, recommended from the beginning the use of half-face, negative-pressure respirators with cartridges effective against ultrafine particles, organic vapors, and acid gases (P100/OV/AG)[13]—the same type recommended by OSHA and EPA onsite. Thousands of samples collected since then confirmed that this initial choice was correct. If properly tested and conscientiously worn, this type of respirator should have been sufficiently protective for workers at the site.

Many organizations were involved in air sampling at the WTC site, including the New York City Department of Health (DOH), the EPA, OSHA, NIOSH, the U.S. Coast Guard, the Bloomberg School of Hygiene and Public Health of Johns Hopkins University, the Operating Engineers National Hazmat Program, and many private firms representing diverse stakeholders. Most samples were collected to determine the exposure in communities near Ground Zero (see Chapter 4).[14] By March 18, 2002, however, OSHA alone had collected 4,496 air samples to determine worker exposures (not including blanks or bulk samples) (Table 5–1).

OSHA began collecting environmental samples on September 13 by having its inspectors, wearing sampling pumps, walk through the financial dis-

TABLE 5–1. OSHA Air Monitoring Results (as of March 18, 2002).

AGENT	NUMBER OF SAMPLES COLLECTED	NUMBER EXCEEDING THE OSHA PERMISSIBLE EXPOSURE LIMIT	PERCENT EXCEEDING THE OSHA PERMISSIBLE EXPOSURE LIMIT
Asbestos	1,144	144[a]	12.6
Carbon monoxide	103	0	0
Total dust	150	5	3.3
Respirable silica	910	60	6.6
Organic compounds	660[b]	1	0.15
Dioxins	10	NA[c]	NA
Polynuclear aromatic hydrocarbons	110	8	7.3
Freon-22, hydrogen fluoride, phosgene	208	0[d]	0
Inorganic acids	173	3	1.7
Metals	1132	13 copper 26 iron oxide 17 lead 1 antimony 2 cadmium 59 total	5.2

[a]Via phase-contrast microscopy.

[b]This total includes the figures for dioxins, polynuclear aromatic hydrocarbons, and Freon.

[c]OSHA does not have a dioxin standard. Only one sample taken on the pile exceeded background levels.

[d]OSHA does not have a standard for Freon. Only one sample had detectable levels of Freon. All samples for decomposition products of Freon, hydrofluoric acid and phosgene, were nondetectable.

(*Source*: United States Department of Labor[15])

trict of New York, which is near the WTC site.[15] They continued this practice for days, working systematically closer to Ground Zero, but they did not conduct personal sampling of workers for fear of slowing the rescue and recovery effort. The first personal sampling of heavy-equipment operators apparently was performed on September 19 by me, while working as an industrial hygienist with the International Union of Operating Engineers Hazmat Unit. From September 18 through October 4, NIOSH collected 1,174 general-area and personal-breathing-zone air samples, focusing on search and rescue personnel, heavy-equipment operators, and ironworkers. They then produced a sampling plan for the site that was turned over to Bechtel to execute. (Recently-reported results of the sampling indicate that most exposures did not exceed NIOSH recommended exposure limits or OSHA permissible exposure limits.[15a])

There was much data-sharing among organizations collecting air and bulk samples. Results sheets were produced daily and distributed at safety meetings; a daily conference call was coordinated by the New York City DOH. These efforts were useful for health professionals, but the disseminated information often did not reach workers. The results verified that most exposures were below limits of detection, and that levels decreased substantially with greater distance from the rubble pile at Ground Zero. For example, the EPA, with real-time monitors, measured benzene levels up to 30 parts per million in the plume of smoke, approximately one foot directly above the smoking pile. But benzene measurements dropped to parts per billion when collected inside the cabs of heavy equipment operating at the rubble pile.

Asbestos measurements caused the greatest concern for workers and the general public and led to the least-coordinated messages from government agencies. Different EPA and OSHA regulations required different measurement methods and referenced acceptable levels that were an order of magnitude (10-fold) apart. The extreme force of the collapse crushed asbestos insulation, releasing fibers that were consistently smaller than the 5.0-micron minimal fiber length defined in the OSHA standard. The overwhelming majority of these fibers were invisible to the optical microscopy method used by OSHA, which had historically worked well in industries producing asbestos products. The EPA used transmission electron microscopy, following its method for assessing asbestos-abatement projects in schools.[14] This method could detect and positively identify the very fine fibers present at the WTC site, but results did not correlate nearly as well with epidemiological data as the OSHA optical method did. OSHA and EPA did not reconcile these differences, which contributed to the confusion and controversy that continued to surround this issue at the WTC site. (See Chapters 2 and 4.)

Industrial hygiene involves both the recognition and evaluation, as well as the control, of workplace contaminants. Sampling is only part of the practice and should lead to implementation of appropriate controls. At the WTC site, there was a disconnect: after 2 weeks of sampling, sufficiently protective control measures (half-face P100/OV/AG respirators) were selected, but sampling continued while workers did not wear respirators.

Despite the chaotic environment, one of the prime contractors arranged for its workers to be quantitatively fit-tested for respirators and medically evaluated during the first week of work at the site. Similarly, the Carpenters Union arranged for fit-testing of approximately 300 of its members. No other significant medical evaluations or respirator fit-testing appear to have been provided on site until October 17, when the Operating Engineers National Hazmat Program made quantitative fit-testing and medical evaluations by a corporation available for any workers onsite. Another corporation later brought a van and fit-tested several thousand more workers.

OSHA provided thousands of respirators, but only taught workers to perform positive and negative fit checks, not the qualitative or quantitative fit-tests that are required under the agency's own respirator standard. Even when quantitative fit-tests were conducted, standard rules were not followed. Workers with beards were reported to have been fit-tested even though this is not permitted under OSHA regulations. Workers with beards often wore respirators within the restricted zone.

The site safety and health plan defined an area, called the "green zone" or "safety zone," within which workers needed to wear respirators. Attempts were made to paint green lines on the affected streets, but the boundaries of the zone were not often clear. Rather than attempting to force hundreds of fire, police, and rescue and recovery workers waiting and watching at the periphery of this zone to wear respirators, safety efforts should have ensured that workers and service personnel in the direct plume wore respirators. Later, the debris pile was demarcated with large median barriers that were painted orange and had signs indicating that respirators were required upon entering the area.

Respirators were routinely worn much like neckties at the site, hanging down below the neck. Compliance at Ground Zero was generally poor, despite the efforts of safety and health professionals. Staff members from the Operating Engineers National Hazmat Program traveled the site daily and, using binoculars, observed every piece of heavy equipment operating within the restricted zone to determine if the operator was wearing a respirator. They found that fewer than half, and often fewer than one-third, of heavy-equipment operators were wearing respirators while working on the pile (Figure 5–6). This percentage was fairly comparable to that of other trades at Ground Zero, according to OSHA records. (At least heavy-equipment oper-

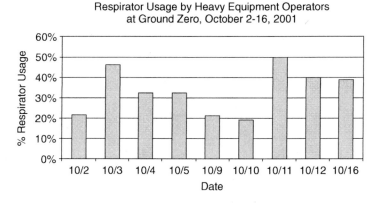

FIGURE 5–6. Respirator usage by heavy-equipment operators at Ground Zero, October 2–16, 2001.

ators could work inside closed cabs, which reduced their exposure.) In strong contrast, the use of respiratory protection at the Fresh Kills dump site on Staten Island was approximately 90 percent.

Compliance at Ground Zero was compromised, in part, because workers received conflicting information, and had poor role models and muddled guidelines that were difficult to follow. Exacerbating the situation, supervisory personnel from many organizations onsite regularly entered the restricted zone without respiratory protection, setting a bad example for workers whom they supervised.

A steady stream of dignitaries and celebrities, including politicians, professional wrestlers, racecar drivers, movie stars—even Miss America—visited the site, but they rarely wore hard hats.[16] In this way, they were poor role models for using safety equipment.

Inadequate Safety Protections

Construction-related safety hazards were the greatest risks to workers at the site. The WTC attack created what the OSHA administrator called "potentially the most dangerous workplace in America."[11] The frenetic pace of the clean-up and the 12-hour shifts contributed to an environment where even safety precautions considered routine for construction work were not followed. Cranes operated regularly without spotters, oxygen and acetylene bottles were misused, and workers in personnel baskets were routinely improperly tied off. No recovery worker died at the WTC site, but there were 30 to 40 near-misses in which someone could have been fatally injured. The most dramatic of these was the fall of a large beam into a pit that had just before been evacuated by 16 firefighters at the request of a safety officer.

Medical Services and Recordkeeping Issues

The New York City DOH, working with FEMA and other organizations, established a worker injury and illness surveillance system for treating workers with job-related injuries. The system included four New York City hospital emergency departments and five Disaster Medical Assistance Teams (DMATs) onsite. DMATs are organized by the U.S. Department of Health and Human Services to provide medical care when normal medical services have been overwhelmed or put out of service by a disaster. DMAT personnel performed admirably from five tents at Ground Zero, working long hours in very difficult conditions, dispensing first aid and providing PPE. They were extraordinarily busy in the first several weeks (Table 5–2). Most common types of reported injuries were eye and lung injuries—primarily irritation from the ubiquitous dust, smoke, and ash—and headaches, blisters, and

TABLE 5–2. Number of Visits to Disaster Medical Assistance Teams (DMATs) and Emergency Departments, by Time after WTC Attack through October 10, 2001.

FACILITY	WEEK 1	WEEK 2	WEEK 3	WEEK 4	TOTAL
All DMAT Sites	1484	2787	1716	800	6787
Emergency Departments	254	84	17	18	373
Total	1738	2871	1733	818	7160

(*Source*: New York City Department of Health[17])

strains and sprains (Table 5–3). There were also 30 fractures and 342 lacerations during the first several weeks. The New York City DOH deserves much praise for generating daily injury reports, which enabled health and safety professionals to modify prevention measures and types of PPE in a timely and appropriate manner.

Results from this system, however, were not directly convertible to parameters routinely used by health and safety professionals. OSHA requires that certain work-related injuries—but not first-aid problems such as headaches and blisters—be recorded by the employer. Since, in contrast, the DMAT incidents include dispensing PPE, an "eye injury" incident may have actually been the provision of safety glasses. Because there was no determination of the number of worker-hours at the site, a true incidence rate could not have been calculated.

Don Elisburg and John Moran, authors of an NIEHS report on safety and health at the site, were criticized for attempting to draw conclusions from these data in their October 6, 2001, report. Their calculations of standard safety and health indices, such as reportable incident rates, resulted in extremely high numbers.[3] OSHA calculated the aggregated lost workday incidence rate (the rate of injuries and illnesses causing lost workdays) at 2.1 per 100 full-time employees per year, for all four prime contractors through December 31, 2001. This rate was lower than the national average rate of 3.6 for heavy construction in 2000. However, the WTC site rate does not include

TABLE 5–3. Most Common Types of Reported Injuries through October 10, 2001.

TYPES	NUMBER	PERCENT
Eye injury	802	11
Headache	664	9
Lung injury	611	9
Blisters	410	6
Sprain/strain	373	5

(*Source*: New York City Department of Health.[17])

any of the incidents reported by firefighters, police, or other emergency responders who were responsible for a major portion of the DOH-reported incidents for the first several weeks.

RECOMMENDATIONS

The following recommendations are made to the planners for future responses, with deep respect for the complexity of the WTC disaster response and for the hard work of thousands of rescue and recovery workers at the site:

Consider the Value of OSHA's Hazardous Waste and Emergency Response Standard (HAZWOPER)

The OSHA standard for hazardous waste operations and emergency response (29 CFR 1910.120) is, arguably, the most proactive standard for protecting workers during disasters. Yet the HAZWOPER standard was purposely and thoroughly avoided during the rescue and recovery operations at Ground Zero. The standard applies to emergency response operations for releases, or substantial threats of releases, of hazardous substances, regardless of the location of the hazard.[18]

The WTC attack released hazardous substances (see Chapter 4). The buildings contained the largest office-chiller plants in the world, with thousands of pounds of Freon-22 in tanks; as many as 50,000 personal computers, each containing lead and mercury; thousands of fluorescent lights containing mercury; several storage tanks of petroleum products; and two electric utility company substations containing approximately 130,000 gallons of transformer oil contaminated with polychlorinated biphenyls (PCBs).[1] Asbestos— perhaps as much as 400 tons—had been sprayed onto structural beams of the first 40 floors of the North Tower during its construction.[19,20]

The HAZWOPER standard should be considered as a framework for organizing future recovery operation because it provides a "comprehensive basis for training of workers, medical surveillance, exposure monitoring, and worker protection levels."[3] Most of the key practices of HAZWOPER, such as creating a site-specific health and safety plan, establishing zones of control, training workers, and decontaminating personnel and equipment, became part of the procedures at Ground Zero. But they were introduced slowly. Some practices, such as personal decontamination, were almost voluntary exercises, and others, such as medical testing, were still being planned as of May 2002. At the Fresh Kills dump site on Staten Island, which functioned as a Level C HAZWOPER site, nearly all workers wore protective clothing and half-face respirators, the degree of protection required under Level C. Workers also routinely decontaminated at the Fresh Kills dumpsite.

The HAZWOPER standard has rightly been criticized for being too focused on chemical hazards. Much greater consideration of basic construction safety should be part of the plan and can be incorporated into it. In addition, training programs for HAZWOPER exist throughout the United States, and those funded by NIEHS are being modified so that they can respond more effectively to terrorist attacks. Under a HAZWOPER-like approach, workers would not be allowed onto the site until they had completed the required training.

Consider Increasing OSHA's Enforcement Responsibility

The Natural Resources Defense Council, in its February 2002 report, recommended that "OSHA, along with appropriate state and city agencies, should immediately undertake stringent enforcement of workplace safety standards for workers at Ground Zero and workers involved in clean-up of dust and debris-filled offices or residences in the vicinity of the Trade Center."[1] OSHA is the obvious choice for quickly and effectively enforcing worker-protection rules. The Federal Response Plan gives that responsibility to FEMA with support from OSHA, but FEMA did not play an active role in safety and health at Ground Zero. OSHA's challenge in future disaster situations will be to focus on major issues, and avoid excessive consideration of minor infractions of the agency's many standards.

Personal Protective Equipment

The recommendations from the participants of a NIOSH/RAND conference in December 2001 are excellent and should be considered in future planning:

- Develop guidelines for the appropriate PPE ensembles for long-duration disaster responses involving rubble, human remains, and a range of respiratory threats. If appropriate equipment is not currently available, address any roadblocks to its development. Such equipment could be used for other major disasters, such as earthquakes or tornadoes, as well as terrorist attacks.
- Define the appropriate ensembles of PPE needed to safely and efficiently respond to biological incidents, threats, and false alarms. Key considerations include providing comparable levels of protection for all responders and addressing the logistical and decontamination issues associated with many responses in short periods of time.
- Explore mechanisms to effectively outfit all responders at large incident sites with appropriate PPE as rapidly as possible.

- Examine any barriers to equipment standardization or interoperability among emergency-responder organizations. Strategies could include coordination of equipment procurement among organizations or working with equipment manufacturers to promote broader interoperability within classes of equipment.

Given the reliance that workers will have to place on respirators in future situations, particularly those involving biological or chemical terrorism, fit-testing of respirators before entering hazardous zones will be critical. Positive and negative fit-testing will not be sufficient and should not be considered.

Air Monitoring

There should be greater use of instruments that provide instantaneous readings. The most critical data are those collected initially when conditions are least understood and most dynamic. Waiting for laboratory analyses is problematic and, in the case of a major attack like that on the WTC, sending specimens to a laboratory may be impossible.

Planning should include criteria for taking action based on actual data obtained. Far too much of the data obtained at Ground Zero did not lead to decisions about control measures. These criteria should also address how to reduce respiratory protection and other PPE requirements when the data indicate that it is appropriate to do so. Forcing workers to wear respirators when contaminant levels are acceptably low is not appropriate.

Planners must consider how to better communicate results of environmental sampling to workers and the general public, with risk communicators and health educators being integral parts of the process. An independent board of experts, working at the site, should review air monitoring data and tell the public whether contaminant levels are acceptable or not.[21] This group would have credibility with the stakeholders in the community before the disaster and would, hopefully, avoid the difficulties experienced by the EPA at the WTC. This same approach might work well for occupational safety and health issues; for example, the board could review data to determine if types of respiratory protection were acceptable and which occupational exposure standards were most applicable.

Training

The following recommendations from the NIOSH/RAND conference should be considered:

- Define mechanisms to rapidly and effectively provide responders at incident sites with useful information about hazards they face and protective equipment. Approaches could include more effective coordination among organizations and the development of technologies that provide responders with real-time environmental information.

- Explore ways to ensure that responders at large-scale disaster sites are appropriately trained to use the protective equipment they are provided.
- Consider logistical requirements of extended response activities during disaster drills and training, which could provide response commanders with information on the logistical constraints.

Using Technology to Protect Workers

There are many innovative technologies being developed by government agencies, especially the U.S. Department of Energy (DOE) Office of Science and Technology (OST), that can provide additional protection for workers. Attempts were made to introduce them at Ground Zero, but with limited success. These technologies should be tested under realistic conditions, and, if found to be useful, made widely available.

The following were suggested to DDC for use at Ground Zero and should be seriously considered for future responses:

Oxy-gasoline torch: This torch is similar to oxyacetylene torches that were used at the WTC site, except that it is fueled by a mixture of gasoline and oxygen. This torch increases cutting speed, especially for metal thicknesses greater than 1 inch; reduces airborne contamination; decreases explosion hazards; increases worker safety; and reduces the cost of operation.

Concrete-dust suppression system: Dust suppression was a major challenge at WTC. This new system is an alternative to traditional methods of controlling dust used at the site: spraying water with a manned fire hose. Mounted directly on an excavator or other piece of equipment, this system consists of a 540-gallon water tank, pump, spray nozzles, and controls. Water is sprayed directly onto debris being lifted. The operator can direct the amount and focus of the spray. This system of focused dust suppression dramatically reduces the amount of water needed.

Remotely operated demolition equipment: The DOE has demonstrated several pieces of heavy equipment that can perform a broad spectrum of demolition tasks while being operated remotely, taking workers out of harm's way.

Personal ice cooling system (PICS): The PICS is a self-contained, core-body-temperature control system that uses ice as a coolant, and circulates cool water through tubing that is incorporated into a durable and comfortable, full-body garment or suit similar to long underwear. The suit is designed to be worn under protective clothing and would have worked well for teams that entered lower levels at the WTC site, where temperatures were elevated for many weeks.

CONCLUSION

The response to the WTC disaster was "the most complex emergency response and management challenge ever faced in the nation."[3] Government agencies, private firms, and labor unions performed admirably in one of the most difficult environments conceivable. There are, however, clear lessons learned from these efforts that will lead to better protection of emergency responders and site workers in the future. Pre-incident planning, particularly for provision of PPE and fit-testing of respirators, is critical. Skilled support personnel in the construction trades need to be trained and equipped to deal with similar emergencies *before* they occur. The response to the WTC disaster demonstrated that the chaos following an attack severely limits any organization's ability to quickly and effectively protect its workers.

REFERENCES

1. Nordgren MD, Goldstein EA, Izeman MA. *The environmental impacts of the World Trade Center attacks, a preliminary assessment.* Natural Resources Defense Council, February 2002.
2. Personal communication with Robert Adams, Director, Site Safety, New York City Department of Design and Construction, March 21, 2002.
3. Elisburg D, Moran J. *National Institute of Environmental Health Sciences Worker Education and Training Program Response to the World Trade Center disaster: initial WETP grantee response and preliminary assessment of training needs,* Contract #273-FH-013264, October 6, 2001.
4. Jackson B, Peterson DJ, Bartis J, et al. Protecting emergency responders: lessons learned from terrorist attacks. National Institute for Occupational Safety and Health/RAND. [On-line] Available at: http://www.rand.org/publications.
5. Personal communication with Robert Adams, March 21, 2002.
6. Code of Federal Regulations. 29CFR Part 1903, Inspections, citations, and proposed penalties.§1903.1, Purpose and scope.
7. Federal Emergency Management Agency. *Concept of Operations from the Basic Plan of the Federal Response Plan, April 1999.* [On-line] Available at: http://www.fema.gov/r-n-r/frp/frpconc.htm March 21, 2002.
8. Personal communication with Ray Master, Safety Officer, Bovis Lend Lease, March 18, 2002.
9. U.S. Department of Labor. Occupational Safety and Health Administration. WTC Recovery Project, joint crane inspection initiative, report and analysis. October 17, 2001.
10. Personal communication with James Platner, March 20, 2002.

11. OSHA. *Chao launches partnership to protect WTC site workers.* OSHA National News Release [On-line] Available at: http://www.osha.gov/media/oshnews/nov01/national-20011120.html, March 21, 2002.

12. Personal communication with Ray Master, December 15, 2001.

13. U.S. Centers for Disease Control, National Institute for Occupational Safety and Health. *NIOSH guide to the selection and use of particulate respirators, certified under 42 CFR 84.* DHHS (NIOSH) Publication No. 96-101, January 1996.

14. U.S. Environmental Protection Agency. *EPA, OSHA update asbestos data, continue to reassure public about contamination fears.* [On-line] Available at: http://www.epa.gov/epahome/headline_091601.htm.

15. U.S. Department of Labor, Occupational Safety and Health Administration. *OSHA sampling results summary as of 3/18/02.* [On-line] Available at: http://www.osha.gov/nyc-disaster/summary.html

15a. CDC. Occupational exposures to air contaminants at the World Trade Center disaster site—New York, September–October, 2001. *Mor Mortal Wkly Rep* 2002; 51:453–456.

16. The Official Site of the Miss America Organization. http://www.missamerica.org/press/travels.html, March 20, 2002.

17. New York City Department of Health. *World Trade Center (WTC) Worker Injury and Illness Surveillance Update, October 11, 2001,* Internal report 10.11.01.

18. 29 CFR 1910.120(a) Scope, application, and definitions.

19. Glanz J, Revkin A. Did the ban on asbestos lead to loss of life? *New York Times,* September 18, 2001.

20. Bates T. The air down there. http://www.poynter.org, quoted in Nordgren MD, Goldstein EA, Izeman MA, *The environmental impacts of the World Trade Center attacks, a preliminary assessment.* Natural Resources Defense Council, February 2002, p. 9.

21. Thurston G. *Dust and air pollution resulting from the World Trade Center disaster,* Presented at the 23rd Annual Scientific Meeting of the Universities' Occupational Safety and Health Educational Resource Center, Mt. Sinai Medical Center, April 5, 2002.

6

The public health response to the anthrax epidemic

PHILIP S. BRACHMAN

HISTORICAL BACKGROUND

The earliest writings about anthrax are found in the Book of Genesis: the fifth of ten plagues was from anthrax that affected the Pharaoh's cattle. There are further references to anthrax involving animals and humans in the writings of the Hindus, Greeks, and inhabitants of the Roman Empire. In the 17th century, an epidemic of anthrax called "the black bane" swept through Europe, reportedly killing 60,000 people and many animals. During this period, an association was observed between human disease and contact with wool and animal hides that were used in clothing.

In the mid-1700s, Maret used the term "the malignant pustule" to refer to cutaneous anthrax. In 1838, Delafond described the organism. Louis Pasteur used anthrax in explaining his germ theory. In 1876, Robert Koch referred to *Bacillus anthracis* in presenting the "Koch postulates," which form the basis of an association between a microorganism and a disease. Pasteur developed an animal vaccine against anthrax, which was first used in 1881. In 1939, Max Sterne developed an attenuated, non-encapsulated, live strain vaccine, which is the animal vaccine that is still used today.[1]

In the 1800s, occupational anthrax was a significant disease in Europe, where it was known as "ragpicker's disease"; in England, it was called "woolsorter's disease." Occupational anthrax was so pervasive in England that a formaldehyde disinfecting station was established in Liverpool in 1921; all wool imported into England had to be decontaminated before being further processed. This decontamination was successful and woolsorter's disease essentially disappeared from England.

There are three forms of anthrax infections in humans: cutaneous, inhalational, and gastrointesinal. In the United States, the main anthrax problem in humans has been cutaneous anthrax. The first case of human anthrax was reported in 1824 in a man in Kentucky who had contact with cattle. Between 1900 and 2000, there were occasional reports of inhalational anthrax in the United States, but no confirmed cases of gastrointestinal anthrax. During the early 1900s, the annual number of human anthrax cases reported in the United States ranged up to 200 cases (Figure 6–1).[2] By the 1950s, this number decreased to 20 to 50 cases. Due to the use of human anthrax vaccine, improved methods of processing imported animal products, and a decrease in the importation of contaminated animal products, the annual incidence decreased in the 1970s to 0 to 6 cases, and then to 0 to 4 cases in the 1980s. The last reported human case, before the bioterrorist event in 2001, occurred in 1992.[3]

EPIDEMIOLOGY

Between 1955 and 1990, a total of 235 human anthrax cases were reported in the United States, of which 203 (86 percent) were cutaneous, 11 (5 per-

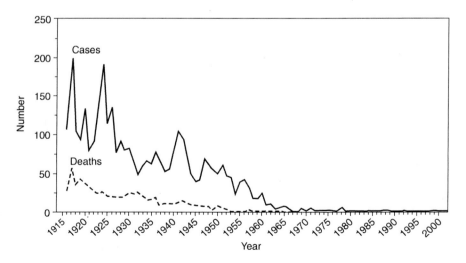

FIGURE 6–1. Anthrax in humans in the United States, 1916–2000. (Adapted from: Centers for Disease Control and Prevention[10].)

cent) inhalational, and 21 (9 percent) of unknown type.[2] Of these 235 human cases, 182 (77 percent) were occupationally related (113 of these cases were associated with goat-hair processing), 43 (18 percent) were associated with animals, and 2 (1 percent) resulted from inadvertent injection of the Sterne-strain animal vaccine into humans; in 8 cases (3 percent), the sources of infection were unknown.

A human anthrax vaccine was developed in the 1950s by George Wright and colleagues in the United States Army Chemical Corps and was field-tested in four goat-hair processing mills in the northeastern United States.[4] The vaccine was shown to be 92.5 percent effective in preventing anthrax. Five cases of inhalational anthrax occurred in one of the mills over a 10-week period during the vaccine trial, two of which occurred in persons who received the placebo inoculations while the other three cases occurred in individuals who had not joined the voluntary vaccination program.[5] The reactogenicity of the vaccine was not considered to be a problem since only 2.5 percent of the recipients developed an adverse reaction that was more than a very mild local reaction.

Since 1900, 18 cases of inhalational anthrax have been reported in the United States, and these have primarily occurred as individual, sporadic cases.[6] In 1957, an epidemic of anthrax took place in a goat-hair processing mill in the northeastern United States, where over a 10-week period nine cases of anthrax occurred among the mill workers—four that were cutaneous and five inhalational. The five inhalational cases (resulting in four deaths) were among employees who had worked in areas shown to be contaminated with *B. anthracis*.

A number of environmental studies performed in goat-hair- and wool-processing factories demonstrated that the environments of these mills could become contaminated with *B. anthracis* due to the processing of contaminated imported animal fibers. Aerosol studies further showed that employees working in this environment would be exposed to airborne *B. anthracis*. In addition to the epidemic cases, only one other case of inhalational anthrax was reported in a mill employee. Air samples taken in two goat-hair-processing mills revealed that employees working in the carding department, which is one of the dustiest areas in such a mill, were exposed to approximately 150 to 1,300 airborne *B. anthracis*-bearing particles less than 5 microns in size during an eight-hour day.[5] No cases of anthrax occurred during these studies. Ninety-one primates were exposed to the air from the carding department in another goat-hair-processing mill; an anthrax case-fatality rate of 10 to 25 percent resulted from a calculated inhaled dose of 1000 to 1500 *B. anthracis*-bearing particles less than 5 microns in size that accumulated over 3 to 5 days.[7]

Of interest are several of the nonoccupational inhalational cases. One case occurred in a 28-year-old male with sarcoidosis, who developed inhalational anthrax in 1957 and died.[8] The only potential source of infection that could be identified was a goat-skin tannery that he passed by daily on his way to and from the bus stop from which he went to his job in a furniture factory. The prevailing winds blew from the rear of the building through the open doors of the receiving area onto the sidewalk where the patient walked each workday. Also of interest is another case of inhalational anthrax that occurred in 1948 in a woman who lived one-and-a-half blocks from the tannery. But, there is no record of whether or not she also may have walked by the receiving area of the tannery.

The last case of inhalational anthrax reported in the United States occurred in a weaving artist who used imported goat-hair yarn in his artwork, and developed inhalational anthrax and died. The yarn he was using was shown to be contaminated with *B. anthracis*. There also were two cases of inhalational anthrax reported in persons who worked in laboratories in which *B. anthracis* had been handled years before.

Two other episodes have added to our knowledge of inhalational anthrax. Both of these episodes clearly demonstrated that *B. anthracis* aerosols could be created that would result in deaths among humans or animals exposed to them. In Sverdlovsk, Russia, in 1979, an explosion in a governmental biological weapons facility discharged *B. anthracis* organisms into the air, resulting in at least 77 cases of inhalational anthrax and at least 66 deaths.[9] Investigations were not conducted until 12 years later when Matthew Meselson and his colleagues were able to examine the remaining records and talk to individuals who were present during this event. Their calculations indicated that the median lethal dose (LD_{50}) for inhaled *B. anthracis* was 4,100 spores. Utilizing data from verbal reports, they projected an incubation period of up to 43 days after exposure. This prolonged incubation period was thought to reflect prophylactic use of oral antibiotics for some exposed individuals that delayed the onset of clinical symptoms until the antibiotics were no longer being taken. This phenomenon has also been demonstrated in experiments with nonhuman primates treated with prophylactic antibiotics. The theory is that as inhaled spores that have been deposited in the regional mediastinal lymph nodes germinate, the vegetative organisms are killed by the antibiotic before they can produce toxin. When the antibiotic use ends, the remaining spores continue to germinate and produce toxin that results in the development of symptoms. This information was very important in designing the recommended prophylactic regimens for people exposed in the anthrax dissemination in 2001.

The second episode that has added to our knowledge of inhalational anthrax was the purposeful exposure of sheep to aerosolized *B. anthracis* on Gruinard Island, Scotland, by the British in the early 1940s. This exposure resulted in a number of the sheep developing fatal anthrax infections.

TERRORIST USE OF ANTHRAX

Over the past several years, the most common bioterrorist threat in the United States has been that of alleged *B. anthracis* in mailed envelopes. All of these events have been hoaxes in which the letters have been opened, a white powder has fallen out, and a note, sometimes enclosed, stated that the individual had been exposed to anthrax. In none of these episodes did the powder actually contain *B. anthracis*—until September 2001.

The anthrax epidemic in 2001 was the first time that *B. anthracis* was successfully used for bioterrorism. There were 18 definite cases (11 inhalational and seven cutaneous) and four suspect cases (Table 6–1).[10,11] There were five deaths among patients with inhalational anthrax. The first diagnosed case was in a 63-year-old graphic artist in Boca Raton, Florida, who worked at a publishing company.[12] It was reported that he opened a letter that contained powder while he was at his computer, with several colleagues present. He subsequently developed inhalational anthrax and died. A colleague who worked in the mailroom in the same building also developed inhalational anthrax, but recovered.[13] *B. anthracis* organisms were recovered from the graphic artist's keyboard and from other locations in his office area, other places in the building, and from the U.S. postal facility in which the publishing company's mail was processed.

Once this case was diagnosed and publicized, it was recognized that there had been five cases of cutaneous anthrax in New York City and New Jersey over the preceding six days. These cutaneous cases occurred at news media offices of the National Broadcasting Company (NBC), the American Broadcasting Company (ABC), the Columbia Broadcasting System (CBS), and the *New York Post*. Each affected person had had contact with a powdered substance in letters that had been delivered through the U.S. mail. One of the cutaneous cases occurred in a seven-month-old infant who had been brought to the ABC building to attend a birthday party and was only in the building for one hour. He had a stormy clinical course, but recovered.[14] This building was the only environmental area related to these cases from which *B. anthracis* was recovered.

A letter addressed to U.S. Senator Tom Daschle and one to U.S. Senator Patrick Leahy were also shown to contain *B. anthracis*. The letter addressed to Senator Daschle was first processed at the U.S. Postal System Hamilton Processing and Distribution Facility in Trenton, New Jersey, and then processed at the Brentwood Postal Facility in Washington, D.C. The letter was then delivered to the Hart Senate Office Building, where it was delivered to Senator Daschle's office and opened, with powder being dispersed into the air. Twenty-eight persons had evidence of exposure to this powder by nasal culture: 13 were in the immediate area when the letter was opened,

TABLE 6–1. Confirmed and Suspected Anthrax Cases (September 16 to November 15, 2001).*

	FLORIDA	NEW YORK CITY	WASHINGTON, D.C.	NEW JERSEY	CONNECTICUT	TOTAL
CONFIRMED						
Cutaneous	0	4	0	3	0	7
Inhalational	2	1	5	2	1	11
(Deaths)	(1)	(1)	(2)	(0)	(1)	(5)
SUSPECTED						
Cutaneous	0	3	0	1	0	4
Inhalational	0	0	0	0	0	0

*A 23rd case of anthrax (cutaneous) was reported in March 2002 in a laboratory worker in Texas who was working with environmental cultures from contaminated facilities. (CDC. Suspected cutaneous anthrax in a laboratory worker—Texas, 2002. *MMWR* 2002; 51:279–281).

nine were in an adjacent area, and six were first-responders.[13,15] Subsequently, it was shown that the powder contained *B. anthracis* spores that had been disseminated through many parts of the building, which resulted in its closure for four months until it was decontaminated.

Subsequently, a similar letter addressed to Senator Leahy, which was also processed through the same two U.S. postal facilities, was uncovered among mail being held for distribution. The Leahy letter was opened at the U.S. Army Medical Research Institute of Infectious Diseases at Fort Detrick, Maryland, under strict isolation conditions. It was reported that it contained a highly purified *B. anthracis* powder, with particles approximately one micron in size—of a higher quality than the powder in the Daschle letter. The powder in the Leahy letter has been described as a "weapons-grade" *B. anthracis* preparation.

After the Daschle letter was shown to contain *B. anthracis* spores and cases of anthrax were diagnosed in employees at the Brentwood U.S. postal facility and the Hamilton postal facility, where the Daschle and Leahy letters had been processed, environmental cultures from both facilities revealed *B. anthracis* throughout the buildings. These facilities were closed and prophylactic antibiotics and anthrax vaccine was offered to all potentially exposed employees.

The last two cases related to this anthrax bioterrorist event were the most difficult ones to explain. The first was in a 61-year-old woman who worked in a New York City hospital.[10] The other case was in a 94-year-old woman who lived in Oxford, Connecticut, and only left her home when accompanied by someone. Neither had any known exposure to *B. anthracis*–containing items or environments. For both cases, comprehensive epidemiological studies failed to identify the source of contamination. Their homes were examined and specimens cultured in detail, including clothing and other materials. The environments in which they went either to or from work and other environmental sites were all examined and cultured, with negative findings.

Months earlier (in January 2001) in Canada, a letter containing a powder was received at a government office—a situation that turned out to be a *B. anthracis* hoax. The Defense Research Establishment, Suffield, a government agency, was concerned about the possibility of the dissemination of *B. anthracis* from an envelope. It performed an experiment in an aerosol test chamber, in which a letter purposely contaminated with *Bacillus globigii* spores (which are approximately the same size as *B. anthracis* spores) was placed in a sealed envelope and, along with other envelopes, handled by an appropriately clothed person.[16] Slit samplers and filters were placed throughout the chamber as the letters were manipulated and then opened by the technician. *B. globigii* spores were disseminated throughout the test chamber. This experiment showed that spores of the same as size as *B. anthracis* spores could be distributed from an envelope as it was opened. But then, how did the environments of postal facilities become contaminated and postal workers infected? It is hypothesized that *B. anthracis*-containing powder can pass through sealed envelopes, either through the spaces that are not sealed at either end of the flap or through the paper of a single-thickness envelope as the letter is being processed through the automated mail sorting system.[13]

One scenario hypothesized to explain the source of infection for the New York City hospital employee and the elderly Connecticut woman has been tertiary contamination of letters that these women received through the mail. Within one minute after the Leahy letter was processed in the New Jersey Hamilton facility, letters were processed for a Wallingford, Connecticut, postal facility, from which letters were distributed to postal routes that included the Connecticut woman's home in Oxford. It is hypothesized that: (a) letters thus contaminated from the Leahy letter went to the Wallingford facility, where (b) they were again processed, which resulted in contamination of mail, which (c) then went to Oxford (and a neighboring community in which a *B. anthracis*–contaminated letter was found in a home, although there were no cases of anthrax among people who had contact with this letter). Thus, it would appear that mail that went to the Connecticut woman's home could also have been contaminated in the Wallingford facility. It is also hypothesized that a similar scenario could explain the source of infection for the New York City woman.

The epidemiological connection with mail is shown in Figure 6–2, which demonstrates that potentially all of the anthrax cases could have been asso-

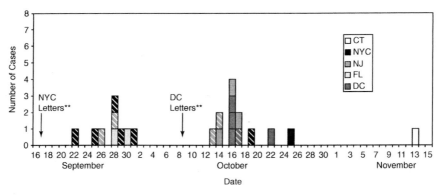

Solid bar = inhalation anthrax
Striped bar = cutaneous anthrax

*Modified from MMWR. November 2, 2001, Vol. 50, No. 43, pp 941-948
**Postmarked date of known contaminated letters.

FIGURE 6–2. Bioterrorism-related anthrax cases, by date of onset and work location (residence for Connecticut case) September 16 to November 15, 2001. (Adapted from: *MMWR*. 2001; 50:941–948.)

ciated with two U.S. postal facilities.[10] These facilities—the Hamilton postal facility in Trenton, New Jersey, and the Brentwood postal facility in Washington, D.C.—had extensive environmental contamination, which necessitated closing the facilities until they could be decontaminated.

The areas within the Hart Senate Office Building in Washington, D.C., that had been shown to be contaminated by environmental culturing were decontaminated with chlorine dioxide. Subsequent samples taken were negative for *B. anthracis*, although in some areas the decontamination had to be repeated several times. No cases of anthrax occurred in people in the Hart Senate Office Building, even though a number of the people who were exposed to the Daschle letter as it was being opened did have positive nasal cultures. The absence of cases among people there may have been a result of the rapid closure of the building and the prophylactic use of antibiotics among exposed individuals. In 1957, Edward Carr and colleagues reported that employees in a goat-hair processing mill could be colonized with *B. anthracis* (14 nasal swabs or pharyngeal washings were positive out of 101 specimens obtained) without developing clinical disease.[17] These individuals were not treated prophylactically, had not been immunized, and did not develop disease.

The Centers for Disease Control and Prevention (CDC) has shown, by molecular subtyping, that all of the patient isolates, environmental isolates, and powder isolates of *B. anthracis* are of the same genotype (62).[18] Additionally, this is the same genotype as the Ames strain, which is used as a stock strain in many laboratories throughout the world.

During the anthrax bioterrorist event in 2001, the CDC recommended, in addition to antibiotic prophylaxis, that some exposed individuals should also be vaccinated with the anthrax vaccine, in order to provide further protection against developing clinical anthrax. This recommendation was based on investigations in nonhuman primates exposed to an aerosol of *B. anthracis* that were treated with antibiotics and/or given anthrax vaccine. The primates that had received both antibiotics and the vaccine had the highest survival rate, compared to those who received the vaccine or antibiotics alone, or nothing.

EVALUATION OF THE PUBLIC HEALTH RESPONSE

Several years ago, the CDC was given the responsibility to develop a public health bioterrorism-preparedness plan for the United States. The plan was developed in collaboration with many individuals and agencies, and was publicized on the CDC website and in printed materials. Table-top exercises were conducted for field-testing of the plan, which outlined responsibilities of federal, state, and local government agencies, nongovernmental organizations, and individual citizens. Some government agencies adapted this plan to their own special needs. The anthrax bioterrorist event was the first application of the CDC plan. Each bioterroist event will be different from others, and thus each will require its own plan.

In evaluating the public health response to the anthrax bioterrorist event in 2001, one may look at the individual major components of the plan, which can be categorized as detection, diagnosis, investigation, therapy, communication, and training.[19]

Detection

Detection refers to public health surveillance and includes the need to develop some novel surveillance systems (Chapter 14). It is necessary to sensitize professional groups and agencies that may be the first to have an opportunity to detect a bioterrorist event. These include clinicians, first-responders, those staffing 911 telephone emergency lines, emergency departments, walk-in clinics, pharmacies, and news-media organizations. The first diagnosed case of anthrax, the inhalational case in Florida, was diagnosed by the clinician who noticed Gram-positive rods in cerebrospinal fluid and considered *B. anthracis*, which was subsequently confirmed by the CDC. When this information was publicized in the *Morbidity and Mortality Weekly Report (MMWR)* and by the news media, the New York City cutaneous anthrax cases that had already occurred were diagnosed.

Diagnosis

Diagnosing the first case of a bioterrorist event and giving it full publicity alerts other health-care providers to potential cases, as occurred in 2001. Had the graphic artist's physician in Florida not made the diagnosis of anthrax, the diagnoses of the New York City cutaneous cases would have been further delayed. Clinical algorithms that take into account the clinical features of anthrax, as seen in the cases in 2001, were important in strengthening the detection system. Soon after the first cases were diagnosed, the CDC placed on its website photographs of cutaneous anthrax lesions (Figures 6–3 and 6–4), chest x-rays of inhalational anthrax cases (Figure 6–5), and microphotographs of Gram-stained *B. anthracis* organisms. It also reported, in the *MMWR* and on its website, other clinical and diagnostic aspects of anthrax infections and treatment regimens.

It is critically important to educate all health professionals about anthrax and other diseases potentially spread by bioterrorism. This education is most efficiently conducted in schools of medicine and other health professional education facilities. Since the curricula will probably not include seeing pa-

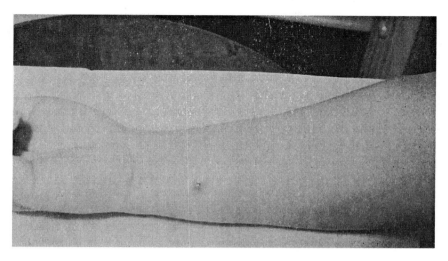

FIGURE 6–3. Cutaneous anthrax lesion on right forearm of a 27-year-old woman who worked in the spinning department of a goat-hair textile mill (day 4) (Photograph by Philip S. Brachman).

tients with these diseases, special components will need to be added to educational programs (see Chapter 10).

The need to have laboratory diagnostic facilities throughout the country was recognized by the CDC, and it has been providing assistance, training, and diagnostic materials to the states to strengthen their laboratory diagnostic capabilities for potential bioterrorist agents (Chapter 14). Since it is not realistic for all laboratories to be able to perform all diagnostic tests, the CDC

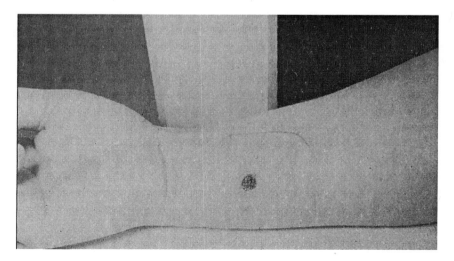

FIGURE 6–4. Same patient as in Figure 6–3 (day 10) (Photograph by Philip S. Brachman).

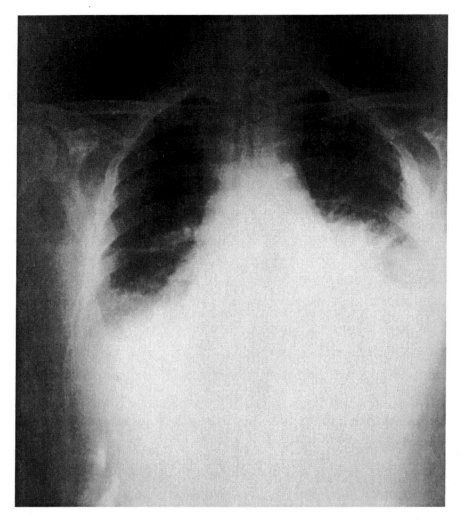

FIGURE 6–5. Chest x-ray of patient with inhalational anthrax. Note markedly widened mediastinum (Public Health Image Library, Centers for Disease Control and Prevention).

is helping selected laboratories serve a regional diagnostic function. Not only did the CDC laboratories provide diagnostic services in a timely and efficient manner, but they also provided advice and diagnostic materials to other laboratories.

Investigation

When the first anthrax case was reported in 2001, the CDC immediately initiated investigations by sending 12 of its people to Florida and subsequently provided hundreds of personnel of many disciplines to other affected areas. In all instances, the CDC worked closely with the involved state and local health professionals as well as with other federal agencies. Although investigators had no previous experience with anthrax, the investigations were conducted carefully, rapidly, and efficiently, which is the standard for the CDC. In some instances, there was concern over jurisdiction, which made it difficult for the CDC to conduct some investigations. This problem was initially compounded by difficulty in receiving the results of environmental cultures taken by other agencies. Another problem was the reporting of environmental culturing results that incorporated testing by methods of unproven quality. In the future, jurisdictional problems must be resolved and mechanisms for the rapid sharing of data must be established if the CDC is to successfully meet its responsibilities. In addition, the technology of testing environmental specimens must be standardized to prevent inaccurate results from being reported.

Therapy

With the diagnosis of the first anthrax case in 2001, treatment recommendations were made by the CDC, based on the past clinical experiences with *B. anthracis*. These recommendations were modified when it was recognized that the agent could have been altered to make treatment more difficult. The CDC then recommended that a different antibiotic, ciprofloxacin, be used in large, intravenous doses and that supportive therapy be more aggressive. The clinical features of the inhalational and cutaneous cases were rapidly publicized in the *MMWR* and on the CDC website.[13] The fact that the case-fatality rate was 40 percent—and not 85 percent, as reported from studies of the previous inhalational cases in the United States—may reflect the implementation of these CDC therapeutic recommendations. The CDC, considering data from the Sverdlovsk epidemic and experimental data from the exposure of nonhuman primates to *B. anthracis*, recommended a prophylactic regimen for persons potentially exposed to the agent, including antibiotics (for 60 days) and anthrax vaccine. (See discussion in Chapter 10.)

Use of anthrax vaccine did cause some concern due to previous publicity about its reactogenicity. In addition, an inadequate supply of vaccine was a problem. When it became available following the licensing of the company that produces it, the U.S. Food and Drug Administration (FDA) rapidly approved its use for prophylaxis as an Investigational New Drug (IND).

A contentious issue was determining which groups of people affected by this bioterrorist event should be offered anthrax vaccine. Laboratory scientists who had been working with materials potentially contaminated by *B. anthracis* comprised a high-priority group. Members of other groups, however, may have had the same risk of becoming infected, such as first-responders, emergency department personnel, field investigators obtaining environmental samples, and those performing decontamination. The CDC should clarify this issue and develop and publicize a plan for addressing this issue if it arises again.

The CDC has been criticized for delays in making recommendations in the fall of 2001 for prophylactic treatment of people with potential exposure to *B. anthracis* in contaminated environments. The CDC was limited in what it could do, however, because (a) it did not have the prime responsibility for the environmental culturing necessary to define the extent of environmental contamination; and (b) it did not have immediate access to the results of cultures taken by other agencies. Thus, until the CDC had all the requisite data, it could not make appropriate recommendations.

Communication

Communication is a critical element in any investigation of a bioterrorist event (Chapter 7). This includes communication among the investigators, communication with state and local health departments, and communication with the public. The routine sharing of data resulting from the investigations conducted by each agency is important for the most efficient use of resources, avoiding duplicating work, and allowing the most expeditious development and implementation of control and prevention measures. During the anthrax investigations in 2001, not all of the participants shared their data as it became available, which created difficulties in making recommendations for prophylaxis and treatment and in developing hypotheses about the source and spread of the agent.

There was also inadequate sharing of data with state and local health departments, which created problems for these agencies in deciding what actions should be taken. The CDC has an electronic communication system with every state and some city health departments, but it was not used to its maximum effectiveness. In addition, the initial lack of regular reports for the public, such as through the *MMWR* or the news media, created a significant public information void, which increased the public's fear and concern. This void made it necessary for the news media to seek information from public officials and private citizens who were not health professionals and/or not adequately informed, resulting in misinformation and vagueness in newspaper, television, and radio reports. This lack of communication with the public for several weeks is not the usual way that the CDC operates during an investigation. Since this investigation included a criminal investigation component, there were some data that could not be immediately released. Yet, not providing *any* data perpetuated fear and inappropriate statements. Daily news-media briefings from a single, authoritative source would have helped allay the public's fear. After the initial delays in the release of information, the CDC did provide updated reports in the *MMWR* and on its website, and then through the news media (see Box 13–1 in Chapter 13). Reports of this bioterrorist event have begun to be published in scientific journals.[20,21]

In the future, public briefings must be held. Information can be provided that does not jeopardize epidemiological or criminal investigations. If the news media have to obtain information indirectly, distortion may occur. Given the opportunity, the news media can be very helpful in providing information to the public that can help calm unnecessary fears.

Training

Even before September 2001, training for bioterrorism preparedness appeared to have been appropriate for what was perceived to be a bioterrorism threat. Since each bioterrorist event is different, no matter how much preparedness training has been accomplished, some areas not covered by such training will be identified. What is learned from a bioterrorist event helps identify and develop new areas for preparedness training. For example, the CDC has initiated educational activities to train health professionals about the clinical features and treatment regimens for other potential bioterrorist agents (see Chapters 10 and 15). This information is also available on the CDC website: www.cdc.gov. The education of health professional students concerning rarely encountered agents that may be used in bioterrorism is vitally important.

CONCLUSION

In summary, the public health response to the anthrax bioterrorist event in 2001 was rapid and comprehensive, and it may have prevented the further spread of anthrax. It is possible that additional cases were prevented by the nature of the investigations, the closing of facilities, and the prophylactic measures recommended and implemented. Although there may have been some delays in promoting and implementing these measures, it is not apparent that these delays had an adverse effect.

For an organization such as the CDC to perform most efficiently and to collaborate most effectively with its partners, there needs to be one authoritative leader. It did not appear that this was the case during the anthrax bioterrorist event in 2001. Although Atlanta-based CDC staff members met regularly to review the progress of the investigations, it did not appear that one authoritative person was knowledgeable about all of the studies, results, and recommendations. Some CDC personnel placed in liaison roles were unfamiliar with this information and with anthrax. These personnel could have been better briefed and provided with daily updates of information.

When the CDC had adequate data, it made appropriate recommendations. With other agencies involved in the investigations, including the Federal Bureau of Investigation (FBI), the U.S. Environmental Protection Agency (EPA), and health departments and other agencies at the state and local level, it was not easy to identify the appropriate and the most efficient lines of authority. The anthrax bioterrorist event dramatically emphasized the need to correct this problem.

The communication problem should not be allowed to occur in the future. A single source of information is important, and that voice must be authoritative, accurate, regular, and comprehensive. Anything less than this will not satisfy the public's need for information to allay its concerns and fears.

There was collaboration between the various agencies with responsibilities in, and knowledge about, the event, but it was not always smooth and spontaneous. Inadequate interagency collaboration can lead to duplicating efforts, redundant investigations, and delays in discovery and in making recommendations for control and prevention. It is human nature to protect one's "turf," but adjustments need to be made when these actions inhibit the progress of investigations or inhibit publicizing and facilitating implementation of control and prevention measures.

Our knowledge of bioterrorism has been extended by the anthrax bioterrorist event of 2001. The CDC has published the results of its investigations and will continue to do so. It also will continue its applied research, including studies to develop more rapid diagnostic techniques for identifying *B. anthracis* and other bioterrorist agents from clinical and environmental specimens. It should evaluate the rapid-identification field kits that were marketed during the investigations in 2001. The CDC has indicated that it will monitor for adverse events the approximately 10,000 people whose exposure histories resulted in their receiving prolonged prophylactic antibiotic treatment and, in some instances, the anthrax vaccine. The CDC has already increased its educational activities on diagnostic and therapeutic recommendations for anthrax, as well as for other potential bioterrorist agents. These educational activities should be extended to the basic education of health professionals.

A disservice will be done if retrospective analyses are used to try to find fault and assign blame. We need to learn what improvements can be made in our ability to respond to a bioterrorist event. If an error was the result of a wrong decision being made when appropriate data were available, adjustments must be made to try to prevent a repetition of this type of error in the future. Using data available *now* to find fault with best-intentioned actions of the past is inappropriate and must not be condoned.

REFERENCES

1. Sterne M. The use of anthrax vaccines prepared from avirulent (uncapsulated) variants of *Bacillus anthracis. Onderstepoort J. Vet. Sci. Anim. Ind* 1939; 13:307–312.

2. Brachman PS, Kaufmann AF. Anthrax. In *Bacterial Infections of Humans.* AS Evans, PS Brachman (eds.) 3rd edition 1998, pp. 95–107.

3. CDC. Summary of Notifable Diseases, United States, 1999. April 6, 2001. *MMWR* 48:53, pp. 1–15.

4. Brachman PS, Gold H, Plotkin SA, et al. Field evaluation of human anthrax vaccine. *Am J Public Health* 1962; 52:632–645.

5. Brachman PS, Plotkin SA, Bumford FH, et al. An epidemic of inhalation anthrax: The first in the twentieth century. *Am J Hygiene* 1960; 72:6–23.

6. Brachman PS. Inhalation anthrax. *Annals of the New York Academy of Sciences* 1980; 353:83–93.

7. Brachman PS, Kaufmann AF, Dalldorf FG. Inhalation anthrax. *Bacteriol Rev* 1966; 30:646–657.

8. Brachman PS, Pagano JS, Albrink WS. Two cases of fatal inhalation anthrax, one associated with sarcoidosis. *N Engl J Med* 1961; 265:203–208.

9. Meselson M, Guillemin J, Hugh-Jones M, et al. The Sverdlovsk anthrax outbreak of 1979. *Science* 1994; 266:1202–1208.

10. CDC. Update: Investigation of bioterrorism-related anthrax and interim guidelines for clinical evaluation of persons with possible anthrax. *MMWR* 2001; 50:941–948.

11. CDC. Update: Investigation of bioterrorism-related inhalational anthrax—Connecticut, 2001. *MMWR* 2001; 50:1049–1051.

12. CDC. Update: Investigation of anthrax associated with international exposure and interim public health guidelines. *MMWR* 2001; 50:889–897.

13. CDC. Update: Investigation of bioterrorism-related anthrax and interim guidelines for exposure management and antimicrobial therapy, October 2001. *MMWR* 2001; 50:909–919.

14. Freedman A, Afonja O, Chang MW, et al. Cutaneous anthrax associated with microangiopathic hemolytic anemia and coagulopathy in a 7-month-old infant. *JAMA* 2002; 287:869–874.

15. Hsu VP, Lukacs SL, Harper S, et al. An anthrax outbreak averted: public health response to a contaminated envelope on Capitol Hill—Washington, D.C. 2001. *Latebreaks II,* International Conference on Emerging Infectious Diseases, 2002.

16. Koournikakis B, Armour SJ, Boulet CA, et al. Risk assessment of anthrax threat letters. *Defence Research Establishment Suffield Technical Report.* DRES TR-2001-048. September 2001. Submitted for publication.

17. Carr EA, Rew RR. Recovery of Bacillus anthracis from the nose and throat of apparently healthy workers. *J Infect Dis* 1957; 100:169–171.

18. Hoffmaster A, Fitzgerald C, Ribot E, et al. Importance of Bacillus anthracis molecular subtyping during the recent multi-state bioterrorism associated anthrax outbreak in the United States. Abstract: *Latebreakers II.* International Conference on Emerging Infectious Diseases 2002, page 22.

19. Bioterrorism Response Plan—DeKalb County. DeKalb County Board of Health, Center for Public Health Preparedness, Decatur, Georgia, 2001.

20. Borio L, Frank D, Mani V, et al. Death due to bioterrorism-related inhalation anthrax: report of 2 patients. *JAMA* 2001; 286:2554–2559.

21. Mayer TA, Bersoff-Matcha S, Murphy C, et al. Clinical presentation of inhalational anthrax following bioterrorism exposure: report of 2 surviving patients. *JAMA* 2001; 286:2595–2597.

7

Educating, informing, and mobilizing the public

MONICA SCHOCH-SPANA

Public reactions to the events of September 11 have changed erroneous preconceptions about the general public on which previous planning and "table-top" (simulated) exercises for terrorism response were often based. The idea that the public has a tendency toward hysteria, panic, and social disorder in such situations was countered by real-life demonstrations of collective resolve and organizational capacity to respond to these emergencies and aid suffering people. During the highly disruptive, though less lethal, dissemination of anthrax, the general public generally displayed a temperate reaction and a practical interest in how to deal with the threat.

Both the earlier expectations of the public's possible responses to terrorism and the actual reactions to the terrorist attacks of 2001 indicate the importance of planning more diligently and thoughtfully for the role of the general population. This chapter is organized around a series of precepts that are meant to stimulate the thinking of public health and other professionals charged with protecting the well-being of people during terrorist attacks. Leaders, policy-makers, and health and safety professionals who are first-responders need to give more attention to communicating with and mobilizing the public.

CONSTRUCTIVE PUBLIC RESPONSE

Simulated Public Responses to Terrorism

Professionals charged with protecting the population's health and safety and serving as first-responders have tended to focus on the potential for widespread psychosocial consequences of a terrorist attack. Terrorism-response literature, discourse, and practical exercises reflect this perspective, which may have perpetuated the image of an emotionally vulnerable public, prone to panic, social disorder, and civil unrest. As a corrective, public health professionals should help devise institutional responses that not only anticipate and protect against the negative psychological and social repercussions of terrorism, but also enhance positive public responses. Relative disregard for the general public's active role in the response to terrorism was characteristic of response planning and policy discussions before the terrorist attacks of 2001.[1,2]

Response scenarios are narratives that depict, in war-game fashion, hypothetical terrorist attacks. They have been valuable in raising basic awareness in various groups about the complexities of medical and public-health management of bioterrorism[3,4] and in stimulating decision-makers and emergency responders to consider the range of challenges that terrorism may pose.[5,6] Important for clarifying the roles and necessary technical expertise of emergency responders and their institutions and for improving coordination among emergency responders, these scenarios have portrayed the public with far less rigor and fidelity. Table-top and field exercises have often employed plot lines that cast the general public in one-dimensional roles as mass casualties and panic-stricken crowds who flee from affected areas or resort to violence to gain access to hospitals or to obtain scarce antibiotics and vaccines. Such typecasting, while arguably preparing responders for the worst case, precludes considering constructive actions by the public and building response systems accordingly. Moreover, it erroneously conveys an image of the public dominated by antisocial behavior, which extensive sociological research into actual responses to natural and technological disasters has refuted.[7]

Guides on the health consequences of biological and chemical weapons have also tended to represent only pathological or maladaptive responses by the public.[8-10] Neglected altogether are possible positive reactions, such as reasoned caution, resourcefulness, resiliency, hopefulness, and humanitarianism, and the frequency with which these occur. Among the psychological responses to a bioterrorist attack that behavioral specialists anticipate are horror, panic, magical thinking about bacteria and viruses, fear of invisible agents and contagion, anger at terrorists and/or the government, scapegoating, paranoia, and demoralization.[11] Foreknowledge of these adverse reactions is necessary for devising ways, such as effective risk communication, to reduce their occurrence and severity. An exclusive focus on negative phenomena, however, may foster an expectation that these will be the dominant responses of a population attacked by terrorists.

The September 11 Terrorist Attacks

Positive responses to crises, such as those that occurred in September 2001, call into question a one-dimensional attitude toward the general public. The positive public response began even before the World Trade Center (WTC) Twin Towers collapsed. Images of heroic police and firefighters dashing into the imperiled buildings captured the popular imagination. But it is critical to remember also the crucial role in the evacuation played by tens of thousands of ordinary people who offered mutual assistance and cooperated with official instructions. Immediately after the WTC attack, some of those in closest proximity acted swiftly to support search and rescue activities, despite the danger and the uncertainty about additional attacks.[12,13]

Skilled and unskilled volunteers from near and far responded quickly to help survivors.[14,15] On September 11, approximately 500 donors arrived at St. Vincent's Hospital and Medical Center, the trauma facility nearest to Ground Zero, and organized themselves by blood type using makeshift cardboard signs.[16] For several weeks afterward, national blood collection rates were two to three times their normal levels, with first-time donors accounting for 50 percent of all contributions, in contrast to the usual 20 percent rate.[17]

These courageous, resourceful, and benevolent acts occurred while those directly affected by the tragedy and many others experienced profound shock, anger, uncertainty, anxiety, and grief. Almost 40 percent of lower Manhattan residents interviewed six to seven weeks after September 11 reported symptoms suggestive of post-traumatic stress disorder (PTSD)—although a later study suggested that the actual rate of PTSD was much lower (Chapter 3).[18] Interviewed three to five days after the attacks, 90 percent of a national sample of people reported experiencing trauma-related symptoms of stress, including upset feelings, disrupted sleep, difficulty concentrating, irritability, short temper, and recurrent disturbing mental images; 44 percent reported experiencing one or more of these symptoms to an extreme degree.[19] Two weeks after the attacks, 60 percent of Americans reported crying; 65 percent, feeling angry; 51 percent, being nervous and tense; and 46 percent, being dazed and numb; and 27 percent wondered if anyone in the United States "could really be safe."[20] New York City respondents experienced each of these reactions more intensely, except for being dazed and numb.

Behaviors present after the terrorist attacks suggested a norm of social cohesion, not disarray. Responding to the national catastrophe, many Americans sought out interpersonal connections and performed acts of charity, perhaps in an attempt to derive comfort and a sense of control in uncertain, tragic times.[19] Among adults surveyed three to five days after the attack, 98 percent reported sharing thoughts and feelings about the events with others; 75 percent, checking on the safety of the people closest to them; 60 percent, participating in a public, commemorative event; 36 percent, donating blood or money, or volunteering; and 32 percent, inquiring about someone who they thought might be injured or missing.[19] Two weeks after the attacks, 59 percent of Americans—and a higher percentage of New Yorkers—indicated that they had donated or attempted to donate blood, made charitable contributions, and/or performed extra volunteer work.[20] By December 16, almost two-thirds of Americans reported having donated money to funds established for the victims of September 11 and their families.[21]

Marring the widespread demonstration of altruism, however, were incidents of suspicion and rage directed at people of the Islamic faith and/or of Middle Eastern origin and at Indian Americans, Latinos, and others presumed to be from offending groups.[22] Hate crimes included sending of hate mail, verbal attacks, physical assault, homicide, and damage to mosques and Arab-American-owned and Muslim-owned businesses (see Box 17–2).

Anthrax Dissemination

Confronted with bioterrorism soon after the WTC and Pentagon attacks, most Americans remained calm and resolute while concerned about personal safety—in contrast to some public officials' expectations of panic. In a September 11 poll, 57 percent of adults in the United States reported being worried that either they or family members would fall victim to terrorism.[23] This percentage dropped in subsequent polls, then spiked again in reaction to the first death from inhalational anthrax (Figure 7–1). After this surge, worry declined steadily,[23–25] despite anthrax contamination of postal service facilities; more anthrax cases and deaths, including two inhalational anthrax deaths with undetermined sources of infection; failure to apprehend the perpetrator of the anthrax attack; the possibility of reprisals in reaction to U.S. military activities in Afghanistan; and nonspecific Federal Bureau of Investigation (FBI) alerts about possible, imminent terrorist attacks.

In this same milieu, levels of anxiety about possible anthrax exposure did not increase (Figure 7–1). The vast majority of people believed that they and their immediate family members were at low risk of contracting anthrax: only 14 percent of those polled following the deaths of two postal workers considered this scenario a likely possibility over the next year[26]; almost three

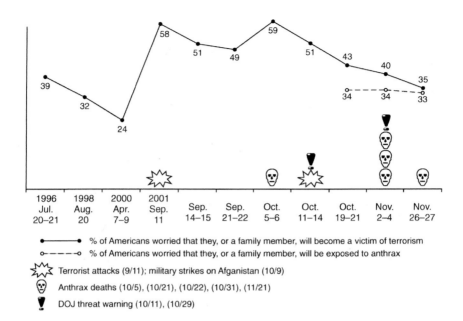

FIGURE 7–1. Public fear of falling victim to terrorism, autumn 2001. Dates shown on x-axis are survey periods. Symbols indicate events that were the backdrop in the relevant survey period. (Survey data adapted from: The Gallup Organization. *Attack on America: key trends and indicators.* December 18, 2001.)

times as many (41 percent) thought injury in an automobile collision likely. After the two additional anthrax deaths for which investigators could not determine a definitive route of exposure, rates of concern declined, with only 9 percent perceiving anthrax infection as a personal or family threat.[27]

Among people living in areas where anthrax was disseminated, especially those whose lives were directly affected, concern was understandably higher. Among Washington, D.C., area residents whose workplaces had been closed due to anthrax or suspected anthrax, who had been exposed to or tested for anthrax, or who had a friend or relative exposed to or tested for anthrax, 26 percent thought that contracting the disease was likely, compared to 15 percent of area residents without any direct experience of the threat and 9 percent of the U.S. population at large.[27] Although individuals with direct experience of the anthrax threat had elevated concerns over possible exposure, this fear apparently did not contribute to erratic or unruly behavior. Reports of mass testing and prophylaxis at affected worksites, such as congressional offices; the American Media, Inc., building in Boca Raton, Florida; and the Brentwood postal facility in the Washington area, indicate that this massive public-health campaign was orderly, with hundreds—sometimes thousands—of people waiting in line for long periods.[28,29]

Overall, the general public exhibited steadfastness in an environment of grave uncertainty and displayed levels of concern commensurate with their proximity to danger. Nonetheless, various leaders exhorted citizens not to panic, and news reports and editorials often featured the public as reactive and hysteria-driven.[30–32] Throughout the fall, the news media frequently reported on citizens hoarding ciprofloxacin and purchasing gas masks and firearms, although the frequency of such reports contrasted with the actual infrequency of this behavior—often presented as "panic buying." These sales increased after the attacks,[33,34] but relatively few people made such purchases. About 70 percent of people surveyed in mid-October 2001 reported not having thought about getting an antibiotic prescription or a gas mask, and only 2 to 3 percent reported having done so.[35] Among those polled after the two postal-worker deaths, 5 percent reported obtaining a prescription for antibiotics and 1 percent reported purchasing a gas mask or other personal protective equipment.[26] Although ill-advised from a public health standpoint, such acquisitions, from the perspective of a concerned person, may seem to represent a reasoned, sensible precaution in the unprecedented context of mass civilian casualties—even though the mass casualties were not due to anthrax.

DEVISING PUBLIC-COMMUNICATION STRATEGIES

Startling evidence of vulnerability to attack, repeated government warnings about the possibility of future assaults, and personal experience with the devastation and disruption of terrorism made many people wonder what to expect and what they and the government should do. Many sought sources of authoritative knowledge. Over three-fourths reported closely following the news coverage of the bioterrorism crisis.[36] Twelve percent of people consulted a website for guidance on personal protection, 6 percent spoke with a personal physician, 4 percent telephoned the health department, and 1 percent telephoned the CDC.[26] Although the public exhibited a strong appetite for candid and personally relevant information, political and public health officials conducted a conservative communications campaign. Designed to avoid fomenting panic, this approach had the unintended consequence of diminishing the credibility of some officials. Learning from this experience, public health practitioners should be prepared to discuss the grave matter of terrorism and its potential consequences with frankness, giving the public as much useful information as possible and, hopefully, breeding confidence in official statements and measures.

A steady stream of criticism regarding restrained public communications by officials on the threat of bioterrorism commenced in late September when

U.S. Secretary of Health and Human Services Tommy Thompson reassured the public that the government was prepared to deal with any type of attack. This reassurance and his characterization, several days later, of the first inhalational anthrax case as an isolated incident that was possibly a natural occurrence suggested the government was employing a strategy to avert public panic by portraying events in the most positive light. Potentially undermining public confidence in this optimistic portrayal was its contrast with the obvious gravity of the September 11 attacks and, later, with the alerts from the federal government telling citizens to be vigilant.[37,38] Evidence that the situation was more serious than officials had first suggested seemed to follow each wave of reassurance.[39] The first "isolated" case of inhalational anthrax was followed by a series of other cases, some fatal, and the recommendation by health officials that mass prophylaxis was not indicated for postal workers was followed by the death of two Brentwood postal facility employees.

The perceived validity of statements was further undermined early in the crisis by the lack of highly visible spokespersons who were expert in health matters and could address the medical and public health implications of the unfolding terrorist incident.[39] Such spokespersons were clearly preferred by the public, as was documented in a poll about whom the general public most trusted.[26] Another problem with the rudimentary public communications campaign was the delay in giving civilians guidelines on how to cope with the threat of additional terrorist attacks. Soon after September 11, the general public shifted its concern to an apparent bioterrorist attack with anthrax (see Chapter 6). Yet people found very few official public health sources of information that addressed the the their most frequently asked questions: Should I buy a gas mask? Should I stockpile antibiotics? Is it safe for me to drink the water? Should I get vaccinated against anthrax or smallpox? Should I set up a "safe room" in my house? How do I protect my children? Although many health agencies eventually prepared public statements on these and other pressing questions, the initial void may have persuaded some to look elsewhere for guidance and lessened the reputation of health agencies as able to respond promptly and meaningfully to the information needs of concerned citizens.

Some individuals directly affected by the attacks were very frustrated in their efforts to obtain prompt, accurate information on how to deal with an immediate problem. For example, the editorial director of American Media, Inc. (AMI), expressed his surprise and anger at having to learn from the Internet and television reports that his co-worker had anthrax because the local health department did not return his repeated calls.[40] Increasing his anger was the lack of consistent advice from authorities about prophylaxis for his son.

PROVIDING PRACTICAL INFORMATION

A high-priority issue for the general public throughout the terrorist events of 2001 was learning what concrete measures people could take to enhance their safety and that of their families. Yet official recommendations on personal precautions were sometimes late, inconsistent, or inscrutable to the intended audience.[41,42] Public health professionals should be prepared to counsel the public immediately and throughout a crisis on which actions individuals should take to help avert danger and which actions they should not take. By being responsive to requests for advice on personal protective strategies, public health professionals can help promote knowledge of the most appropriate measures, foster people's sense of control in a threatening and bewildering context, and enhance public confidence in government measures to deal with the threat.

Polled several days following the WTC attack and several times throughout the anthrax crisis, a national sample of Americans reported engaging in a wide range of protective behaviors.[19,20,26,27] Most commonly, people stocked up on essentials, such as food, gasoline, and cash; avoided "risky" locations, such as government buildings, downtown areas, and public events; and consulted the Internet. Less frequently, they talked to their physicians, sought and sometimes filled prescriptions for antibiotics, and spoke with health professionals about anthrax and/or smallpox vaccines. More rarely, they purchased firearms, bought gas masks and other personal protective equipment, constructed bomb shelters,[43] and enrolled in anti-terrorism classes.[44] The most frequently reported behavior, mentioned by more than one-third, was exercising caution when opening the mail, including 30 percent who washed their hands afterward and 6 percent who wore gloves.[27] Residents in the metropolitan areas disrupted by the anthrax scare, with interrupted mail service, closed workplaces, and mass testing and prophylaxis of employees, practiced greater vigilance in handling their mail.[27] Only 2 percent of people in the national sample completely avoided opening the mail—an extreme approach to personal safety.[27]

Although it was relatively infrequent behavior, public attempts to obtain gas masks and antibiotics received much news-media coverage and troubled health officials. Officials worried that individuals self-medicating with antibiotics could suffer side effects and develop resistance to these medications, thus reducing their potential future efficacy. Unregulated and unwarranted demand for antibiotics could prevent their reaching people who needed them. Gas masks, which promised little protection from a covert biological attack because people would not be told when to wear them, had the potential, albeit unlikely, to asphyxiate the wearer. Businesses marketing personal protective equipment and easy access to antibiotics were exploiting a worried population. Physicians freely writing antibiotic prescriptions for people without a medical condition that warranted their use were engaging in an ethically questionable practice that could have affected antibiotic supplies, contributed to resistance of microorganisms, and conveyed an inappropriate message to patients. Yet public debate raged as to whether the National Pharmaceutical Stockpile had sufficient supplies that could be distributed rapidly enough to communities faced with large-scale attacks, and whether individuals should indeed take such matters into their own hands.

Public health practitioners should recognize that some protective behaviors that appear, from their professional viewpoint, over-reactive, unnecessary, ill-advised, useless, dangerous, or constituting a misapplication of scarce medical resources, may represent, from the individual's perspective, a sensible, prudent attempt to achieve security. This underlines the responsibility of public health officials to convey sufficient information on the protective value and potential adverse effects of a protective measure.

EDUCATING THE PUBLIC TO USE HEALTH SERVICES WISELY

Though there were no panicked masses in 2001, the actions of cautious, vigilant, and/or frightened citizens put excessive burdens on hospitals, law enforcement agencies, and public health and safety institutions. Remedying this problem in the future will require adjustments in both supply and demand. By providing the public with a better flow of information about threats to health, public health practitioners can sharpen the public's ability to make appropriate and judicious requests for information from medical, public health, and public safety professionals and institutions. The ability of health departments and other public health entities to increase public education and outreach operations during a crisis is critical. Meeting the demands of the public for information may then contribute to a more effective use of material resources, such as anthrax antibody tests, vaccines, antibiotics, and antidotes, and the capacities of medical care and of hazardous-materials handling.

During October 2001, the FBI responded to more than 2,500 suspected anthrax attacks—10 times the number of all purported attacks by weapons of mass destruction that it typically investigates in a year.[45] Anthrax attacks, hoaxes, and frights consumed vast amounts of time and money, as ambulances, emergency medical personnel, and teams of hazardous-materials experts and investigators responded to suspected threats.[46] Public health agencies grappled with a level of demand they were unaccustomed to. They fielded many calls from the public, collected and evaluated suspicious material, and performed massive testing and prophylaxis and/or treatment of people possibly exposed to anthrax.[46] Staff members at public health laboratories, many of whom were diverted from other duties to assist in bioterrorism response, worked around the clock, sometimes setting up residence in facilities to keep up with the workload. A rapid survey by the Association of State and Territorial Health Officials, which one-half of state health departments responded to, revealed that, on average, state health agencies expected to spend $1 million to $5 million each on anthrax-specific costs from the start of the crisis through January 2002—a large unbudgeted expense.[46] Physicians' offices and emergency departments experienced an influx of patients asking to be tested for exposure to anthrax. Most of the people were at little or no risk (Chapter 6).[29,47,48]

Four percent of respondents to a national survey in late October noted that they or other household members had telephoned a state or local health department to obtain information on anthrax or smallpox, and one percent had contacted the CDC.[26] Calls by even this very small percentage of the population put very heavy burdens on health agencies. Nevertheless, some health professionals judged their responsiveness to the public's need for practical guidance and reassuring words as having the secondary benefit of helping to reduce demands on scarce emergency services. In Montgomery County, Maryland, adjacent to Washington, D.C., health officials established a round-the-clock hotline with taped information, a live hotline staffed by public health professionals daily from 7:00 a.m. to 10:00 p.m., and a walk-in health-risk assessment center in order to provide counseling, education, and referrals for anthrax and other concerns and to reduce demands on local hospitals for tests for anthrax exposure.[48] Similarly, the county fire department developed a triage system to deal with the growing number of reports of suspicious substances and packages. Conversing with callers, officials attempted to discern grounds for suspicion and to exercise discretion in deploying the bomb squad and hazardous-materials team.

In addition to preparing to meet a large volume of demand, public health practitioners should be prepared to deliver the kinds of information that represent priorities to the public. This requires being attentive to the questions most frequently posed by the public and actively surveying a community for what it needs to know. The New York City Department of Health, for example, interviewed lower Manhattan residents to determine unmet physical and mental health needs of people living next to the WTC disaster site.[18] This survey revealed a strong desire for more information on potential health risks associated with exposure to the dust and debris emanating from the WTC site and guidance on proper cleaning of contaminated building interiors, exteriors, and air conditioners. Also of concern to residents was information about mental health, the welfare of their children, and eligibility for relief funds.

ACTIVATING CIVIL-SOCIETY ORGANIZATIONS

Having witnessed the devastation wrought upon the WTC and the Pentagon, members of the general public, including highly specialized professionals, organized themselves to aid the search-and-rescue efforts and the longer-term recovery process. Unions, churches, tenant associations, professional societies, businesses, and many other organizations galvanized existing social ties, leadership structures, and communication links to channel a collective desire to help.

Public health professionals can benefit from establishing and improving partnerships with civic groups whose organizational capacities can be similarly marshalled during a terrorist crisis. Public health agencies, for example, can move critical health information to diverse sectors of society by fully utilizing the communication networks of civil-society organizations—through meetings, phone trees, e-mail list services, and on-line and print newsletters—and by interacting with the leaders of these organizations to reach their members. As evidenced by the broad range of assistance that civil-society organizations provided in response to the September 11 attacks, these organizations have a valuable role to play as potential collaborators with public health and safety agencies in responding to the consequences of future terrorist incidents. Locally-based community groups capitalized on their proximity to disaster sites and their wealth of local knowledge to act promptly and help tailor their own response efforts and those of health and safety agencies to actual needs. Associations with regional or national networks were capable of drawing in distant resources to help address needs at disaster sites.

The tenants' association for the Independence Plaza housing complex just north of the WTC played a significant role in maintaining the well-being of residents.[49] Immediately after the attack, members helped direct the streams of people running away from the collapsed buildings through the Independence Plaza area, thus performing a critical public safety function when many police had been called away to the WTC site. The association organized an "urgent needs" team to canvass homebound residents to determine who needed assistance, such as disabled and elderly individuals unable to obtain food and medicine on their own, and then to provide that assistance. In addition, the group worked with local businesses to maintain resident access to critical sites, such as by acting as volunteer cashiers at groceries and pharmacies when paid employees could not get into the area. Responsive to residents' air quality concerns, the tenants' association conducted an independent environmental review of city-devised procedures for removing materials from the WTC site and successfully advocated changes to reduce the environmental impact on residents in the Tribeca area near the disaster site.

Professional societies were critical in alerting health professionals to the possibility of mass casualties in New York City, broadcasting a national call for members' expertise and services. Within hours of the attack, for example, the 290,000-member American Medical Association contacted state and local medical societies and specialty organizations to request volunteers.[15] More than 1,700 medical personnel, including 700 physicians, responded to requests for critical-care specialists. The Healthcare Association of New York State identified local physicians, nurses, and other emergency medical personnel to help treat the anticipated mass casualties. The group also responded to more than 8,000 telephone calls during the initial 24-hour period from health-care workers throughout the United States who were offering to help.[15] This generous outpouring of assistance met with the grim reality that there were few survivors who needed acute care. The American Psychological Association and the American Public Health Association, among other organizations, similarly contacted their members seeking to identify mental health experts willing to counsel New York City residents affected by the attacks.[50]

Community organizations that reacted constructively to the crisis included unions, churches, libraries, and businesses, large and small. Building-trades labor unions immediately gathered crews of operating engineers, ironworkers, laborers, Teamsters, and others; set up equipment; and sought out architectural drawings in order to perform the dangerous work of searching through the rubble for survivors.[13] One union hall located in Tribeca was converted into a Red Cross Disaster Service Center that helped connect affected residents with relief services.[49] The Seamen's Church Institute of New York and New Jersey, whose headquarters was located near the perimeter of the site, dedicated its cooking facilities to feeding rescue and recovery workers, and members of Episcopal churches in the area took turns staffing the kitchen.[49] In the immediate aftermath of the Pentagon attack, Virginia's Arlington County libraries posted regular on-line traffic updates and police and fire department briefings to meet critical information needs of the nearby community.[51]

UTILIZING VOLUNTEERS

The humanitarian volunteer response in New York City involved diverse individuals and organizations, from large, well-established associations, to smaller groups arising in response to an emergent need. A wide array of goods was donated; they were usually put to effective use, but occasionally were not congruent with the needs of the affected communities.

In the future, public health practitioners, anticipating what volunteers can contribute, may wish to plan more systematically to incorporate and capitalize upon the humanitarian response to a terrorist attack. By developing protocols for integrating volunteers and by developing partnerships with volunteer organizations, public health agencies can enhance their responsiveness to community needs in two ways: First, public health agencies can help assure that sufficient personnel are available to carry out critical public health functions during the crisis. Second, they can offer the general public a positive and active role during a period of grave uncertainty and insecurity, thus countering the terrorizing effects of an attack.

Volunteer efforts in New York City were indicative of the resourceful ways people used existing social institutions and relationships to organize collective humanitarian efforts. For example, prominent organizations, such as the Red Cross and the Salvation Army, activated their trained, highly structured volunteer membership and coordinated with the local people who volunteered to help (Figure 7–2). Civil-society organizations, such as churches, unions, and tenants' associations, organized their members to help. Less formal relationships among friends, neighbors, relatives, and co-workers facilitated smaller efforts. For example, the family owners of a restaurant near Independence Plaza freely distributed nonperishable goods to lower Manhattan residents who were without food because of interrupted supply chains, from their restaurant, which was closed to business.[49] In some instances, individuals and groups that were brought together by chance filled a perceived need;

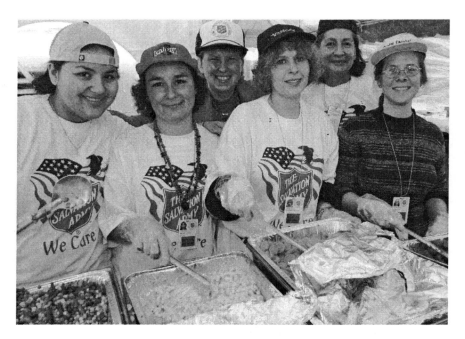

FIGURE 7–2. Volunteers from the Salvation Army feeding workers near Ground Zero in October 2001 (Photograph by Andrea Booher/FEMA News Photo).

for example, attendees at an emergency medicine and critical care conference in Brooklyn obtained supplies from a nearby pharmacy, established a
triage unit in the conference hotel, and posted lookouts at the foot of the
Brooklyn Bridge to direct the "walking wounded" to assistance.[15]

Donated goods and services for those affected ranged from the ordinary to
the high-tech. While New York area hospitals readied themselves for mass
casualties, area restaurants pledged food and cleaners pledged laundry services. Residents donated clothes, bottled water, and money. Medical equipment companies sent imaging equipment and engineers to provide technical
support.[14–16] Businesses and individuals donated workboots, shoe inserts,
gloves, socks, respirators, heavy-duty apparel, and food and water to help
outfit and feed rescue and recovery workers, emergency responders, and security personnel working at the disaster site.[49] During the recovery period,
information-technology companies donated hardware, software, and technical support to aid charitable organizations struggling with rudimentary information systems and an overwhelming amount of data on donations, volunteers, and requests for help.[52]

Not everyone wanting to volunteer, however, found an opportunity to do
so. In addition, a surplus of material donations presented serious logistical
challenges. Within two hours of the WTC attack, for example, the Community Assistance Unit (CAU) of Mayor Giuliani's office received calls from
100 potential volunteers. Although CAU was able to use a few volunteers,
the many calls over the next several days prompted the office to collect contact and skills information for most volunteers, intending to use this information for future needs that never materialized.[49] Many volunteers asking
city officials how they could help were directed to the Red Cross, as there
were few alternatives.[49] Individuals and groups who had traveled long distances were often frustrated to find that they were not needed.[53] Well-
meaning appeals by leaders for donations, such as dog food for search-
and-recovery canines, sometimes led to waves of contributions that far
exceeded real needs and caused practical problems of inventory management
and disposal.[49]

Alongside the strong volunteer presence in New York arose health and
safety concerns for the volunteers and the people they were assisting (see
Chapters 3 through 5). Physical hazards, poor air quality, and emotional stress
prompted actions by health and safety officials to protect rescue and recovery workers.[13] Some of the many first-time blood donors, giving in response
to the terrorist attacks, were informed unexpectedly that they had syphilis or
HIV, hepatitis B virus, or hepatitis C virus infections.[17] Concerned about
food-handling techniques of volunteers and the possibility of rats in food-
preparation areas, the New York City Department of Health deployed numerous food inspectors to oversee preparation and distribution of donated

food items. Their presence, though operating in an educational rather than an enforcement mode, fostered resentment among some volunteers who expressed concern over wastage when questionable food was thrown out.[49] Some mental health professionals criticized the quality of counseling provided by the wide variety of credentialed and noncredentialed persons presenting themselves to those in need.[49]

The New York experience after the WTC attack demonstrated the broad range of volunteered human and material resources potentially available in a terrorist crisis, and the challenges in managing these resources. For the future, public health professionals should devise ways to access volunteers should they be needed to support a public health response to a terrorist crisis, by cultivating relationships with community and relief organizations before a crisis and by creating an organizational system that enables individuals and groups to assist. They should also develop processes for promptly collecting and communicating information about what human and material resources are needed in such a crisis. In addition, they will need to attend to potential needs of volunteers, such as training, health and safety protection, and acknowledgement of the volunteers' work.

CONCLUSION

The wide range of positive public responses to the consequences of terrorist attacks in 2001 indicates that health and safety professionals need to reassess their assumptions about the public's capacity to respond constructively after a terrorist attack.

Health and safety professionals should consider the public and civil-society organizations as capable partners in responding to the consequences of terrorism and should provide information and organizational resources that enable people to protect themselves and their families and to volunteer their assistance.

REFERENCES

1. Dobbs M. A renaissance for U.S. civil defense? *Journal of Homeland Security* 2001. Available at: http://www.homelandsecurity.org/journal/Articles/Dobbs_July01.htm. Accessed 7 July 2001.
2. Taylor ER. Are we prepared for terrorism using weapons of mass destruction: government's half measures. *Policy Analysis* 2000; 387:1–19.
3. O'Toole T. Smallpox: an attack scenario. *Emerg Infect Dis* 1999; 5:540–546.
4. O'Toole T, Inglesby TV. Epidemic response scenario: decision-making in a time of plague. *Public Health Rep* 2001; 116(Suppl 2):92–103.

5. Johns Hopkins Center for Civilian Biodefense, Center for Strategic and International Studies, Analytic Services, Inc. (ANSER), & the Memorial Institute for the Prevention of Terrorism. Dark winter: bioterrorism exercise, Andrews Air Force Base, June 22–23, 2001. Available at http://www.hopkins-biodefense.org/DARK%20WINTER.pdf. Accessed July 1, 2001.

6. Inglesby TV, Grossman R, O'Toole T. A plague on your city: observations from TOPOFF. *Clin Infect DIs* 2001; 32:436–445.

7. Quarantelli EL. The sociology of panic. In Smelser N, Bates PB, eds. *International Encyclopedia of the Social and Behavioral Sciences.* New York, NY: Pergamon, 2001: 11020–30.

8. Norwood AE, Holloway HC, Ursano RJ. Psychological effects of biological warfare. *Mil Med* 2001; 166(Suppl 2):27–28.

9. DiGiovanni C. Domestic terrorism with chemical or biological agents: psychiatric aspects. *Am J Psychiatry* 1999; 156:1500–1505.

10. World Health Organization (WHO). Health aspects of chemical and biological weapons. Geneva, Switzerland: WHO, 1970.

11. Holloway HC, Norwood AE, Fullerton CS, et al. The threat of biological weapons: prophylaxis and mitigation of psychological and social consequences. *JAMA* 1997; 278:425–7.

12. Barry D. Determined volunteers camped out to pitch in. *New York Times.* 23 September 2001: B,1.

13. Rubin DK. Building trades lend hand and heart to WTC site recovery and cleanup. *Engineering News-Record* 2001; 247(25):31.

14. Shute N, Howe J, Sobel RK, et al. Amazing grace. *US News & World Report.* 14 September 2001; 50.

15. Romano M. Medical personnel respond. *Modern Healthcare.* 17 September 2001; 24.

16. Becker C, Galloro V. An overwhelming response; within hours of disaster, medical supplies were on their way to N.Y., D.C. *Modern Healthcare.* 17 September 2001; 18.

17. Villarosa L. A nation challenged: the volunteers; out to do good, some first-time blood donors get bad news. *New York Times.* 20 December 2001; B,6.

18. Community HealthWorks, NYC Department of Health. A community needs assessment of lower Manhattan following the World Trade Center attack. December 2001. Available at http://www.ci.nyc.ny.us/html/doh/pdf/chw/needs1.pdf. Accessed 11 January 2002.

19. Schuster MA, Stein BD, Jaycox LH, et al. A national survey of stress reactions after the September 11, 2001, terrorist attacks. *N Engl J Med* 2001; 345(20)1507–1512.

20. Smith TW, Rasinski KA, Toce M. America rebounds: a national study of public response to the September 11th terrorist attacks—preliminary findings. 25 October 2001. National Opinion Research Center, University of Chicago. Available at http://www.norc.uchicago.edu/projects/reaction/pubresp.pdf. Accessed 8 January 2002.

21. The Gallup Organization. Poll topics & trends: terrorist attacks and the aftermath. Available at http://www.gallup.com/poll/topics/terror.asp. Accessed 7 January 2002.

22. Southern Poverty Law Center. Raging against the other: September's terrorist strikes trigger a violent outbreak of American xenophobia. *Intelligence Report.* 2001 Winter; 104. Available at http://www.splcenter.org/cgi-bin/printassist.pl?page=/intelligenceproject/ip-4t6.html. Accessed 16 January 2002.

23. Gallup Poll News Service. Attack on America: key trends and indicators. 18 December 2001. Available at http://www.gallup.com/poll/Releases/Pr010926c.asp. Accessed 9 January 2002.

24. The Pew Research Center for the People and the Press. No rise in fears or reported depression: public remains steady in face of anthrax scare. October 2001. Available at http://www.people-press.org/midoct01rpt.htm. Accessed 7 January 2002.
25. The Pew Research Center for the People and the Press. Ratings of government effort slips: worries about terrorism subside in mid-America. 8 November 2001. Available at http://www.people-press.org/110801rpt.htm. Accessed 7 January 2002.
26. Blendon RJ, Benson JM, DesRoches CM, et al. Harvard School of Public Health/Robert Wood Johnson Foundation survey project on Americans' response to biological terrorism, tabulation report, October 24–28, 2001. 31 October 2001. Available at http://www.hsph.harvard.edu/press/releases/blendon/report.pdf. Accessed 12 November 2001.
27. Blendon RJ, Benson JM, DesRoches CM, et al. Harvard School of Public Health/Robert Wood Johnson Foundation survey project on Americans' response to biological terrorism, Study 2: national and three metropolitan areas affected by anthrax, November 29–December 3, 2001. 9 December 2001. Available at http://www.hsph.harvard.edu/press/releases/blendon/report2.pdf. Accessed 7 January 2002.
28. Povich E, Brune T. America's ordeal: anxiety on Capitol Hill. *Newsday*. 18 October 2001; A,2.
29. Riddle A. FBI probing workers' exposure to anthrax, hundreds seek tests. AP State & Local Wire. 9 October 2001.
30. Szegedy-Maszak M. Infected letters spread a contagion of fear that goes far beyond germs; mass hysteria. *US News & World Report*. 5 November 2001; 47.
31. Siegel M. You can't cure fear of terrorism with antibiotics; the main risk from anthrax is still psychological. *Los Angeles Times*. 29 October 2001; P2,11, op ed.
32. Robbins A. Confusing medicine with public health. *Boston Globe*. 17 November 2001; A,15, op. ed.
33. Witt A. Area families try to prepare for unknown; shoppers grab cell phones, gas masks, life insurance. *Washington Post*. 24 September 2001; B,1.
34. Petersen M. With anthrax fears, Bayer is to lift antibiotic output. *New York Times*. 11 October 2001; C,2.
35. Jones JM. Nine in 10 Americans are going about business as usual. Gallup News Service. 26 October 2001. Available at http://www.gallup.com/poll/releases/pro11026.asp. Accessed 7 January 2002.
36. The Pew Research Center for the People and the Press. Attacks at home draw more interest than war abroad. 22 October 2001. Available at http://www.people-press.org/102201.htm. Accessed 7 January 2002.
37. Kiely K. Americans confused: should we worry or go about our business? *USA Today*. 30 October 2001; A,6.
38. Editorial. Life in a time of terror. *New York Times*. 31 October 2001; A,14.
39. Schwartz J. The truth hurts; efforts to calm the nation's fears spin out of control. *New York Times*. 28 October 2001; S4,P1.
40. Steve Coz, interview by Elizabeth Vargas. *Good Morning America*, ABC, October 12, 2001.
41. Quinn S. What we need to know. *Washington Post*. 3 October 2001; A,31.
42. Quinn S. I asked, but I couldn't find one. *Washington Post*. 9 December 2001; B,1.
43. Sager B. Backyard bomb shelters a stylish trend. *Atlanta Constitution*. 23 November 2001; D,18.
44. Cobb K. America responds: civil defense 101, class teaches students how to act if caught in terroristic situation. *Houston Chronicle*. 18 October 2001; A,26.

45. Levine S. Disseminating dread; pranksters, disgruntled Americans perpetrate hoaxes. *Washington Post.* 26 October 2001; A,1.
46. Dembner A. Fighting terror; infectious agents funding civil defense; fear, testing drain health department budgets. *Boston Globe.* 23 October 2001; A,16.
47. Daniel M. Health officials work to avoid outbreak of fear; many false alarms in anthrax reports. *Boston Globe.* 20 October 2001; B,5.
48. Ly P, Becker J. County officials move to ease fear of bioterrorism; phone, web information available, counseling center established. *Washington Post.* 25 October 2001; T,3.
49. Schoch-Spana M, Young B, Kwik G, Lien O. The people's role in biodefense: Guidelines for incorporating volunteers into large-scale bioterrorism response. Manuscript in preparation.
50. Stoil MJ. Behavioral health's "finest hour." *Behav Health Management* 2001; 21(5):8–10.
51. Will BH. The public library as community crisis center. *Library Journal* 2001; 75.
52. Khirallah DR. Charities in need of IT—vendors collaborate to build a central database to help victims of the Sept. 11 attack. *New York Times.* 19 November 2001; 20.
53. Lueck TJ. A nation challenged: the volunteers; good intentions lead to a bad ending. *New York Times.* 18 October 2001; B,11.

8

Responding to the public health crisis in Afghanistan

PETER SALAMA, JENNIFER LEANING, AND ANNALIES BORREL

The Al Qaeda organization, which carried out the September 11 terrorist attacks, was based in Afghanistan and closely associated with the Taliban government there, which had ravaged the Afghan people, violated their human rights, and further worsened their health and quality of life—already seriously damaged by decades of war and civil strife. In response to the terrorist attacks of September 11, the U.S. military, allies, and in-country opposition forces brought down the Taliban government in October 2001. The new political situation has led to increased opportunities to respond to the public health crisis in Afghanistan. This chapter describes that crisis and the response to it.

BACKGROUND

Afghanistan is a landlocked country of 652,225 square kilometers—slightly smaller than Texas—that shares its borders with Turkmenistan, Uzbekistan, and Tajikistan to the north, China to the northeast, Pakistan to the east, and Iran to the west. Rugged mountainous terrain, large deserts, limited arable land, and a shortage of water characterize its geography. Climactic conditions are extreme, with hot, dry summers and harsh winters, which furnish the snow that feeds its five major river systems, providing water for irrigation.

The predominantly rural population comprises more than 20 ethnic groups. Pashtuns, the largest group, live mainly in the south and east, Tajiks in the northeast, and Uzbeks in the northern plains. Other important groups are the Hazara in the central highlands, and the Kuchi, a pastoralist group. The population of Afghanistan was estimated to be 13.8 million in 1979 and by extrapolation is now estimated to be more than 24 million.[1]

Because of its strategically important location, Afghanistan has been subjected to invasions throughout its history. Its geopolitical importance peaked during the Cold War; in 1979, Soviet troops intervened to support the People's Democratic Party of Afghanistan, triggering an intense armed rebellion by the mujahideen. The Soviets concentrated their forces in urban areas and, in their attempt to undermine support for the mujahideen, targeted rural areas for indiscriminate bombing. In response, with increasing support from the West, the mujahideen became more militarized. By the time Soviet forces withdrew in 1989, an estimated 1.5 million people had been killed and more than 7 million Afghans had been displaced from their homes, 4.5 million of whom became refugees in Pakistan and Iran.[2] (Many more continued to be displaced[2] during the next 12 years.) (Figures 8–1 and 8–2).

The first decade of civil war produced an increasing socioeconomic divide between the more secular cities, where access to government services, in-

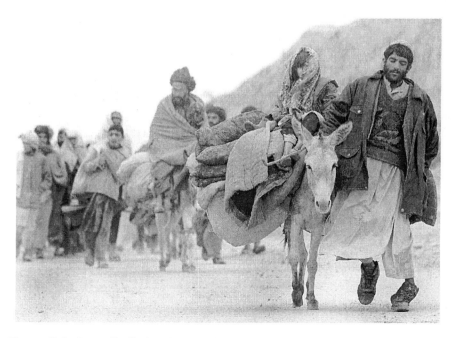

FIGURE 8–1. Internally displaced persons from Kunduz arrive at the front line near Khanabad in northern Afghanistan on November 20, 2001 (AP/Wide World Photos).

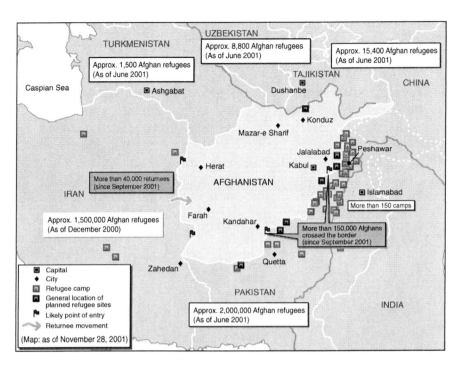

FIGURE 8–2. Even by the middle of 2001, millions of refugees had fled Afghanistan, mainly to Pakistan and Iran. (United Nations High Commissioner for Refugees.)

cluding tertiary education for women, had improved, and the devastated rural areas. The second decade of civil war (between 1990 and 2000), however, resulted in the destruction of the urban infrastructure. As the mujahideen forces became increasingly divided, a new force, the Taliban, appeared in 1994. It was composed largely of traditional religious students from southern Pashtun tribes, who had been trained and equipped in Pakistan. The Taliban implemented their own strict interpretation of Islamic sharia law, which included edicts forcing men to grow beards to a prescribed length, closing girls' schools, and banning television, music, photographs, and employment of women. Penalties for infringements were severe, including amputation of a limb for theft and execution for adultery.

By the year 2000, the Taliban controlled 90 percent of the war-weary country.[2] As the war increasingly targeted noncombatants, the Taliban were isolated by the international community. It was not until after the events of September 11, 2001, however, that the links between the Al Qaeda network and the Taliban regime became more clear to the Western world. Afghanistan became the focus of the Western political and military establishment's "war on terrorism." By the end of 2001, following an American-led military campaign, the Taliban regime had collapsed. In early 2002, an interim authority led by Chairman Hamid Karzai took control of the country.

Perhaps due to the political instability of the country for more than 20 years, development of the social sectors, such as health and education, has never been given a high priority in Afghanistan. The World Bank noted in 1978 that for few countries was the health situation as serious as it is in Afghanistan, where disease and illness were rampant, and the infant mortality rate was among the highest in the world. As of early 2002, all health indicators, although based on unreliable data, pointed to an acute public health crisis, especially among women and children. A description of lives and livelihoods in Afghanistan is provided in Box 8–1.

CHILDREN'S HEALTH

The infant mortality rate in Afghanistan of 165 deaths per 1,000 live births and the under-5 mortality rate of 257 per 1,000 live births are, in each category, the fourth highest in the world.[3] Major causes of mortality among children and adults include measles, diarrhea, acute respiratory infection, malaria, tuberculosis, and war-related trauma, including injuries from landmines and unexploded ordnance (see Boxes 8–2 and 9–1).[4] Furthermore, mortality surveys performed during periods of crisis have shown that under-5 mortality rates have remained elevated for many months.[5] This pattern contrasts with that of most other humanitarian crises, where under-5 mortality rates are high for the first 2 to 3 months and then drop sharply, once the most vulnerable have died and humanitarian services are being provided.[6] The pattern in Afghanistan suggests that the public health crisis is due to chronic factors, rather than merely due to acute food shortages or epidemics of communicable disease. In one recent study, more than 50 percent of deaths among children less than 5 years of age occurred among infants (less than one year of age) (SCF-US/CDC unpublished data, 2001). Prevalence of acute wasting was also significantly higher in infants than in older children, suggesting a relationship between poor breastfeeding and complementary feeding practices, and wasting.

As in all developing countries, communicable diseases account for a large proportion of mortality among children in Afghanistan, and the risk of death from these diseases is increased if associated with malnutrition. The relationship between communicable disease and malnutrition has become increasingly important in the past 12 months (April 2001 through March 2002), when the effect of three consecutive years of drought has been seen in moderately elevated rates of acute malnutrition. Case-fatality rates for measles are particularly high among malnourished children, and large outbreaks of

Box 8–1. Lives and Livelihoods in Afghanistan.

Vulnerability in Afghanistan is a combination of political, economic, and climatic risks. Decades of armed conflict have limited the available coping strategies, while the post-Taliban persistence of commander-dominated enclaves has produced varying degrees of stability and administrative capacity. These factors have important implications for food security because they limit mobility, discourage investment, and threaten the capacity of humanitarian actors to provide assistance. In late 2001, the Afghan currency appreciated sharply, inducing price declines and a loss of purchasing power that was devastating for all who held debt in the local currency, the Afghani. This was hardest on shopkeepers who held their stocks on short-term credit and for people who had borrowed money or mortgaged their lands, orchards, or water rights. Debt burdens have limited people's access to new credit in some areas and served as a crippling source of shame.

In the most drought-affected areas, control over water influences the household's ability to preserve food security and to avoid destitution or death. Water is required for drinking; for maintaining hygiene and, hence, health; for preserving livestock herds, orchards, and vineyards; for producing crops and vegetable gardens; and for maintaining shelter. Shortages of water, therefore, are creating health and food security crises, contributing to both death and destitution. Death results when limited water supplies translate into threats to people's health.

A typical destitution pathway is: drought leading to crop failure; leading to loss of livestock, orchards, gardens, and vineyards; leading to mortgage of assets and further indebtedness; leading to loss of assets (land, house, family members, savings, and other assets); and, ultimately, to destitution. Malnutrition, especially stunting, is widespread and serves as an important link between the health and food crises. Families with sick members forgo consumption, incur debt, and deplete assets to pay for health care, threatening the nutritional status of other family members. Food crises can lead directly to malnutrition, decreasing immunity and increasing risk of health crisis and death.

The primacy of water, the stresses on the institutions of credit, and the need to increase physical security and political stability all require authorities and humanitarians to carefully consider policies to promote food security. Where water is scarce, it must be prioritized to preserve human life, even if crop production must be delayed until the drought cycle breaks. Interventions are needed to ensure that adequate food is available through both commercial and humanitarian channels, including interventions to support purchasing power. Strategies to promote physical security are required in order to ensure access to markets and protection of livelihoods.

—Sue Lautze

140

Box 8–2. Landmines and Unexploded Ordnance in Afghanistan.

Afghanistan is one of the most densely mined and unexploded ordnance (UXO)-affected countries in the world. Lacking a recognized government up until now, Afghanistan is not a signatory to the international treaty to ban landmines. In Afghanistan, approximately 10 million landmines are still present—10 percent of the estimated 100 million mines laid in 64 countries throughout the world. In 1997, the vast majority of the country's land remained contaminated by mines, approximately half of that land classified as high-priority areas—agricultural lands, waterways, schools, clinics, and commercial thoroughfares. Since 1992, an estimated 20,000 people have been killed by landmines and 400,000 injured. Of these, 80 percent are estimated to be civilians and 40 to 50 percent women and children. The nomadic Kuchi are particularly at risk. It is estimated that 50 percent of landmine victims die shortly after the injury occurs due to lack of medical attention and facilities.[1] Landmine and war injuries comprise 18 percent of admissions to hospitals in some areas.[2] (See also Box 9–1 in Chapter 9.)

Recent U.S.-coalition bombardments have added to the problem of unexploded ordnance (UXO) and contributed to war-related injuries. New areas have been contaminated by coalition UXO, and the targeting of ammunition depots in cities resulted in UXO often being scattered over a circular area with a five-kilometer radius. It is also estimated that 10 to 30 percent of the cluster bombs and missiles used by coalition forces failed to detonate due to mechanical reasons. In addition to causing human and livestock deaths, mine and UXO contamination inhibits the return of refugees and internally displaced persons, decreases the area of arable land, hinders access to shelter and water resources, and prevents the rehabilitation of essential infrastructure, such as roads and bridges.

There is an urgent need to collect data on contamination by landmines and UXO in the country; especially to document new areas of contamination. Such information is critical as refugees unfamiliar with current patterns of contamination begin to return to the country. In addition, an integrated national surveillance system to collect, analyze, and disseminate data on landmine injuries in a timely fashion is needed. These data need to be used to prioritize areas for mine-clearance and mine-awareness programs. Studies investigating the risk factors for landmine injury need to be performed, and such information should be used for mine-awareness campaigns that are integrated with childhood education.

Finally, mine clearance is a development priority for Afghanistan. The UNOCHA Mine Action Programme for Afghanistan (MAPA) is one of the largest and most cost-effective mine-clearance organizations in the world, employing almost 5,000 Afghan workers. From 1990 to 1999, MAPA found and destroyed 9,000 anti-tank mines, 202,000 anti-personnel mines, and 985,000 pieces of UXO. Mine clearance costs US$0.77 per square kilometer in Afghanistan, and MAPA estimates that, given

(continued)

Box 8–2. *(continued)*

adequate resources, Afghanistan could be free of the impact of mines and UXO within seven years.

—Muireann Brennan

BOX REFERENCES
1. Landmine Monitor Research 2000, Afghanistan. Afghan campaign to ban landmines.
2. UNDP/World Bank 2000. Health services delivery in Afghanistan. Present and future perspectives.

---

measles have been documented in Afghanistan in the past.[7] Due to the remote location of many villages and poor immunization services, a large proportion of rural children may reach adolescence or adulthood without being exposed to either wild measles virus or measles vaccine virus. Consequently, measles outbreaks have been reported among adolescents and adults in Afghan refugee camps, where measles vaccination coverage in 2001 was greater than 90 percent among children 6 months to 15 years of age (CDC/MSF unpublished data, 2001).

Other vaccine-preventable diseases also pose a threat in Afghanistan. Coverage for routine Expanded Program on Immunization (EPI) antigens in Afghanistan is between 30 and 40 percent.[8] Outbreaks of diphtheria have been reported in the past.[9] Polio, which is a leading cause of disability in Afghanistan, remains endemic; polio eradication activities began in Afghanistan in 1974, but drought, civil war, poor transportation infrastructure, extremes of climate, massive population shifts, and recent bombardment have hampered efforts to interrupt virus transmission.[10] Despite these factors, coverage by National Immunization Days in 2001 was very high.[10a]

Deaths due to diarrhea and acute respiratory infection (ARI) have a seasonal pattern in Afghanistan, with diarrhea deaths peaking during the summer and ARI deaths peaking during the winter. Large epidemics of cholera have also been reported in Afghanistan. Only 13 percent of households are estimated to have access to safe drinking water, and 12 percent to adequate sanitation.[8]

Other communicable diseases are also important causes of mortality and morbidity, especially among children. The epidemiology of malaria in Afghanistan has changed in recent years: (1) Malaria is being reported from more districts, including the central highlands, and malaria transmission in Afghanistan may be contributing to the reemergence of malaria in countries of the former Soviet Union and increasing malaria incidence in eastern Iran.[11] (2) Drug resistance is increasingly reported; up to 70 percent of cases of falciparum malaria in eastern Afghanistan may now be chloroquine-resistant.[12] Case-fatality rates for falciparum malaria are highest among children less than 5 and pregnant women. Another important cause of communicable disease morbidity among children is cutaneous leishmaniasis; first reported in 1964, its incidence has increased steadily in Kabul,[13] and WHO estimates that more than 270,000 people, including 120,000 children under 14 years of age, had active leishmaniasis in the year 2000.[14]

WOMEN'S HEALTH

Health conditions for women in Afghanistan appear to be among the worst in the world. The situation for women has been deteriorating for many years, beginning with the onset of war and political instability in 1979. Invasions of homes, pillaging of towns and villages, and shelling of major urban areas placed women and their families in grave danger throughout the period of the war against the Russians and then the mujahideen civil conflicts. The ascendancy of the Taliban regime in 1996, first welcomed as restoring order and security, imposed a new set of oppressive measures that restricted women's access to education, health care, and economic activity. Although quantitative information is lacking, these measures, along with increasingly predatory Taliban behavior towards women and ethnic minorities in the North, contributed to a worsening of health status and access to health services for women. Surveys conducted by nongovernmental organizations (NGOs),[15] the United Nations,[16] and human rights organizations[17,18] all point to increasing levels of poverty, depression, and isolation among women who had been forced to live under Taliban rule. An especially vulnerable subset of women are the approximately one million war widows,[16] who cannot rely on husbands to support them or their children. Observers during the Taliban period noted a marked increase in the number of women and children begging on the streets in urban areas.[19,20]

More specifically, reported incidence and prevalence rates of tuberculosis (TB) are much higher among women than among men in Afghanistan; an estimated 12,000 to 13,000 of the 15,000 TB deaths each year occur among women.[21] Further investigation into the gender distribution and the risk factors for TB among women in Afghanistan is needed. Particular attention should be given to investigating the barriers that are faced by women when they seek health care. Data relating to nutritional status and children's health, as noted earlier in this chapter, are consistent with the overall assessment that the health of women in Afghanistan has reached a critical stage.

Maternal mortality is perhaps the most important indicator demonstrating that life is extraordinarily difficult for women in Afghanistan; the maternal mortality ratio (MMR) is estimated to range from 820 to 1700 maternal deaths per 100,000 live births. In Afghan refugee camps in Pakistan, the MMR is approximately 290 deaths per 100,000 live births, but maternal and neonatal (first month of life) deaths are still the leading cause of death in the camps, accounting for more than 22 percent of all mortality.[22] Although abortion appears to have been underreported, causes of maternal death in Afghan refugee camps have been otherwise similar to those reported globally: hemorrhage, sepsis, and pregnancy-induced hypertension. As an outcome measure, the high maternal mortality probably has many causes, including: high fertility as a result of poor education and poor access to contraception; poor nutrition (with resulting anemia, maternal stunting, and poor uterine muscle tone); inadequate or nonexistent prenatal care; and an inability to access emergency obstetric care when needed. The last of these causes most likely occurs due to failure to recognize pregnancy complications, an inability to access obstetric care because of transportation difficulties, sociocultural barriers to services or the absence of services, and delays in obtaining appropriate services after reaching facilities.

FOOD SECURITY AND NUTRITION

Today, Afghanistan is facing the consequences of three years of drought compounded by the chronic effects of more than 20 years of civil conflict. Precarious security conditions, lack of government structures, lack of long-term resources, and problems of access have hampered the collection of high-quality information on the current crisis. Nonetheless, it is widely recognized that the food crisis in much of the whole country has worsened over the past three to four years.[4,23] The effects of the drought and conflict, however, are not homogenous, with the worst-affected areas being in the north, north-western, and western regions of the country.[24,25]

Changes in availability of food and, to a lesser extent, in access to food, explain the severe food shortage that the population of Afghanistan faces. Afghanistan is largely an agricultural country, in which over 80 percent of the cultivated land is used to produce wheat.[26] Wheat production capacity has decreased sharply because of a decrease in area under cultivation as well as crop failure; crop loss as a percentage of seed utilization was an estimated 57 percent in 1999–2000, and rain-fed wheat production is likely to be 40 percent less in 2002 than it was in 2000. From 1999 to 2002, therefore, Afghanistan has continued to face massive food deficits in its food production; the national food deficits in 1998–1999 were an estimated 226,000 metric tons (MT); in 1999–2000, an estimated 1,047,000 MT; and in 2000–2001, an estimated 1,032,000 MT.

While food production has been dramatically affected, access to food in the short term has remained comparatively more resilient. In many parts of Afghanistan, rural populations have become increasingly reliant on markets for obtaining food.[25,27] For example, in Kohistan district in the north, where crop cultivation is the predominant form of subsistence, only 5 to 10 percent of people were reported to be consuming food from their own production during April 2001. The market price of wheat, however, generally a good indicator of food access, has remained relatively stable in most major towns.[28] A number of economic factors have contributed to the reliance on markets for food: (a) the well-developed and functioning market system that continues to exist in Afghanistan, including the capacity of regional traders to respond to increases in demand; (b) relatively stronger-than-expected purchasing power; (c) remittances sent from relatives living abroad; and (d) coping strategies, such as the sale of livestock.[29] The existence and persistence of a resilient and functional market system, characteristic of Afghanistan, has raised questions as to whether cash assistance or food assistance is the most effective form of intervention.[30]

Despite the functioning markets, however, chronic poverty and three years of consecutive drought have depleted many people's assets. In response to the deteriorating situation, many households have engaged in various coping strategies. While these coping strategies have prevented many from becoming destitute in the short term, people's livelihoods have become seriously threatened. Strategies to increase household income include: (a) collection and sale of wild foods, such as cumin; (b) increased male labor migration to Pakistan and Iran (not generally preferred because it is viewed as degrading, poorly paid, and difficult); (c) child labor; and (d) sale of household items, such as carpets and jewelry.[27] In addition, livestock losses of up to 70 to 80 percent of total stock numbers have been reported in the worst-affected areas in the north.[25] Sales of livestock have been reported throughout Afghanistan, and disease and shortages of animal fodder have resulted in high mortality rates, decreased milk yields, and reduced market value.[31] Pastoralists, especially the Kuchi, have been most affected by the significant losses in livestock.

High-risk coping strategies, characterized by low returns and long-term negative consequences, have become more common in Afghanistan. For example, borrowing food at interest—sometimes as high as 350 percent — has increasingly been reported.[27] Daughters are given in marriage at younger ages and at lower bride prices, sometimes 20 percent of normal. Furthermore, inability to pay bride prices has resulted in many women and girls marrying men in other parts of the country, an unusual practice, which is of concern to many.[25] As a last resort, many families have sold their land since the year 2000, moving to refugee camps outside the country or to one of the many internally displaced persons (IDP) camps inside Afghanistan.

During the drought, the nutritional situation in Afghanistan has been characterized by extremely high levels of chronic malnutrition or stunting (45 to 59 percent, < -2 SD z-score height for age), high mortality rates among children under five years of age, and widespread occurrence of micronutrient deficiency diseases.[32,33] However, despite widespread and severe food insecurity, the prevalence of acute malnutrition (or wasting), although increasing, remained relatively low (6 to 12 percent, < -2 SD z-score weight for height) from 2000 to 2002,[34–36] except in certain IDP camps, from which higher rates of acute malnutrition have been reported.[37] This pattern of high mortality and relatively low levels of acute malnutrition, which was also observed among the Kurdish refugees in Iraq in 1992,[38] is very different from the pattern of high mortality and high prevalence of acute malnutrition seen in African famines, such as the recent food security crisis in Ethiopia.[39] One contributing factor may be that food shortages in parts of Africa occur regularly and perhaps more gradually, allowing time for physiological adaptation to the decreased caloric intake. Another factor may be that in parts of Afghanistan, mortality and wasting may be high before the age of six months, which is the *minimum* cut-off age for registration into nutrition surveys. Such surveys, therefore, may underestimate acute malnutrition. Results from recent surveys, which have assessed both maternal and infant nutritional status, suggest that mothers and infants younger than six months may be at particular nutritional risk in Afghanistan.[32]

The general micronutrient status of the population is poor, largely as a result of the lack of diversity of food in the diet and overreliance on the staple food, wheat, which is eaten as a leavened bread (*naan*). Vegetables are rarely produced and not a priority in much of the central highlands. Outbreaks of Vitamin C deficiency (scurvy), locally known as seialengia (black legs), occurred in 2001 in Faryab province and in 2002 in Ghor province in northwestern Afghanistan and resulted in many deaths.[25,40] Symptoms of angular stomatis and other Vitamin B deficiencies have also been reported in the northern drought-affected areas.

Other major micronutrient deficiencies in Afghanistan are more chronic. Iron-deficiency anemia is widespread, occurring in 72 percent of pregnant women and 89 percent of nonpregnant women.[41] Iodine deficiency is common and results from low iodine levels in the soil of one-third of the provinces, especially in the north and in the central highlands. It can result in low birthweight, deafness, and cretinism. As yet, salt-iodization programs have not achieved a wide coverage.

Poor complementary feeding and breastfeeding practices and lack of nutrient-dense weaning foods are likely to be important factors in the etiology of acute and chronic malnutrition. Less than one-third of women practice exclusive breastfeeding, and food taboos, reinforced by traditional elders, have a strong influence on feeding practices. For example, after childbirth, women are often encouraged not to breastfeed for the first three days and to discard the colostrum (initial breast secretions). The high prevalence of chronic malnutrition among children in Afghanistan is probably explained by poor maternal nutritional status, leading to poor intrauterine growth and low birthweight, and by poor complementary feeding practices, micronutrient deficiencies, and high incidence of diseases such as diarrhea. This cycle of malnutrition will only be broken by comprehensive public-health, nutrition, and food-security interventions that effectively address these causes.

PROGRAM STRATEGIES AND RECOMMENDATIONS

There is virtually no remaining health infrastructure in Afghanistan. There is no national network of community health workers, no functioning health information system, few skilled health workers at any level in the rural areas, and public buildings are in shambles (Figure 8–3). And the land is still heavily mined.[42] The World Health Organization (WHO) estimates that people in more than 50 of the 330 districts in Afghanistan do not have access to basic health services. Clearly, if child and maternal mortality indicators are to improve in Afghanistan, a basic package of health services should be extended to all people in Afghanistan. Such a package would include: immunizations; nutrition interventions; antenatal, delivery, and postnatal care, including emergency obstetric services; treatment for communicable diseases at the community level; and a basic referral service. In the emergency phase in 2001–2002, United Nations agencies, in partnership with NGOs, have initiated wide-scale interventions to reduce mortality. These interventions, such as the mass measles campaign led by the United Nations Children's Fund (UNICEF), which targets nine million children, have the added advantage of demonstrating to the rural population that the interim authority is committed to delivering services to all Afghans. Distribution of a general food ration or asset protection programs will need to continue in parts of the country until the drought is over and people are able once again to meet their own household food requirements through production or trade.

In addition to the basic maternal and child health programs, other priorities will need to be addressed at a national level. The national program to interrupt transmission of polio remains a priority and is part of a regional and global campaign to eradicate polio. Malaria, leishmaniasis, and TB are the other national communicable disease programs that will be a priority. As hundreds of thousands of refugees return to Afghanistan from Pakistan and Iran, all communicable disease programs will need to consider the epidemiologi-

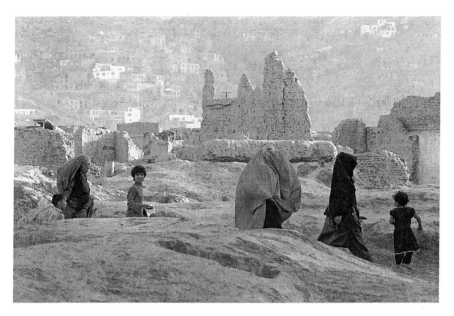

FIGURE 8–3. Afghan women and children walk through the ruins of Kabul's old town on May 24, 2002. (AP/Wide World Photos).

cal effect on disease transmission of large population movements and of treatment interruption. Other national priorities will include micronutrient programs, such as the prevention and treatment of iron deficiency anemia, and the distribution of iodized salt to prevent iodine deficiency.

A program that produces a sustainable reduction in mortality and distributes these gains in health equitably, however, will require a broader focus than merely the delivery of basic health services. The interim authority will need to make important policy decisions about how and by whom health services will be delivered in Afghanistan. NGOs and the private sector currently deliver most services. Ministry of Public Health workers have not been paid salaries for months or years. Many have been trained in the Soviet system and may prioritize the delivery of hospital-based services by a centralized government-run system over the delivery of basic primary health care.

Before determining such policies definitively, the Afghan government will need to learn the lessons from other post-conflict settings, such as those in Cambodia, East Timor, Kosovo, and Mozambique, and adapt successful policies for the unique setting of Afghanistan. After 20 years of war, data upon which to base such policy decisions are scarce. The government needs to determine a research agenda for informing such policy decisions and for programmatic and scientific purposes. This formative research will provide the basis for determining health education messages needed to improve breast-feeding and complementary feeding practices, optimal landmine injury prevention programs, the best strategies for reducing maternal mortality, and treatment protocols for malaria and tuberculosis.

From the perspective of women's health, this fragile post-conflict period poses several challenges and opportunities.[43-45] Dire health conditions for women need to be addressed within an overall strategy of community stabilization and development. International and national relief and development strategies for Afghanistan can finally, after years of distortion imposed by domestic political constraints, give an appropriate level of attention to the significant, longstanding needs of women.[46]

A major determinant of infant and maternal mortality in Afghanistan is the social status of women. This, in turn, determines girls' access to education and household resources, such as food and money, which, in turn, affects maternal nutrition as well as breastfeeding and complementary feeding practices. Programs aimed at improving female literacy and employment opportunities will also improve the health status of women and children. In fact, health and nutrition strategies will need to be multisectorial. Diarrheal disease prevention will be addressed most effectively by an emphasis on the provision of safe drinking water, sanitation facilities, and hygiene education and promotion.

There are many constraints to achieving a sustained improvement in the health of Afghans. The security situation in Afghanistan remains fragile. As of March 2002, coalition forces are still actively engaging Al Qaeda forces in eastern Afghanistan. Reports of discrimination and human rights abuses against Pashtun communities in the north and west are ominous signs for the future. The chief early challenge will be restoration of security throughout the country to prevent the fighting among rival warlord factions, which wrought havoc on local populations and infrastructure from 1992 to 1996. If such conditions of lawlessness are permitted to prevail, women will be driven into further penury and distress.

Human resources are another key constraint. Recent data suggest that there is not a lack of doctors in Afghanistan, but there is a critical lack of female health workers, especially skilled birth attendants, nurses, and midwives. Opportunities now exist (a) to bring women back into the workforce, (b) to train a broad range of health professionals who can reach out to women (with priority given to skilled birth attendants and midwives), and (c) to open the educational system at all levels in order to draw on the reservoir of female talent and expertise that has so long been suppressed and excluded (Figure 8–4). Culturally appropriate strategies to attract female health workers to rural areas are urgently required. One method that has been effective in some parts of the country has been to employ couples. Collaborations with Western institutions with expertise in training as well as health policy and research will be critical for building the capacity of Afghan institutions over the next few years. The Afghans with needed expertise who are living in neighboring coun-

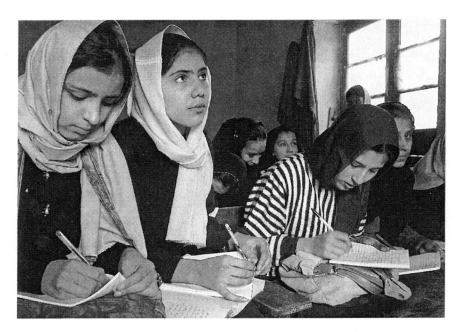

FIGURE 8–4. Some of the more than 600 Afghan schoolgirls at the Manu Chera school for girls in Kabul on December 31, 2001. After 5 years of being denied education, girls have returned to school in Afghanistan (AP/Wide World Photos).

tries and in the West should be given the opportunity to assist in rebuilding Afghanistan.

The final important challenge is to mobilize funds to support a country-wide reconstruction effort, organized according to social priorities and human needs. In the absence of a government with strong technical capacity, and as many donors and humanitarian agencies begin funding or implementing programs in Afghanistan, the need for a coordinated approach to international assistance is critical, if duplication and wasting of resources is to be avoided. Women in both rural and urban areas need to be included at all stages of this endeavor so that their concerns can be voiced and their interests integrated into the overall strategy. Priorities in health and nutrition programs of Afghanistan must be determined by public health priorities of the country and not by the competing agendas of foreign agencies. Programmatic decisions must be evidence-based. The current urban bias in health service concentration should be urgently addressed.

The current government of Afghanistan may have the best opportunity in 20 years to improve the health status of its citizens. The international community should make the required financial and human resources available to the government so it can accomplish this goal. Reconstructing the health system and achieving measurable gains in infant, under-5, and maternal mortality in Afghanistan may take 5 to 10 years of sustained effort; the gains, however, will be measured in political, epidemiological, and human terms.

REFERENCES

1. Government of Afghanistan. Final results of the first population census of Afghanistan. Ministry of Central Statistics, 1979.
2. Global movement for children, Afghanistan working group. Lost chances: the changing situation of children in Afghanistan, 1990–2000. June 2001.
3. UNICEF. State of the World's Children, 2001.
4. Assefa F, Jabarkhil MZ, Salama P, Spiegel P. Malnutrition and mortality in Kohistan District, Afghanistan, April 2001. *JAMA* 2001; 286:2723–2728.
5. Gessner B. Mortality rates, causes of death, and health status among displaced and resident populations of Kabul, Afghanistan. *JAMA*, 1994; 272:382–385.
6. Burkholder B, Toole MJ. The evolution of complex emergencies. *Lancet* 1995; 346:1012–1015.
7. Ahmad K. Alarming measles epidemic kills hundreds in Afghanistan. *Lancet* 2000; 355:998.
8. UNICEF. Multiple Indicator Cluster Survey, 1997.
9. Singh M, Saidali A, Bakhtiar A, Arya LS. Diptheria in Afghanistan—a review of 155 cases. *J Trop Med Hygiene* 1985; 88:373–376.
10. Progress towards poliomyelitis eradication, Afghanistan, 1999–2000. *MMWR* 2001; 50(08); 144–7.
10a. Progress towards poliomyelitis eradication, Pakistan and Afghanistan, January 2000–April 2002. *MMWR* 2002; 51:521–524.
11. WHO. Afghanistan annual report, 2000.
12. Rab MA, Freeman TW, Durrani N, et al. Resistance of Plasmodium falciparum malaria to chloroquine is widespread in eastern Afghanistan. *Ann Trop Med Parasitol* 2001; 95:41–46.
13. Ashford RW, Kohestany KA, Karimza MA. Cutaneous leishmaniasis in Kabul: observations on a "prolonged epidemic." *Ann Trop Med Parasitol* 1992; 86:361–371.
14. Afghanistan in the 21st Century. A health sector analysis. WHO Afghanistan, 2000.
15. Relief International. Survey of women in Taloquan area, December, 2001. Unpublished.
16. United Nations. UN Document E/CN.4/2000/33. Report on the situation of human rights in Afghanistan. United Nations, New York, 2000.
17. Physicians for Human Rights. Women's health and human rights in Afghanistan. PHR, Boston, September 2001.
18. Human Rights Watch. Humanity denied: systematic violations of women's rights in Afghanistan. *Human Rights Watch.* New York, October, 2001.
19. Goodwin J. Buried alive: Afghan women under the Taliban. *The Progressive Woman's Quarterly* 1998; 7:1.
20. Physicians for Human Rights. The Taliban's war on women: a health and human rights crisis in Afghanistan. Boston: PHR, August, 1998.
21. WHO. Health in Afghanistan: Situation analysis. Available at www.who.int/disasters/country.cfm

22. Bartlett L, Jamieson DJ, Kahn T, et al. Maternal mortality among Afghan refugees in Pakistan, 1999–2000. *Lancet* 2002; 359:643–649.
23. Matheou A. Natural disasters and complex political emergencies: responding to drought in Afghanistan. *Humanitarian Exchange* 2001; 19:8–10.
24. World Food Programme, Afghanistan. Food Security Assessment July–August 2001. WFP Vulnerability Assessment Mapping Unit, Islamabad. October 2001.
25. Save the Children (USA). Nutritional Survey Report: Kohistan District, Faryab Province, northern Afghanistan. SC, Islamabad. April 2001.
26. Food and Agricultural Organization and World Food Programme. *Report for Crop and Food Supply Assessment Mission.* FAO/WFP Afghanistan. June 2001.
27. Concern Worldwide. Nutritional anthropometry, health, food security and agriculture assessment in Badakshan and Takhar Provinces, Afghanistan. October 2001.
28. *Strengthening Food Security in Afghanistan.* Islamabad, Pakistan. Church World Service. November 2001.
29. Pain A. Livelihoods under stress in Faryab Province, Northern Afghanistan: opportunities for support. A report to Save the Children (USA). October 2001.
30. Lautze S, Stites E, Nojumi N, Najimi F. Qaht-E-Pool—"A cash famine." Food insecurity in Afghanistan 1999–2002. The Feinstein International Famine Center, Friedman School of Nutrition Science and Policy, Medford, Mass., May 2002.
31. Food and Agricultural Organization, *Afghanistan. Livestock Development for Food Security: Afghanistan.* Islamabad, 1996.
32. Action Contre le Faim. Nutritional survey in Kabul city: assessment of children under five years and infants less than 6 months old. February 2000.
33. Medecins Sans Frontières. Nutritional Survey in Faryab Province. September 2000.
34. United Nations Office for Project Services, United Nations Development Programme, and Save the Children, United Nation. *Women's Health in the Central Highlands.* Bamyan, Afghanistan. June 1998.
35. Action Contre le Faim. *Nutritional Survey in Kandahar city.* May 2000.
36. Action Contre le Faim. *Nutritional Survey in Herat city.* July 2000.
37. Nutritional survey in internally displaced persons (IDPs) camps and settled populations in Baghlan Province, northern Afghanistan. *Focus*, July 2001.
38. Yip R, Sharp TW. Acute malnutrition and high childhood mortality related to diarrhea: lessons from the 1991 Kurdish refugee crisis. *JAMA* 1993; 270:587–90.
39. Salama P, Assefa F, Talley L, et al. Malnutrition, measles, mortality, and the humanitarian response during a famine in Ethiopia. *JAMA* 2001; 286:563–571.
40. WHO. Investigation in Halri village, Ghor province, March 2002.
41. *Multiple Indicator Cluster Survey in Afghanistan.* UNICEF, Islamabad, 2000.
42. Afghanistan and Central Asia: Priorities for reconstruction and development. November 27, 2001. *ICG Asia Report* No. 26. Osh/Brussels.
43. Symposium on reconstruction of the health system in Afghanistan: Challenges and opportunities. World Health Organization. 22 January 2002, London. Available at www.who.int/disasters/country.cfm.
44. Humanitarian policy and conflict research. Central Asia policy brief no. 3, v. 2. hpcr@hsph.harvard.edu.
45. Preliminary needs assessment for recovery and reconstruction. World Bank. December 2001. www.Inweb.18.worldbank.org/SAR/sa.nsf.
46. Verdirame G. Testing the effectiveness of international norms: UN humanitarian assistance and sexual apartheid in Afghanistan. *Human Rights Quarterly* 2001; 23:733–768.

II

Terrorist weapons

9

Small arms, explosives, and incendiaries

WENDY CUKIER AND ANTOINE CHAPDELAINE

Small arms, explosives, and incendiaries are the weapons used in most terrorist acts. While the use of nonconventional weapons—weapons of mass destruction—must not be ignored, small arms, explosives, and incendiaries have had a more significant impact so far, as recorded terrorist events in recent years demonstrate.[1,2] The World Health Organization (WHO) set a priority on violence and injury prevention in 1996[3] because studies projected that injury, violence, and war will be among the leading causes of death until the year 2020.[4] From a public health perspective, these injuries have one factor in common[5]: they are caused by the inappropriate discharge of energy from a small arm, explosion of a bomb, or incendiary device—whether an AK-47, a Molotov cocktail, or a fuel-laden commercial airplane.

Most injuries are caused by abnormal energy transfers or interference with energy transfers:[6] mechanical or kinetic energy (which accounts for three-fourths of all injuries), such as from missiles, bullets, shrapnel, debris, and motor-vehicle crashes; thermal energy, such as a Molotov cocktail or napalm; chemical energy, such as a chemical blast; radiation energy, such as from "dirty bombs" (Chapter 12); electrical energy, like that released from a cattle prod or a stun gun used as a weapon; or the absence of essentials—such as oxygen, due to carbon monoxide poisoning after a blast. Injury-prevention strategies rest on understanding the factors contributing to the injury, the causal links, and the ways of intervening.

SMALL ARMS

It has been estimated that small arms are used to kill over 500,000 people each year,[7] and for every death many more people are injured and traumatized. The mortality associated with these weapons varies in different contexts. Suicide attempts with firearms are almost always fatal (92 percent of the time), while assaults are less frequently fatal.[8] War injury rates are at least twice war mortality rates and may be 13 times as high. When military weapons are used in a confined space against civilians, such as in terrorist attacks and other mass murders, however, the injuries-to-deaths ratio decreases to less than 1:1.[9]

Worldwide, the percentage of small-arms deaths in what are deemed terrorist acts is quite small. Nevertheless, small arms are stockpiled by terrorist organizations around the world to support a wide range of activities— robberies, kidnappings, armed conflicts, and massacres. Not only does terrorist violence cause death, injury, and psychological stress, but it also impedes economic development and the provision of essential services. Small arms are the principal tools of terrorists. For example, in Colombia, where fighting among factions considered to be terrorists has resulted in the highest reported homicide rate in the world, 80 percent of these deaths have been caused by small arms. In Afghanistan, Al Qaeda fighters have been well equipped with military-specification small arms. In Northern Ireland, the decommissioning of small arms of the Irish Republican Army (IRA) proved to be one of the major stumbling blocks to peace. Although comprehensive data are not available, an analysis of 400 recorded "terrorist" incidents from 1997 to 2001 revealed that small arms were clearly used in 119 (30 percent) of them and probably used in another 40 kidnappings and abductions.[10]

Many terrorist acts occur in the context of sustained political conflict, but acts of violence regarded as terrorism are generally defined by their deliberate targeting of civilians (see Chapter 1). Small arms have been used in many mass attacks against civilians over the past 30 years.[11] One of the first highly publicized attacks occurred on September 5, 1972, at the Munich Olympics, when eight members of Black September, a Palestinian Liberation Organization (PLO) splinter group, killed two Israeli athletes and took nine more as hostages, whom they eventually killed. Other high-profile attacks on civilians in recent years have included:

- February 1994: Hebron Kach-militant and Jewish extremist Dr. Baruch Goldstein killed 39 worshippers in a mosque at the Tomb of the Patriarchs in the West Bank and was hailed by some as a hero;
- November 1997: In Luxor, Egypt, 62 tourists were killed and 26 injured with small arms—while no group claimed responsibility, Al-Gama'a Al-Islamiyya is considered the possible perpetrator; and
- August 2000: Right-wing "paramilitaries," using small arms, attacked two villages in Colombia, killing 22 people.

Research has shown that death and injury rates due to small arms are linked to the accessibility of these weapons. In industrialized countries, death rates are strongly correlated with firearms ownership.[12–14] In post-conflict situations, the presence of small arms in a society fuels violence even after formal conflicts have ceased. A study that compared injuries in one region during conflict and peace revealed that weapons injury declined only 20 to 40 percent after "peace" was established. Another study that contrasted two areas in one country—one where there was "peace" and one where there was armed conflict between factions—revealed a high rate of noncombat injury, even in the peaceful region: 80 deaths per 100,000 people, half of which were related to small arms.[15] It follows that where small arms are readily available, the risk of terrorists' gaining access to them rises.

Types of Small Arms

Small arms are lightweight and "person-portable" weapons, including revolvers and self-loading pistols, rifles and carbines, light machine-guns, sub-machine-guns (the Uzi), and assault rifles (the AK-47). Some might include hand grenades, landmines, and small mortars.[16] Military assault weapons, which are characterized by large-capacity magazines and semi- or fully-automatic fire, are particularly efficient and require little skill. A single gunman can slaughter dozens of people in a short period of time.

Small Arms, Bullets, and Penetrating Trauma[17,18]

High-velocity bullets create a permanent cavity, cause hemorrhaging, and produce a temporary cavity that expands and contracts three to four times after the bullet has passed through. This cavity can be 30 to 40 times larger than the bullet, damaging both tissue and structures far from the wound track. A handgun with a standard round can produce a cavity five to six times the diameter of a bullet. In comparison, knife injuries result in little or no cavitation. When a small arm is used in an assault, it is 12 times more lethal than a knife.[19]

Bullets are designed to kill and injure efficiently, and some have been designed specifically to maximize tissue exposure and damage. For example, hollow-point bullets are designed to present a large frontal area, to mushroom, and to slow immediately upon impact, delivering maximum energy to tissue. The (U.S.) M-16 assault rifle bullet slows down when it strikes tissue, causing it to tumble over and over, thus widening the wound track. Some bullets are constructed so that once they hit tissue, they break into many pieces that disperse. Shotguns disperse upon firing to cause a cone of particles that produce high damage at close range, but have low energy thereafter.[9,20]

The main suppliers of military small arms include Russia (AK-47 assault rifle and its derivative, the AK-74), China (Norinco AK-47 look-alikes), Belgium (FAL assault rifle), Germany (G3 rifle), the United States (M-16 rifle), Israel (Uzi submachine gun), and France (FAMAS assault rifle). The United States, Austria, and Germany are leading manufacturers of handguns.

The United States sold or transferred $463 million worth of small arms and ammunition to 124 countries in 1998. Of these countries, about 30 were at war or experiencing persistent civil violence in 1998. In at least five of these countries, U.S. or U.N. soldiers on peacekeeping duty have been fired upon or threatened with U.S.-supplied weapons; this is called "the boomerang effect." Covert military operations have also fueled the illicit supply of weapons that are now being used against the very countries that initially provided them. For example, during the 1980s, in an effort to topple the Soviet-backed government of Afghanistan, the U.S. government provided at least $2 billion worth of arms and military training to Islamic rebel groups (the mujahideen). The U.S. Congress approved the transfer of a limited number of Stinger missiles in 1985[21]—about 1,000 were transferred, of which several hundred are still at large. The Central Intelligence Agency (CIA) primarily funnelled arms and money through the Pakistan Army Inter-Services Intelligence (ISI). The Taliban were armed with weapons left by the Soviets, weapons left over from the U.S. arms pipeline of the 1980s, and arms recently sent by Pakistan, which has leftover stores from the 1980s and acquires other items on the international black market. The CIA allocated $65 million in the 1990s to try to purchase the Stinger missiles back from the black market, with limited success.[21]

There are also many documented cases of military weapons, police weapons, and weapons recovered in crime re-entering the secondary market through theft or illegal sales.

Worldwide, there are as many small arms in the possession of individuals as there are in the possession of states. Diversion of these small arms also fuels the illicit supply. In many countries, most small arms recovered in crime appear to have been legally owned at one time by states or by individuals.

In countries where legally owned small arms are more readily available, civilian weapons fuel the illegal markets.[22] In the United States, where there are 260 million people with an estimated 200 million firearms, it has been estimated that 500,000 firearms are stolen each year—thereby entering the illegal market. Inadequate controls over gun sales also fuel illegal markets.[23] Approximately 50 percent of illegal handguns in Canada, 80 percent of illegal small arms in Mexico, and many small arms of the Irish Republican Army (IRA) originated in the United States. Weapons sold at unregulated U.S. gun shows have also been linked to terrorists. The circuitous routes through which legal arms have been diverted to terrorists are exemplified in the incidents below:

- A Danish citizen and a British arms dealer bought a Russian cargo plane in Latvia and had it flown to Bulgaria, where it was loaded with 77 cases of weapons, including 300 assault rifles, ammunition, pistols, hand grenades, and rocket launchers. The plane then flew to India, where the weapons were parachuted down over the village of Purulia. The deal was financed out of Hong Kong. The intended recipient was a violent religious sect.[24]
- Members of the IRA allegedly arranged arms transfers with rogue intelligence officers in South Africa. The IRA members were later arrested for shipping AK-47s from Mozambique.[25]
- Four Irish citizens were arrested on the charge of buying more than 50 guns and hundreds of rounds of armor-piercing ammunition and mailing them to IRA sympathizers. A gun dealer from Boynton Beach, Florida, admitted supplying them with dozens of weapons and, for an extra $50 per gun, agreeing not to file the federal paperwork.[26]
- A Canadian dealer was charged with smuggling more than 40,000 mislabeled military small arms and components into the United States that were bound for the Middle East.[27]

All illegal small arms begin as legal small arms. The diversion of weapons from "licit" to "illicit" markets has been a major concern, because gun runners do not distinguish between petty criminals, organized-crime participants, insurgents, freedom fighters, or terrorists. They simply follow the money. Consequently, efforts to prevent terrorist acts involving small arms are part of a much larger effort to prevent the misuse of small arms. While gun running is linked to drug trafficking, it is very different. Most illicit drugs are illegal from production to consumption, whereas most small arms begin as legal products, but may end up being used or possessed illegally through a variety of channels. Licit small arms are diverted to illicit distribution networks and purposes through illicit or covert state transfers, diversion from state stockpiles, theft, loss, "straw" purchases, falsification of documents, "cloning," and illegal transactions by dealers and brokers. Reactivating weapons that had been deactivated or disabled and reassembling weapons from components that are often available by mail order are also problems. Consequently, in order to discourage diversion and assist in detection and enforcement, efforts to reduce illicit trafficking in small arms depend on improved controls of the legal movements of small arms.

Countermeasures

As noted above, there has been extensive work that has established the strong link between mortality and morbidity and the proliferation of small arms. This work provides general support for measures aimed at improving controls over legal small arms in order to reduce the risk of misuse and diversion. At the same time, considerably more research is needed in order to better understand the contextual factors and to assess the effectiveness of particular forms of interventions. For example, the priorities assigned to measures by governments and NGOs are not necessarily tied to empirical evidence of their relative effectiveness. Rather, political expediency and symbolic significance are often dominant factors in policy-making at the national and international levels.

There are a number of international agreements that are aimed at reducing the illicit trade in small arms to conflict and crime, including:

- The United Nations Convention on Transnational Organized Crime establishes standards for import, export, transfer, marking, and tracing of firearms (excluding state-to-state transfers);
- A resolution passed in 1997 by the United Nations Commission on Crime Prevention and Criminal Justice, which recommended that countries ensure minimum standards of domestic regulation, including standards on licensing of firearm owners, recordkeeping of firearms sales and possession, and safe storage; and
- A program of action established by the United Nations 2001 Conference on the Illicit Trade in Small Arms in All Its Aspects.

Regional agreements include:

- The Economic Community of West African States (ECOWAS) Moratorium on the Import, Export and Manufacture of Small Arms;
- The European Union (EU) Code of Conduct, which establishes criteria for the export of small arms and recordkeeping aimed at preventing sales to conflict zones and to states likely to violate human rights; and

- The Organization of American States (OAS) Convention, which defines standards for import, export, and transit controls on commercial shipments as well as marking of firearms and model regulations.

Many states and most nongovernmental organizations (NGOs), including the International Action Network on Small Arms (IANSA),[28,29] have maintained that much more needs to be done to prevent the proliferation and misuse of small arms. In addition to encouraging states to ratify existing international agreements, many other measures are being promoted. Given the nature of the illicit trade and the misuse of these weapons, the proposed measures are similar, regardless of whether the concern is conflict, crime, injury, or terrorism. These measures include:

- Strengthening export and import license authorizations, such as by ensuring that there are reciprocal measures so that both the importing and the exporting countries must approve transactions;
- Concluding a legally binding global agreement on the marking and tracing of weapons, to include systems for adequate and reliable marking of arms at manufacture and/or import;
- Adequate recordkeeping on arms production, possession, and transfer;
- Agreeing on international definitions of arms brokers and shipping agents, and developing legally binding controls on their activities; and
- Establishing, on an international basis, a set of standards and measures to strengthen controls governing the legal transfer of weapons to both state and non-state actors, in order to prevent the transfer of weapons that might be used for repression or aggression or might contribute to escalation of conflict or regional destabilization.

Despite continued opposition by the United States,[30] strong domestic regulation of civilian possession and use is critical.[31] Measures that allow legitimate civilian uses of small arms, but reduce the risk that small arms will be misused or diverted from legal to illegal markets, include licensing, regulation, implementing standards for safe storage, and banning civilian possession of fully automatic military assault weapons, which are not needed for legitimate sporting activities. Efforts of the international community to establish norms for domestic regulation have been consistently blocked by the United States, largely because of the influence of the National Rifle Association. The draft Programme of Action for the UN 2001 Conference on the Illicit Trade in Small Arms in all its aspects contained measures to encourage nation-states to ensure adequate regulation of the civilian use and possession of small arms, and also suggested a prohibition of civilian possession of military assault weapons. The United States, however, forced the removal from the final version of Programme of Action any reference to the responsibility of states to adequately regulate civilian possession of firearms.[32] More recently, in a move that was widely regarded with disbelief, U.S. Attorney General John Ashcroft detained more than 1,000 individuals suspected of terrorist activities without charge, but refused to allow the Federal Bureau of Investigation (FBI) to check whether they had tried to purchase firearms, because that would be a "violation of [their] constitutional rights" (see Chapter 17).[33] While the United States pressures countries such as Canada to address problems that it believes represent a threat to its security, it takes little responsibility for its role as the principal supplier of illegal small arms worldwide.

Attention has also been focused on measures to collect and destroy surplus weapons. International standards have been proposed for the destruction of confiscated or surplus small arms and light weapons. Weapons-collection programs in post-conflict areas are critical to the establishment of lasting peace—otherwise the risk of high levels of violence remains.[34] Although decommissioning the IRA was part of the peace agreement in Northern Ireland, the IRA's refusal to comply with this requirement was a significant impediment to the peace process.[35] The value of weapons-collection programs in other contexts varies. In some cases, especially where these programs are mandatory and accompanied by incentives and/or criminal sanctions, such as in Australia or Great Britain, they have resulted in many weapons being collected and destroyed. In other contexts, their impact appears to be largely educational and associated with efforts to build a culture of peace. Improvements to recordkeeping, tracing, information exchange, and enforcement have also been emphasized by the international community.

There has been renewed emphasis on local measures, such as more strictly controlling access to small arms in public places. Some countries, such as South Africa, have legislated "gun-free zones" to reduce risk. There have also been efforts directed at manufacturing "smart guns," which can be activated only with codes or biometric information, and at developing technologies to reduce the impact of bullets, such as Kevlar vests. In addition, measures to address factors that create the demand for small arms are needed—for preventing terrorism, as well as crime and conflicts. From a public-health perspective, injury prevention must be also supported by injury control. Timely and appropriate treatment of injuries from small arms can significantly reduce mortality rates. Consequently, improved emergency services and training should be critical components of an overall strategy for injury control and prevention.

One approach that will not keep civilians safer—in the air or on the ground—is increasing access to small arms. The recent surge in civilian firearm purchases in the United States, for example, should be a major cause for concern among health professionals, as should the rush to arm pilots and "sky marshalls."[36]

EXPLOSIVES AND INCENDIARIES

The WTC attack had the most fatalities of any single documented terrorist event (Chapter 2).[37,38] While hijacking and bombs on airplanes have previously been identified as risks, this was the first time an airplane was used as a missile, an explosive, and an incendiary device, raising the specter of other terrorist acts and threats, including attacks on nuclear reactors (Chapter 12).

Between 1980 and 1990, there were 12,216 bombings in the United States, causing 1,782 injuries, 241 deaths, and almost $140 million in property damage. Between 1990 and 1994, there were 8,567 bombings and nearly 2,000 additional bombing attempts in the United States.[39] Most of these explosions involved pipe bombs (53 percent in 1990), charged with a low-velocity filler such as black powder, and packed with fragments that extended fragmentary and thermal injuries.[40]

While only a small proportion of these attacks were classified as terrorism, explosives and incendiaries are the weapons of choice used by terrorists throughout the world. An analysis of 400 documented incidents between 1997 and 2001 reveals that more than 250 of them involved bombs, explosives, or incendiaries.

When bombs are successfully planted on airplanes, there are few survivors. Canada was, and remains, the site of the single worst terrorist act in aviation history—the Air India bombing in 1986, which claimed 329 lives. In 1988, a bomb planted on Pan Am Flight 103 exploded over Lockerbie, Scotland, killing all of its 259 passengers.[41] Plastic and volatile explosives such as SEMTEX are the predominant weapons used by terrorists in aviation-related incidents.[42]

In most bombings, however, many more are injured than killed. For example:

- In the 1993 bombing of the WTC, six people were killed, but more than 1,000 were injured.[43]
- In the 1995 Oklahoma City bombing, 167 people were killed and 759 injured (Figure 9–1).[44]
- In the 1998 bombing of the U.S. embassy in Nairobi, Kenya, 253 people were killed (83 percent of whom were income-earners) and over 5,000 were injured (3,600 needed plastic surgery and 1,000 needed major reconstructive surgery).[45]

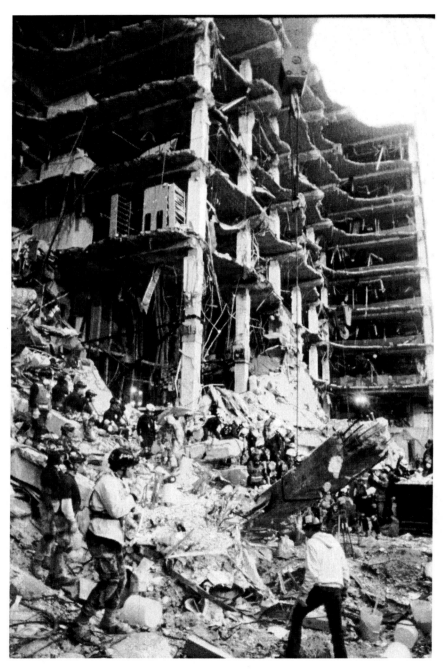

FIGURE 9–1. The Murrah Federal Building in Oklahoma City after being bombed in 1995 (FEMA News Photo).

- In the 1998 car bombing in Omagh, Ireland, 29 were killed and 330 injured.
- In the 1998 bombing of an oil pipeline in Antioquia, Colombia, 71 were killed and 100 injured.
- In 2000, in Rajwas, India, a grenade thrown on an open fire in a community kitchen killed 30 and injured 47.[46]

The impact of bombs goes beyond the mortality and morbidity. The main objective is to create psychological terror, which, in turn, can cause chaos and panic.[37] Letter-bombs only kill about 3 percent of those affected. Nevertheless, they create widespread fear.[47] Secondary devices render an area insecure, thereby hampering rescue efforts and so injury control.[48]

An explosion is defined as "a rapid increase of pressure in a confined space, generally caused by the occurrence of exothermic chemical reactions in which gases are produced in relatively large amounts." A simpler or broader definition is "a rapid release of energy."[49] Powerful explosions have the potential to inflict many different types of injuries on victims, although the pattern of injury inflicted on the body is relatively consistent, regardless of the context.[50] Whatever the type of explosion—chemical, diffuse vapor, mechanical, or nuclear—four main types of injuries result: primary, secondary, tertiary, and miscellaneous.[51]

Primary injuries are caused by the blast pressure wave, a sphere of compressed gas molecules that rapidly expands outward from the center of the blast at thousands of pounds per square inch. The blast wave lasts no more than five milliseconds, but the massive change in air pressure causes enormous damage, including myocardial contusion and shearing of the large heart vessels, detachment of the small intestine and colon from their supporting structures; tearing of the bowel wall; and rupture of the eardrums. The respiratory system can be seriously injured by a blast wave: lungs can hemorrhage or rupture, leading to hemothorax or pneumothorax; embolisms can occur from air entering the pulmonary circulation; and the diaphragm and tracheobronchial tree can tear. Secondary blast injuries are those caused by bomb fragments and nearby debris propelled into the air at missile-like speed, commonly 4,500 feet per second. These injuries include lacerations, abrasions, contusions with fractures, and penetration of body parts. Tertiary injuries are caused by the blast wind, which can reach speeds of 940 miles per hour, the result of the blast waves displacing air molecules. It can cause amputations, compound limb-fractures, and skull fractures. Miscellaneous injuries are caused by the aftermath of the explosion, such as injuries from falls, broken bones, amputations that occur when buildings collapse, and burns from fires and chemicals.[52]

TABLE 9–1. Favored Explosive Charges.

SEMTEX (used in Pan Am 103 explosion over Lockerbie)
RDX (Cyclonite or Hexogen, depending on form)
PETN (raw form of RDX)
C4 (plastic explosive)
TNT (Trinitrotoluene; common Drano can be used as a base)
Common fertilizer (used as a base)
Dynamite

Specific types of injuries are associated with specific explosives. For example, the Molotov cocktail burn syndrome occurs when people in cars are struck: they sustain massive smoke inhalation and disfiguring burns from the combination of gasoline ignition and synthetic fumes inside the car.[53] In addition, those with close exposure to the traumatic event, especially when threatened with possible injury or death, are likely to have adverse psychological responses.[54] Those who have lost loved ones or friends in a disaster, and rescue, recovery, and mortuary workers are also at risk for post-traumatic stress disorder (PTSD) (Chapter 3). Knowledge of the potential mechanisms of injury, early signs and symptoms, and natural courses of these problems will greatly aid the management of blast-injured patients.

Simple explosive devices are often made from readily available substances (Tables 9–1 and 9–2). Although many explosive materials, such as dynamite and nitroglycerin, are controlled in most countries, the diversion of materials from legal to illegal markets is very difficult to control. Most bombs assembled by terrorists are improvised. The raw material required for explosives is stolen or misappropriated from military or commercial blasting supplies, or made from fertilizer and other readily available household ingredients. Such assembled "homemade" bombs are known as Improvised Explosive Devices (IEDs). IEDs have a main charge, which is attached to a fuse. The fuse is attached to a trigger. In some types of IEDs, these three components are virtually integrated into a single whole. The trigger activates

TABLE 9–2. Methods and Triggers Used to Detonate Explosives.

Pressure activation (physical, water, or atmospheric)
Electronic signal (remote control or radio frequency)
Electronic pulse (detonator box)
Photoelectric cell ("when dawn breaks")
Motion or heat detector
Radiation trigger
Circuit connection (anti-handling device)
Electronic time switch
Acid-activated time switch
Fuse wire

the fuse, and the fuse ignites the charge, causing the explosion—a violent pulse of blast and shock waves. The purpose of most IEDs is to kill or maim.[55] Some IEDs, known as incendiaries, are intended to cause damage or destruction by fire. The pipe bomb is the most common type of terrorist bomb and usually consists of low-velocity explosives inside a tightly capped piece of pipe. Pipe bombs are very easily made using gunpowder, iron, steel, and aluminum or copper pipes and are sometimes wrapped with nails to cause even more harm. The Molotov cocktail is an improvised weapon that is extremely simple to make and can cause considerable damage. Materials such as gasoline, diesel fuel, kerosene, ethyl or methyl alcohol, lighter fluid, and turpentine are placed in a glass bottle, which breaks upon impact. A piece of cotton serves as a fuse, which is ignited before the bottle is thrown at the target. Fertilizer truck bombs consist of ammonium nitrate; hundreds of kilograms may be required to cause major damage. The Irish Republican Army, the Tamil Tigers in Sri Lanka, and some Middle Eastern groups have used the ammonium nitrate bomb.

Antipersonnel landmines are another type of explosive weapon that has been used to injure, maim, and kill—and terrorize—civilian populations. While they are often directed against opposing military forces, they can be considered to be terrorist weapons (see Figure 9–2 and Box 9–1).

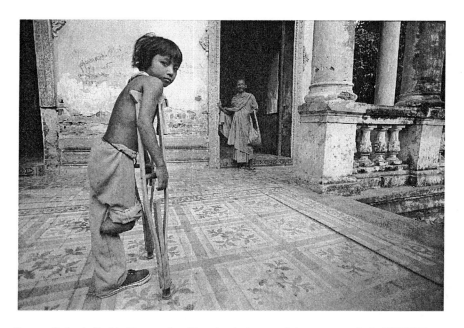

FIGURE 9–2. A disabled boy maimed by a landmine stands in a courtyard of a UNICEF–assisted rehabilitation center located in the Wat Tan Temple in Phnom Penh, Cambodia (Photographer: UNICEF/5907/Roger Lemoyne).

Box 9–1. Landmines.

Antipersonnel landmines are explosives and are considered by many to be weapons of indiscriminate mass destruction, one person at a time. Some analysts consider them terrorist weapons because they frequently kill and injure civilians.

There are an estimated 100 million landmines that have been strewn in more than 60 countries (including many in Afghanistan; see Box 8–2 in Chapter 8), and an estimated 230 to 245 million mines are stockpiled by about 100 countries.

Annually, antipersonnel landmines are estimated to injure or kill between 15,000 and 20,000 people, primarily civilians. Landmines are also render large areas of land uninhabitable. The people most likely to encounter landmines are the rural poor, including peasants tilling fields or foraging for food and wood, and children herding livestock.

In 1997, the Convention on the Prohibition of the Use, Stockpiling, Production, and Transfer of Anti-Personnel Mines and On Their Destruction (the Mine Ban Treaty) was opened for signature; it entered into force in 1999. For developing and leading the International Campaign to Ban Landmines, Jody Williams received the Nobel Prize for Peace in 1997. As of April 2002, there were 142 nations that had signed the Mine Ban Treaty, including all nations in the Western Hemisphere, except for the United States and Cuba, and all nations in the North Atlantic Treaty Organization (NATO), except for the United States and Turkey. Other nations that had not signed the treaty included Russia, most of the former Soviet republics, most nations in the Middle East, and many Asian nations, including China, India, and Pakistan. As a result of the treaty, there is less use of antipersonnel mines, a dramatic decrease in production, an almost complete end to trade in landmines, rapid destruction of mines that have been stockpiled, fewer mine victims in critically affected countries, and more land de-mined, although an enormous amount of expensive and dangerous de-mining remains to be done.

—Barry S. Levy

BOX REFERENCES
1. International Campaign to Ban Landmines. *Landmine Monitor Report 2000: Toward a Mine-Free World.* New York: Human Rights Watch, 2000.
2. Stover E, Cobey JC, and Fine J. The Public Health Effects of Land Mines: Long-Term Consequences for Civilians. In: *War and Public Health.* BS Levy and VW Sidel (Eds.). New York: Oxford University Press, 1997, pp. 137–146.

Countermeasures

Countermeasures need to be informed by good research on the impact of explosions and the causal factors. In particular, understanding the full range of injuries and disorders, including PTSD, is critical.[56,57] Epidemiological surveillance of victims of terrorist attacks can be valuable for both effective countermeasures and proper care and rehabilitation of victims.[58] The Hostile

Action Casualty System determines the magnitude of each explosion and the distance of victims from the explosion in order to assess, for example, the protective value of wearing armor near a blast.

As with small arms, explosives serve legitimate purposes, but are often diverted to illegal purposes for criminal or terrorist acts. Although many explosive materials are regulated, theft is a major problem. Interventions have been proposed to reduce the risk that explosives will be misused by terrorists or criminals. These interventions include the regulation of commercial explosives, the use of technology to detect explosive materials and to tag and track explosive materials, information-sharing, and investigative support. Efforts have also been directed at "target-hardening," such as by making access to buildings more difficult and thereby reducing the probability they can be bombed. Increased public awareness and watchfulness can help prevent injuries (Figure 9–3).

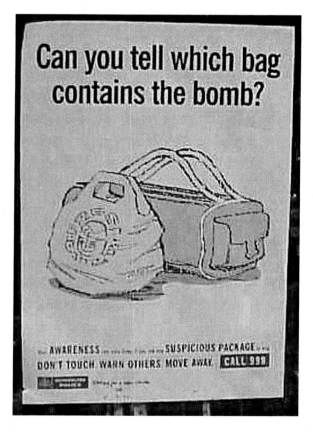

FIGURE 9–3. Increased public awareness and watchfulness is critical to remaining safe at scenes of explosions or explosive threats. In the United Kingdom, as shown here, the general public is enlisted through a public awareness campaign and poster placement in areas of public assembly (Photograph by Paul Maniscalco).

Laws vary among jurisdictions regarding the regulation of explosive materials and devices, but there are international conventions and agreements aimed at establishing minimum standards.[59] The United Nations Economic and Social Council (UNESCO) resolution of 1998, for example, made the following recommendation: "Recognizing that, with the increasing dimensions and scale of international transport and the growing sophistication of transnational illicit trafficking in explosives, States which have not already done so may consider reviewing the legislation and administrative regulations concerning explosives and their component parts to make those instruments more effective in combating crime."[60] But studies have indicated that many of the regulations in place are poorly enforced. For example, in the United States, there are regulations to tightly control commercial explosives, but there are variations in achieving this goal among the states, and evidence of poor storage and inadequate inspection and enforcement. There have been proposals in the United States for extending regulatory requirements and broadening the Bureau of Alcohol, Tobacco and Firearms' authority to conduct inspections in order to reduce misuse and diversion.

More recently, there have been discussions among governments about using "taggants" (coded materials) that provide better detection, tracing, and control of explosives.[61] In the United States, as a result of the U.S. Anti-Terrorism Act of 1996, taggants must be added to all plastic explosives "to make them visible to detection." There is also research underway to explore ways to render inert the fertilizer chemicals that have been used to manufacture explosives.

The investment in screening is often an issue of cost-benefit analysis. Airport security has been increased in response to the September 11 attacks and other incidents involving airlines, and airport passengers are being screened for explosives and other weapons. Research studies are in progress to improve screening and detection,[62] including direct imaging of explosives with a nitrogen camera to detect SEMTEX and other concealed explosives with high nitrogen concentrations.[63] Medical computed tomography (CT) scan technologies can also be used to detect explosives. Preboarding "shoe checks" are being performed on some passengers after the attempt by a terrorist in December 2001 to ignite explosives hidden in his shoe during a Paris-to-Miami flight. Some airlines are considering installing closed-circuit television cameras on aircraft to monitor passengers' behavior during flights.

In order to reduce the impact of explosions, especially secondary explosions, efforts are also being directed at developing blast-resistant structures and various types of armor to protect those detecting and defusing threats. For example, an oatmeal-type absorbing fabric called TABRE (Technology for Attenuating Blast-Related Energy) blocks flying fragments (shrapnel) and eliminates approximately 90 percent of the shock wave that is released in an explosion. TABRE can be used below vehicles to protect against landmines, in trousers designed to protect the legs and genitalia of minesweepers, in blastproof airline baggage containers, and in urban garbage containers.[64]

Hardened luggage containers in airplanes, for which the U.S. Federal Aviation Administration (FAA) has developed a standard, can neutralize explosives. Hardened containers can also be used for small bags that are difficult and expensive to scan with x-rays.[41] This shock-absorbing and shock-deflecting technology can be utilized in blastproof and bulletproof cockpit doors on commercial aircraft. Finally, efforts have been directed at raising awareness of some risks, such as by encouraging the public to identify and report suspicious packages or suspicious behaviors in public places.

CONCLUSION

The public-health approach, in part, addresses environments that give rise to problems. In order to prevent terrorism with small arms, explosives, and incendiaries, we must reduce the diversion of legal small arms and explosives to illegal markets, improve information exchange and investigations, "harden" targets, and strengthen injury control and emergency preparedness. We must also ensure that there are well-developed alarm systems as well as evacuation and emergency procedures in public buildings. The public-health approach brings together professionals of various health, safety, and security disciplines and their agencies and organizations. Liaisons with various communities are critical for collecting information and implementing countermeasures. Finally, the focus must be not only on managing terrorism, but also on managing anxiety and fear of terrorism, which are often disproportionate to risks and sometimes accompanied by backlash against specific communities and by hate crimes. We must also address the root causes of terrorism (Chapter 18).

REFERENCES

1. Parachini J. Comparing motives and outcomes of mass casualty terrorism involving conventional and unconventional weapons. *Studies in Conflict and Terrorism* 2001; 24:389–406.
2. Mascrop A. Mass hysteria the main threat from bioweapons. *Br Med J* 2001; 323:2–5.
3. WHO, Resolution WHA 49.25, "The Prevention of Violence: A Priority for Public Health." Geneva: World Health Organization, 1996: http://www.who.int/violence_injury_prevention/pdf/WHA49en.pdf. Internal document quoted as: WHA 49/1996/Rec/1.

4. Murray CJL, Lopez AD. *Global Burden of Disease Studies: The Global Burden of Disease. (Projections for 2020).* Cambridge, Mass.: Harvard University Press; 1996.

5. Kellerman AL, Lee RK, Mercy JA, Banton J. The epidemiologic basis for the prevention of small arm injuries. *Annu Rev Public Health* 1991; 12:17–40.

6. Haddon W Jr, Baker SP. Injury control. In: Clark D, MacMahon B, eds. *Preventive and Community Medicine.* Boston: Little Brown & Company, 1981:109–140.

7. Cukier W. International fire/small arms control. *Canadian Foreign Policy* 1998; 6:73–89.

8. Cukier W, Chapdelaine A. Small arms: a major public health hazard. *Medicine and Global Survival* 2001; 7:25–28.

9. Coupland RM, Meddings DR. Mortality associated with use of weapons in armed conflicts, wartime atrocities, and civilian mass shootings: literature reviews. *Br Med J* 1999; 319:407–410.

10. Bureau of Public Affairs, United States State Department, "Patterns of Global Terrorism": http://www.state.gov/s/ct/rls/pgtrpt/

11. Mastrapa AF. Political Terrorism Database: http://polisci.home.mindspring.com/ptd/

12. Cukier W. Small arm regulation: Canada in the international context. In: *Chronic Diseases in Canada* 1998; 19:25–34.

13. Van Dijk JJM. Criminal victimization and victim empowerment in an international perspective. Ninth International Symposium on Victimology, Amsterdam, the Netherlands, 25–29 August 1997. See also Mayhew P, van Dijk JJM. Criminal victimization in eleven industrialized countries. WODC, 1997: http://www.minjust.nl:8080/b_organ/wodc/summaries/ob162sum.htm.

14. Killias M. Gun ownership, suicide and homicide: an international perspective. *Can Med Assoc J*, April 1993: http://www.unicri.it/icvs/publications/understanding files/1 9 GUN%20OWNERSHIP.pdf.

15. Meddings D. Weapons injuries during and after periods of conflict: retrospective analysis. *British Medical Journal* 1997; 315:1417–1421.

16. Adapted from the United Nations' *Experts' Report*, Note #5, p. 24: http://www.un.org/Depts/dda/CAB/rep54258e.pdf.

17. Armstrong JF. Bullets: damage by design. *RN* 1999; 62:38–39.

18. American College of Surgeons, Committee on Trauma. *Advanced Trauma Life Support (ATLS) for Doctors,* 6th edition, 1997:360–363.

19. Saltzman LE, Mercy JA, O'Carroll PW, et al. Weapon involvement and injury outcomes in family and intimate assaults. *JAMA* 1992; 267:3043–3047.

20. Swiss Armed Forces, *Global Arms Control and Disarmament.* International Workshop on Wound Ballistics, Interlacken: October 1997.

21. "India: Arms and Abuses in Indian Punjab and Kashmir." Human Rights Watch 1994; 6: http://www.hrw.org/campaigns/kashmir/1994/kashmir94-02.htm.

22. Webster DW, Vernick JS, Hepburn LM. Relationship between licensing, registration, and other gun sales laws and the source state of crime guns. *Injury Prevention* 2001; 7:184–189.

23. Cukier W. Vuurwapens: legale en illegale kanalen, translation of Firearms: licit/illicit links. *Tijdschrift voor—Criminologie,* edited by Frankie HJ and de Wijs ES, 43(1), March 2001:27–41.

24. Bonner R. Murky life of an international gun dealer. *New York Times,* 14 July 1998.

25. IRA linked to African arms deal. London *Sunday Times,* 15 March 1998.

26. Lebowitz L. 4 suspects in arms deal face new charges. *Miami Herald,* 25 January 2000: 1B.

27. Gun-runners used Toronto store: Owner admits rifles likely bound for Mideast passed through his premises. *Globe and Mail*, 20 December 2001.
28. International Action Network on Small Arms (IANSA), Focusing Attention on Small Arms: Opportunities for the UN 2001 Conference on the Illicit Trade in Small Arms and Light Weapons. IANSA, 2000.
29. *Biting the Bullet Briefings, International Alert, Saferworld*. London: BASIC, 2001.
30. Goldring N. A Glass Half Full. The UN Small Arms Conference, Council on Foreign Relations, Roundtable on the Geo-Economics of Military Preparedness, 26 September 2001.
31. Cukier W, Bandeira A, Fernandes R, et al. Combatting the illicit trade in small arms and light weapons: strengthening domestic regulations. *Biting the Bullet Briefing 7, International Alert, Saferworld*. London: BASIC, 2001.
32. United Nations Foundation. Despite U.S. resistance, states agree on pact. 27 July 2001.
33. Butterfield F. Background checks: Justice Dept. bars use of gun checks in terror inquiry. *New York Times*, 6 December 2001.
34. International Committee of the Red Cross (ICRC). Arms Availability and the Situation of Civilians in Armed Conflict, June 1999.
35. Sagramoso D. The proliferation of illegal small arms and light weapons in and around the European Union: instability, organized crime and terrorist groups. *Saferworld*, July 2001.
36. Harrison D. *Daily Telegraph* (UK), 6 January 2002.
37. Stein M, Hirshberg A. Medical consequences of terrorism. *Surg Clin North Am* 1999; 79:1537–1552.
38. McCarthy M. Attacks provide the first major test of USA's national anti-terrorist *medical* response plans. *Lancet* 2001; 358:941.
39. U.S. Department of Justice, FBI Bomb Data Center, Bomb Summary. Washington, D.C., 1990.
40. BATF, Statistics 1990–1998. Washington, D.C., 1998.
41. McMullin D. Lockerbie insurance, air security, hardened luggage containers can neutralize explosives. *Scientific American* 2002; 266:15–16.
42. Safeer HB. Aviation security research and development plan. N.J.: U.S. Department of Transportation, Federal Aviation Administration, March 1992.
43. Parachini JV, *op. cit.*
44. Spengler C. The Oklahoma City bombing: a personal account. *J Child Neurol* 1995; 10:392.
45. Hollander D. Nairobi bomb blast—trauma and recovery. *Tropical Doctor* 30, 2000: 47–48.
46. Mastrapa AF. Political Terrorism Database: http://polisci.home.mindspring.com/ptd/; Bureau of Public Affairs, United States State Department, "Patterns of Global Terrorism"; http://www.state.gov/s/ct/rls/pgtrpt/.
47. Missliwetz J, Schneider B, Oppenheim H, Weiser I. Injuries due to letter bombs. *J Forensic Sci* 1997; 42:981–985.
48. Christen HT, Walker R. Weapons of mass effect: explosives. In *Understanding Terrorism and Managing the Consequences*, Manisclaco PM, Christen HT, eds. Upper Saddle River, NJ: Prentice Hall, 2002.
49. Nedved M. Explosion prevention and control. *Occup Health* 1980; 32:358–62.
50. Stein, Hirshberg. Medical consequences of terrorism, 1537–1552.
51. Armstrong JF. Bombs and other blasts. *RN* 1998:26–29.

52. Ibid.
53. Benmeir P, Lusthaus S, Talisman R, et al. Terrorist bombing with a "Molotov cocktail" inside traveling cars: an old weapon for a new burn syndrome? Department of Plastic Surgery, Hadassah University Hospital, Jerusalem, Israel.
54. Stephenson J. Medical, mental health communities mobilize to cope with terror's psychological aftermath. *JAMA* 2001; 286:15.
55. United Nations Office for Drug Control and Crime Prevention (UNODCCP), "Conventional Terrorist Weapons." Available at http://www.undcp.org/terrorism weapons conventional.html.
56. Abenhaim L, Dab W, Salmi LR. Study of civilian victims of terrorist attacks (France 1982–1987). *J Clin Epidemiol* 1992; 45:103–109.
57. Dab W, Abenhaim L, Salmi LR. Epidémiologie du syndrome post-traumatique chez les victimes d'attentat et politique d'indemnisation (Épiter). *Santé publique* 1991; 3:36–42. In French.
58. Mellor SG, Cooper GJ. Analysis of 828 servicement killed or injured by explosions in Northern Ireland 1970–1984: the Hostile Action Casualty System. *Br J Surg* 1989; 76:1006–1010.
59. The Inter-American Convention against the Illicit Manufacturing of and Trafficking in Firearms, Ammunition, Explosives and other Related Materials, 13 November 1997.
60. United Nations, Economic and Social Council. Regulation of explosives for the purpose of crime prevention and public health and safety, Resolution 1998/17.
61. U.S. Alcohol, Tobacco and Firearms Administration, Explosives Study Group, 1998 Progress Report. Available at http://www.atf.treas.gov/pub/treas pub/taggant/98.
62. Gowadia HA, Settles GS. The natural sampling of airborne trace signals from explosives concealed upon the human body. *J Forensic Sci* 2001; 46:1324–1333.
63. Knapp EA, Moler RB, Saunders AW, Trower WP. Direct imaging of explosives. *Appl Radiat Isot* 2000; 53:711–716.
64. Cropley E. New boot could lessen land-mine impact. From Reuters News Agency, Derby, England, in *Globe & Mail* 1999; 13:A-19.

10

Biological weapons

VICTOR W. SIDEL AND BARRY S. LEVY

Of all the forms of terrorism, bioterrorism may inspire the most fear—perhaps because of the public perception that biological agents may not be visible, are easy to disseminate, can spread easily from person to person, and can cause horrific diseases. While not all of these perceptions are necessarily accurate, much public and professional attention has focused on bioterrorism. Before the 1990s, public concern about bioterrorism centered on the types of biological weapons that might be used by *nation-states* that had the capability to produce such weapons.[1,2] During the 1990s, the potential for bioterrorist attacks by *individuals* and *nongovernmental groups* was widely publicized in the United States, and the U.S. government began developing policies and programs to address the threats posed by bioterrorism.

Bioterrorism began to be perceived as a greater threat in the United States following the attacks on the World Trade Center (Chapter 2) and the Pentagon on September 11, and especially following the dissemination of anthrax spores through the mail in September and October of 2001 (Chapter 6). Five people died of inhalational anthrax, six more people developed and survived confirmed cases of inhalational anthrax, and 11 others had confirmed or suspected cutaneous anthrax. In addition, thousands of postal workers, news-media workers, and others received prophylactic treatment, and millions more feared that they, too, could be at risk of developing anthrax.

The extent to which additional incidents involving biological weapons, such as the dissemination of anthrax or smallpox, will occur in the future in the United States or elsewhere is unknown, in part because terrorist attacks with biological weapons have been extremely rare. In comparison, terrorist attacks with small arms, explosives, or incendiaries have occurred much more frequently (Chapter 9).

The United States and other countries indeed need to be prepared for future potential bioterrorist actions and threats. This preparedness should not, however, (a) lead to inappropriate responses, (b) draw resources away from preparedness programs for other, much more likely, forms of terrorism, or (c) draw resources away from programs that address other urgent problems of public health importance.[3–5] In addition, responses to bioterrorist acts and threats should neither compromise the principles and practice of public health, nor damage the trusting relationships that public health professionals and their agencies and organizations have with the communities that they serve.

PROLIFERATION AND USE

Biological weapons are living organisms—usually microorganisms—or their toxic products used intentionally to cause illness or death in humans, animals, or plants. They are produced or used with the goal of causing illness or death in humans, limiting food supplies or agricultural resources, and evoking fear in populations.

History of Use

Biological weapons were first used thousands of years ago. Assyrians poisoned enemy wells with rye ergot in the sixth century B.C. Persia, Greece, and Rome attempted to contaminate sources of drinking water with diseased corpses. In 1347, when some of the Mongols who were attacking the walled city of Caffa in Crimea (now Feodosiya, Ukraine) died of the plague, the surviving attackers catapulted the corpses into the city.[6]

In the best-documented case, Sir Jeffrey Amherst, commander-in-chief of the British forces in North America in 1763 during the French and Indian Wars, suggested to the besieged commander at Fort Pitt that smallpox be used: "You will Do well to try to Inoculate the Indians by means of Blanketts, as well as to try Every other Method that can serve to Extirpate this Execrable Race." Apparently officers at Fort Pitt had already executed a similar plan a few months earlier. The commander of the local militia, William

Trent (who gave his name to Trenton, which coincidentally appears to have been a city from which anthrax spores were mailed about 250 years later), recorded in his diary that he had given a delegation of Delaware Indians who had visited the fort seeking its surrender "two Blankets and a Handkerchief out of the Small Pox Hospital." A severe epidemic of smallpox subsequently occurred among the besieging Native Americans, but it is not clear whether this was the result of purposeful infection.[7]

During World War I, Germany is alleged to have used the bacteria that cause glanders, a highly-infectious animal disease, against horses and mules, and the bacteria that cause anthrax against cattle.[8] In the 1930s, Japanese troops used planes to drop rice and wheat mixed with plague-carrying fleas in China, resulting in plague in areas that previously had been plague-free.[9] During World War II, according to testimony at the Nuremberg trials, prisoners in German concentration camps were infected during tests of biological weapons.[8] Great Britain and the United States, fearing the Germans would use biological weapons during the war, developed their own: the British tested anthrax spores off the coast of Scotland on Gruinard Island, which remained uninhabitable for decades; the United States developed anthrax spores, botulinum toxin, and other agents as biological weapons. But Great Britain and the United States did not use these weapons.[8]

During World War II, Japanese laboratories conducted extensive experiments on prisoners of war, testing many organisms selected for possible use as biological weapons, including those that cause anthrax, plague, gas gangrene, encephalitis, typhus, typhoid, hemorrhagic fever, cholera, smallpox, and tularemia.[9] Unlike the Soviet Union, which in 1949 prosecuted 12 Japanese prisoners for involvement in this work, the United States never prosecuted any of the participants. Instead, U.S. experts urged that the Japanese experts be "spared embarrassment" so the United States could benefit from their knowledge.[10]

After World War II

Development, production, and testing of biological weapons continued in several nations after World War II, but despite numerous allegations, no offensive use of these weapons has been substantiated or even fully investigated. The U.S. biologic weapons program was based at Fort Detrick, Maryland (Figure 10–1). In the 1950s and 1960s, U.S. Navy ships released in the San Francisco Bay area large numbers of different bacteria as simulants (materials believed to be nonpathogenic that mimic the spread of biological weapons) to test the efficiency of their dispersal. Some subsequent infections and deaths were attributed to one of these organisms. During this period, the U.S. government conducted 239 top-secret, open-air disseminations of simulants, in-

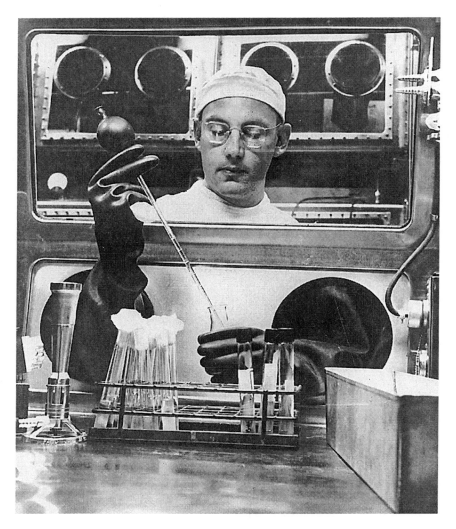

FIGURE 10–1. Researcher in laboratory of the biological weapons program at Fort Detrick, Md., in the 1950s. Scientists turned at least seven biological agents, including anthrax, into weapons during the program's three-decade history at the fort, which served as headquarters for the U.S. biological weapons program from World War II until the program ended in 1969 (AP/Wide World Photos).

volving such sites as the New York City subway system and Washington National Airport. The University of Utah conducted secret, large-scale field tests at the U.S. Army Dugway Proving Ground of biological weapons, including the agents that cause tularemia, Rocky Mountain spotted fever, plague, and Q fever.[11] The U.S. military developed a large infrastructure related to biological weapons, consisting of laboratories, test facilities, and production plants. By the end of the 1960s, the United States had stockpiles of at least ten different biological and toxin weapons.[10] Similar development of offensive biological weapons continued in the Soviet Union.[12] (An accidental release of smallpox virus from the Soviet bioweapons program in 1971 caused three deaths.[12a])

In 1969, the Nixon administration, with the concurrence of the U.S. Department of Defense, which had previously declared that biological weapons lacked "military usefulness," unconditionally renounced U.S. development, production, stockpiling, and use of biological weapons, and announced that the United States would unilaterally dismantle its biological weapons program.[13] In 1972, the Soviet Union ended its opposition to a separate biological weapons treaty, and with the United States and other nations negotiated the Convention on the Prohibition of the Development, Prevention and Stockpiling of Bacteriological (Biological) and Toxin Weapons and on Their Destruction (the Biological Weapons Convention, or BWC). The BWC prohibits—except for "prophylactic, protective and other peaceful purposes"— the development or acquisition of biological agents or toxins, as well as weapons carrying them, and the means of their production, stockpiling, transfer, or delivery. The U.S. Senate ratified the BWC in 1975, and it entered into force during the same year. As of 2002, there were 144 states parties (nations) that had ratified or acceded to the BWC (see Box 10–1). There is evidence that the Soviet Union continued extensive development and testing of biological weapons after the BWC went into force.[13] There is credible evidence that the Soviet bioweapons program employed 42,000 scientists and that it weaponized anthrax, missile-mounted smallpox, developed antibiotic-resistant plague and anthrax, and mass-produced hemorrhagic fever viruses.[13a]

Outbreaks of Anthrax and Salmonellosis

Two outbreaks during the past quarter-century, an anthrax outbreak in the Soviet Union in 1979 and a salmonellosis outbreak in the United States in 1984, provided additional information on the adverse health effects of a potential bioterrorist attack. In 1979, an accidental release of anthrax spores from a Soviet biological weapons factory caused an outbreak of inhalational anthrax with at least 77 (and perhaps 1,000) cases, at least 66 of which were fatal (see Chapter 6).[13,13a,14] In 1984, the first bioterrorist attack occurred in the United States. In Central Oregon, members of a cult intentionally contaminated local restaurant salad bars with *Salmonella* bacteria. Over 700 people became ill, but there were no reported deaths in this outbreak[15] (see Box 10–2).

Invoking the specter of possible new biological weapons and unproven allegations of aggressive biological weapons programs in other countries, the Reagan administration during the 1980s initiated intensive efforts to conduct

Box 10–1. International Control of Biological Weapons.

The Convention on the Prohibition of the Development, Production and Stockpiling of Bacteriological (Biological) and Toxin Weapons and on Their Destruction ("the Biological Weapons Convention" or BWC) was the first multilateral disarmament treaty banning the production and use of an entire category of weapons. Negotiated following President Nixon's renunciation of the use of biological weapons by the United States in 1969, the BWC was opened for signature in 1972 and entered into force in 1975. By 2002, a total of 144 states parties (nations) had ratified or acceded to the BWC.

The BWC bans the development, production, stockpiling, or acquisition of biological agents or toxins of any type or quantity that do not have protective, medical, or other peaceful purposes, or any weapons or means of delivery for such agents or toxins. Under the treaty, all such material was to have been destroyed within nine months of the BWC's entry into force. The absence of any formal verification regime to monitor compliance has limited the effectiveness of the convention.

Recognizing the need to strengthen the BWC, a group of governmental experts was established at the Third Review Conference of the BWC in 1991 in order to identify and examine potential verification measures. At a special conference in 1994 in Geneva, the states parties agreed to establish an ad hoc group in order to negotiate and develop a legally binding verification regime for the Convention. The ad hoc group was mandated to consider four specific areas: definitions of terms and objective criteria; incorporation of existing measures and further enhanced confidence-building and transparency measures, as appropriate, into the regime; a system of measures to promote compliance with the Convention; and specific measures designed to ensure the effective and full implementation of Article X, which deals with peaceful purposes, including scientific activities and disease prevention.

In 1996, the ad hoc group was instructed to conclude its work on the future protocol at the latest by the Fifth Review Conference. In July 2001, the United States rejected the draft protocol and ruled itself out of further negotiations. At the Fifth Review Conference in late 2001, the United States proposed that the Conference's final declaration terminate the ad hoc group's mandate, angering many other states parties. The Fifth Review Conference was scheduled to reconvene in November 2002 in Geneva, when the states parties were to have before them a nearly finalized draft Final Declaration to strengthen verification of the BWC.

—Merav Datan

Box 10–2. A Community Salmonellosis Outbreak Caused by Intentional Contamination of Restaurant Salad Bars.

In 1984 in a community in central Oregon, 751 people were identified with *Salmonella* typhimurium gastroenteritis that was related to working or eating at 10 restaurants in the area. Their dates of onset of symptoms occurred in September and October, with a peak in late September. Epidemiological investigations, which were performed on employees of all 10 restaurants and customers at four of the restaurants, determined that eating food from the salad bars was the major risk factor. The specific food items served at the salad bars varied from one restaurant to another. No other common source, such as the water supply, a specific food item, or a supplier of food items, could be identified. There was no indication that ill restaurant workers started the outbreak.

A criminal investigation by the Federal Bureau of Investigation (FBI), with technical assistance from the Oregon Public Health Laboratory, was conducted after epidemiological and environmental studies were performed, and found that members of a religious commune in the area contaminated these restaurant salad bars deliberately. A strain of *S.* typhimurium discovered in a commune laboratory could not be distinguished from the strain that caused the outbreak.

The authors of the article advised that "if investigation of a large and cryptic outbreak implicates a mechanism of contamination that does not resemble established patterns, then the possibility of intentional contamination should be considered and law enforcement agencies should be asked to consider undertaking an independent investigation."

(Adapted from Török TJ, Tauxe RV, Wise RP, et al. A large community outbreak of salmonellosis caused by intentional contamination of restaurant salad bars. *JAMA* 1997; 278:389–395.)

"defensive research," which is permitted under the BWC. The budget for the U.S. Army Biological Defense Research Program (BDRP), which sponsored programs in a wide variety of academic, commercial, and government laboratories, increased dramatically during this period. Much of this research was medical, including the development of immunizations and treatments against organisms that might be used as biological weapons.[16] Research and development of new biological weapons, which is outlawed by the BWC, may nevertheless have still occurred.[13,17–19] Defectors from Russia have stated that the Soviet Union and then Russia continued work on offensive biological

weapons despite the BWC,[12,20] and there is some evidence that Iraq also may
have in recent years produced biological weapons.[21] Novel dangers lie in new
genetic technologies, which permit development of genetically altered organisms not known in nature. Stable, tailor-made organisms used as biological weapons could travel long distances and remain infectious, become resistant to antibiotic treatment, and rapidly infect a population and cause
widespread illness and death.

POTENTIAL BIOTERRORIST WEAPONS AND
THEIR ADVERSE HEALTH EFFECTS

There are many biological agents that might be used for bioterrorism. Protocols for diagnosis, treatment, and prevention are now widely available, with
frequent updates from the CDC and elsewhere. The CDC website on bioterrorism, www.bt.cdc.gov, is an extremely useful source of information.
Other useful sources are listed in the background reading at the end of Chapter 1. (See also Chapters 6, 15, and 16.)

The CDC has developed three categories of biological agents, prioritized
according to their likelihood of bioterrorist use and the severity of the diseases they produce:

- Category A (high-priority) agents include "organisms that pose a risk to national security because they can be easily disseminated or transmitted from
  person to person; cause high mortality, and have the potential for major public health impact; might cause public panic and social disruption; and require special action for public health preparedness."
- Category B (second-highest-priority) agents include "those that are moderately easy to disseminate; cause moderate morbidity and low mortality; and
  require specific enhancements of CDC's diagnostic capacity and enhanced
  disease surveillance."
- Category C (third-highest-priority) agents include "emerging pathogens that
  could be engineered for mass dissemination in the future because of availability, ease of production and dissemination, and potential for high morbidity and mortality and major health impact."

The diseases and agents in each of these three categories are listed in Table
10–1. In 1999, the General Accounting Office, the investigative arm of Congress, analyzed the likelihood of a bioterrorist attack by several bacterial and
viral agents. Its conclusions are shown in Table 10–2. (Note that neither Table

TABLE 10–1. Categories of Diseases and the Biological Agents that Cause Them.

CATEGORY A

Anthrax (*Bacillus anthracis*)
Botulism *(Clostridium botulinum* toxin)
Plague (*Yersinia pestis*)
Smallpox (*Variola major*)
Tularemia (*Francisella tularensis*)
Viral hemorrhagic fevers (filoviruses, such as Ebola and Marburg; and arenaviruses, such as Lassa and Machupo)

CATEGORY B

Brucellosis (*Brucella* species)
Epsilon toxin of *Clostridium perfringens*
Food safety threats (such as *Salmonella* species, *Escherichia coli* O157:H7, and *Shigella*)
Glanders (*Burkholderia mallei*)
Melioidosis (*Burkholderia pseudomallei*)
Psittacosis (*Chlamydia psittaci*)
Q fever (*Coxiella burnetii*)
Ricin toxin from *Ricinus communis* (castor beans)
Staphylococcal enterotoxin B
Typhus fever (*Rickettsia prowazeki*)
Viral encephalitis (alphaviruses, such as Venezuelan equine encephalitis, eastern equine encephalitis, and western equine encephalitis)
Water safety threats (such as *Vibrio cholerae* and *Cryptosporidium parvum*)

CATEGORY C

Hantaviruses
Multidrug-resistant tuberculosis
Nipah virus
Tickborne encephalitis viruses
Tickborne hemorrhagic fever viruses
Yellow fever

(Centers for Disease Control and Prevention. Accessed at www.bt.cdc.gov/Agent/Agentlist.asp on March 30, 2002.)

10–2 nor Table 11–3 includes one of the CDC Category A agents: botulinum toxin.)

The remainder of this section deals with the six CDC Category A diseases and the agents that cause them: three that are caused by bacteria (anthrax, plague, and tularemia); one that is caused by a bacterial toxin (botulism); and a disease (smallpox) and a group of diseases (viral hemorrhagic fevers) that are caused by viruses (see Chapter 15). Category B and Category C diseases and the agents that cause them are briefly described in Tables 10–3 and 10–4. In addition to their direct effects, bioterrorist agents can produce psychological effects.[22–24]

TABLE 10-2. Characteristics of Selected Potential Bioterrorist Weapons.

BACTERIAL AGENTS	EASE OF MANUFACTURE	STABILITY	LETHAL EFFECTS	LIKELIHOOD OF AN ATTACK
Anthrax	Virulent stock is hard to obtain and process.	Spores are very stable. Resistant to sunlight, heat, and some disinfectants.	Very high for pulmonary anthrax.	Possible, but requires sophistication to manufacture and disseminate.
Plague	Very difficult to acquire seed stock and to process.	Can be long-lasting, but heat, disinfectants and sunlight render it harmless.	Very high.	Possible, but not likely, as it is difficult to acquire suitable strain and to weaponize and disseminate it.
Glanders	Difficult to acquire seed stock; moderately difficult to process.	Very stable.	Moderate to high.	Potential, but difficult to acquire, produce and disseminate it.
Tularemia	Difficult to acquire correct strain; moderately difficult to process.	Generally unstable in environment. Resists cold; killed by mild heat and disinfectants.	Moderate if untreated, low if treated.	Possible, but difficult to stabilize.

Brucellosis	Difficult to acquire seed stock; moderately difficult to process.	Very stable. Long persistence in wet soil or food.	Very low.	Not likely because of difficulty of getting stock, long incubation period and low lethality.
Q Fever	Difficult to acquire seed stock; moderately difficult to process and weaponize.	Stable. Persists for months on wood and in sand.	Very low if treated.	Not likely because of low lethality.
VIRUSES				
Hemorrhagic fevers (Ebola and Marburg)	Very difficult to obtain and process. Unsafe to handle.	Relatively unstable.	Depending on strain, can be very high.	Unlikely because of difficulty of acquiring pathogen, safety considerations, and relative instability.
Smallpox	Difficult to obtain stock and to process. Only confirmed sources are in the U.S. and Russia.	Very stable.	Moderate to high.	Questionable because of limited availability. But consequences of an attack are deemed especially serious.

(General Accounting Office. Risk assessments: the biological threat. As reported in the *New York Times*, November 1, 2001, p. B7.)

TABLE 10–3. Brief Descriptions of CDC Category B Diseases and the Agents That Cause Them.

Brucellosis (*Brucella* species): Systemic bacterial disease with acute or insidious onset, with fever, headache, weakness, profuse sweating, chills, joint pain, depression, weight loss, and generalized aches. Transmission by contact with tissues, blood, urine, vaginal discharges, aborted fetuses, and especially placentas, and by ingestion of raw milk and dairy products from infected animals. Airborne transmission can occur. No evidence of person-to-person transmission.

Epsilon toxin of *Clostridium perfringens*: *Clostridium perfringens* causes intestinal disorders with sudden onset of colic followed by diarrhea. Nausea common, but vomiting and fever usually absent. Type C strains cause necrotizing enteritis. Transmission typically through the ingestion of food contaminated by soil or feces and then held under conditions that permit multiplication of organism.

Food safety threats (such as *Salmonella* species, *Escherichia coli* O157:H7, and *Shigella*): Food can be contaminated by microorganisms or toxins. These contaminants cause illness with varying symptoms, most often characterized by some combination of nausea, vomiting, abdominal pain, and diarrhea.

Glanders (*Burkholderia mallei*): Highly communicable disease of horses, mules, and donkeys. Human infection occurs rarely and almost always in workers with contact with animals or who work in laboratories, such as veterinarians, equine butchers, and pathologists.

Melioidosis (*Burkholderia pseudomallei*): Bacterial infection with range of clinical manifestations, from no disease or asymptomatic pulmonary consolidation to necrotizing pneumonia and/or a rapidly fatal septicemia. May simulate tuberculosis or typhoid fever. Clinical picture may include pulmonary cavitation, empyema, chronic abscesses, and osteomyelitis. Transmission usually by contact with contaminated soil or water through overt or inapparent skin wounds, by aspiration or ingestion of contaminated water, or by inhalation of dust from soil.

Psittacosis (*Chlamydia psittaci*): Acute, generalized chlamydial disease with variable clinical presentations. Fever, headache, rash, myalgia, chills, and upper or lower respiratory tract disease common. Respiratory symptoms often disproportionately mild when compared with the extensive pneumonia demonstrable by x-ray. Transmission by inhaling agent from desiccated droppings, secretions, and dust from feathers of infected birds. Imported psittacine birds most frequent source of exposure, followed by turkey, squab, and duck farms. Processing and rendering plants have been sources of disease. Person-to-person transmission rarely reported to occur.

Q fever (*Coxiella burnetii*): Acute febrile rickettsial disease, often with sudden onset with chills, retrobulbar headache, weakness, malaise, and severe sweats. A pneumonitis is sometimes found on x-ray, but respiratory signs and symptoms not prominent. Abnormal liver function tests common, and acute and chronic granulomatous hepatitis reported. Transmission commonly by airborne dissemination of organisms in dust from premises contaminated by placental tissues, birth fluids, and excreta of infected animals. Airborne particles containing organisms may be carried downwind for one-half mile or more. Direct transmission from person-to-person occurs rarely, if ever.

(continued)

TABLE 10–3. (continued)

Ricin toxin derived from *Ricinus communis* (castor beans): Potent cytotoxin that can cause necrosis of the respiratory tract, if inhaled; severe gastrointestinal tract irritation, if ingested; and local tissue and muscle necrosis, if administered parenterally.

Staphylococcal enterotoxin B: Potent toxin that causes gastrointestinal and other symptoms.

Typhus fever (*Rickettsia prowazeki*): Rickettsial disease with variable onset, often sudden and marked by headache, chills, prostration, fever, and general pains. Macular rash appears on the 5th to 6th day, initially on the face, palms, or soles. Transmission is the body louse, which is infected by feeding on the blood of a patient with acute typhus fever. Inhalation of infective louse feces in dust may account for some infections.

Viral encephalitis (alphaviruses, such as Venezuelan equine encephalitis, eastern equine encephalitis, and western equine encephalitis): This group of acute inflammatory viral diseases of short duration involves parts of the brain, spinal cord, and meninges. Signs and symptoms vary. Most infections are asymptomatic. Mild cases may be associated with fever and headache or aseptic meningitis. Severe infections usually marked by acute onset, headache, high fever, meningeal signs, stupor, disorientation, coma, tremors, occasional convulsions, and spastic paralysis. Can be spread by mosquitos. No evidence of direct transmission from person to person.

Water safety threats (such as *Vibrio cholerae* and *Cryptosporidium parvum*): Cholera is an acute bacterial disease characterized in its severe form by sudden onset, profuse painless watery stools, nausea and vomiting early in the course of illness, and, in untreated cases, rapid dehydration, acidosis, circulatory collapse, hypoglycemia in children, and renal failure. Transmission occurs through ingestion of food or water contaminated directly or indirectly with feces or vomitus of infected persons.

Cryptosporidiosis is a parasitic infection of medical and veterinary importance that affects the epithelial cells of the gastrointestinal, biliary, and respiratory tracts. Asymptomatic infections common and constitute source of infection for others. Major symptom in humans is diarrhea, which may be profuse and watery, preceded by loss of appetite and vomiting in children. Diarrhea associated with cramping abdominal pain. Malaise, fever, anorexia, nausea, and vomiting occur less often. Transmission by fecal-oral route, which includes person-to-person, animal-to-person, waterborne, and foodborne transmission.

(Adapted from: Chin J [ed.]. *Control of Communicable Diseases Manual* [17th Edition]. Washington, D.C.: American Public Health Association, 2000.)

Anthrax

Anthrax is a highly virulent infectious disease of animals that can infect humans, but there is no evidence of person-to-person transmission. The route of exposure determines the type of infection in humans. In the cutaneous form, anthrax spores or bacteria enter the body through breaks in the skin,

TABLE 10–4. Brief Descriptions of CDC Category C Diseases and the Agents That Cause Them.

Hantaviruses: Infect rodents worldwide. Several species infect humans, with primary effect on vascular endothelium, resulting in increased vascular permeability, hypotensive shock, and hemorrhagic manifestations. One syndrome is acute zoonotic viral disease, with abrupt onset of fever, lower back pain, hemorrhagic manifestations, and renal involvement. Another syndrome is acute zoonotic viral disease, with fever, muscle pain, and gastrointestinal complaints, followed by abrupt onset of respiratory distress and hypotension. Both syndromes presumably transmitted mainly by aerosol transmission from rodent excreta.

Multidrug-resistant tuberculosis: Tuberculosis is a mycobacterial disease. Initial infection usually goes unnoticed, but skin-test sensitivity appears within 2 to 10 weeks. Early lung lesions commonly heal. In 5% of apparently normal hosts and as many as 50% of persons with advanced HIV infection, initial infection may progress directly to pulmonary tuberculosis or, by lymphohematogenous dissemination to pulmonary, miliary, meningeal, or other extrapulmonary involvement. Exposure to tubercle bacilli in airborne droplet nuclei produced by people with pulmonary or laryngeal tuberculosis during expiratory efforts, such as coughing, singing, or sneezing, is primary mode of transmission.

Nipah viral disease: Zoonotic viral disease manifested primarily as encephalitis. Symptoms range in severity from mild, to coma and death, and include fever, headache, sore throat, dizziness, drowsiness, and disorientation. Transmission appears to be primarily through direct contact with infected swine or contaminated tissues. No evidence for person-to-person transmission.

Tickborne encephalitis: Group of viral diseases clinically resembling the mosquito-borne encephalitides, except some are associated with focal epilepsy, flaccid paralysis, and other residua. Transmission by the bite of infective ticks or by consumption of milk from certain infected animals. No direct transmission from person to person.

Tickborne hemorrhagic fever: Viral disease with sudden onset of fever, malaise, weakness, irritability, headache, severe pain in limbs and loins, and marked loss of appetite. Occasionally vomiting, abdominal pain, and diarrhea occur. Flush on face and chest and injection of conjunctivae develop early. Hemorrhagic enathem of soft palate, uvula, and pharynx, and a fine petechial rash spreading from the chest and abdomen to the rest of the body generally associated with the disease. Possible bleeding from gums, nose, lungs, uterus, and intestine. Transmission by bite of adult tick. Nosocomial infection of medical workers, occurring after exposure to blood and secretions from patients, important in recent outbreaks; tertiary cases occurred in family members of medical workers.

Yellow fever: Acute viral disease of short duration. Mild cases have sudden onset, with fever, chills, headache, back ache, generalized muscle pain, prostration, nausea, and vomiting. Pulse may be slow and weak out of proportion to the elevated temperature. Jaundice moderate early in the disease and intensified later. Some cases progress to a more severe stage, with hemorrhagic symptoms and liver and renal failure. Transmission by the bite of mosquitos. Highly communicable where many susceptible people and abundant vector mosquitos coexist. Not transmitted by direct contact or common vehicles.

(Adapted from: Chin J [ed.]. *Control of Communicable Diseases Manual* [17th Edition]. Washington, D.C.: American Public Health Association, 2000.)

causing itching, boils, and the formation of a black scab, which can mimic a spider bite (see Figures 6–3 and 6–4 in Chapter 6). Severe skin infections can result in sepsis and microangiopathic hemolytic anemia. In the rare gastrointestinal form, eating infected meat or drinking contaminated water can result in nausea, vomiting, and diarrhea. In the most serious form, inhalational anthrax, inhalation of the organism causes fever, chest pain, and difficulty breathing due to hemorrhagic mediastinitis, usually fatal once the patient develops resultant symptoms (see Figure 6–5 in Chapter 6). Symptoms usually start within two to seven days, but may begin several weeks after exposure. Standard universal precautions should be used in the care of patients infected with anthrax; special isolation precautions are not required. Treatment for anthrax includes high-dose penicillin, ciprofloxacin, or doxycycline. All forms of the disease must be treated promptly.[25] (See Chapter 6.)

Preventive measures are indicated if an exposure has occurred: Spores can be washed off with soap and water. Clothes should be changed if contaminated. Oral ciprofloxacin or doxycycline should be given to everyone exposed. In the United States in the fall of 2001, fears of anthrax exposure fed demand for ciprofloxacin, which was partially balanced by physicians' limiting unnecessary prescriptions for antibiotics in order to help prevent antibiotic resistance from developing. In such situations, physicians should counsel patients against overreacting, and prescribe medications on the basis of sound clinical judgment. This is particularly true because of the number of hoaxes of anthrax dissemination that occurred following the dissemination of anthrax in the mail in 2001.[26]

The anthrax vaccine is of uncertain efficacy against inhalational anthrax. First developed during the 1950s, and reformulated in the 1960s, it was approved by the U.S. Food and Drug Administration (FDA) for general use in 1970. The vaccine has been given to some veterinarians, those who work with livestock or animal products, anthrax researchers, and U.S. troops during the Persian Gulf War and some U.S. military personnel since then. Despite endorsement in 2002 in a report by a committee of the U.S. Institute of Medicine, the evidence that this vaccine will be effective in protecting against airborne infection with anthrax remains questionable. The only published human efficacy trial of an anthrax vaccine is a study performed 40 years ago in a mill that processed contaminated, raw, imported goat hair, where clinical anthrax infections occurred.[27] Some protective value against cutaneous anthrax was noted, but there were not enough cases of inhalational anthrax to reach any conclusions about vaccine efficacy. Vaccine experiments on monkeys and guinea pigs exposed to inhalational anthrax have yielded contradictory results. The Senate Veterans' Affairs Committee examined the issue of the efficacy and safety of the vaccine in 1994 and recommended that "the vaccine should be considered investigational when used as a protection against biologic warfare."[28] More recent experiments using rhesus macaques have led to greater conviction by the military that the vaccine may be effective against the strain of anthrax the macaques were exposed to,[29,30] but the military has not been able to predict which strain, if any, will be used.

Further complicating the question of efficacy is the evidence that new strains of anthrax may have been developed specifically to make the current vaccine ineffective.[31–34] Despite warnings by concerned groups,[35] the U.S. Department of Defense began an extensive immunization program in 1997.[36,37] Concerns by military personnel about adverse reactions to the vaccine led to a number of refusals, with severe punishment of the refusers.[38] The American Public Health Association adopted a policy statement urging suspension of the program,[29] but it was not until an inspection by the U.S. Food and Drug Administration of the sole facility producing the vaccine found numerous deficiencies in the production process that immunizations were suspended for several years.[39–41] Production has now resumed, and U.S. military personnel are again receiving mandated immunizations. In March 2002, the Institute of Medicine reported that the current anthrax vaccine, although "far from optimal," is safe and likely to be effective, even against strains of the bacterium that have been engineered as weapons.[41a]

Plague

Plague is caused by the bacterium *Yersinia pestis*, which is found in rodents and the fleas that infest them. Pneumonic plague occurs when this bacterium infects the lungs. This form of plague can spread from person to person through the air via organisms suspended in respiratory droplets, although this usually requires close contact with the affected person. Transmission could occur in a bioterrorist attack with aerosolized *Y. pestis* bacteria. The first symptoms are usually fever, headache, weakness, shortness of breath, chest pain, cough, and sometimes bloody or watery sputum. Over 2 to 4 days, the pneumonia progresses, possibly causing respiratory failure, shock, and death. Antibiotics should be given within 24 hours of the first symptoms in order to decrease the likelihood of death. Streptomycin, gentamicin, tetracyclines, and chloramphenicol are all effective against this form of the disease.[42]

Plague also occurs in two other forms. Bubonic plague, the most common form, occurs when an infected flea bites a person or when contaminated materials enter through a break in the skin. Symptoms include swollen, tender lymph nodes (buboes), fever, headache, chills, and weakness. There is no person-to-person transmission of this form of the disease. Septicemic plague occurs when plague bacteria multiply in the blood—usually a complication of either of the other two forms of the disease. Septicemic plague also is not transmitted from person to person.[42]

Tularemia

Tularemia is caused by the highly-infectious bacterium *Francisella tularensis*. People can become infected in many ways, including bites of infected arthropods, handling of infectious animal tissues or fluids, direct contact with or ingestion of contaminated food, water, or soil, and inhalation of infective aerosols. There is no person-to-person transmission. In recent years in the United States, the case–fatality rate has been 1.4 percent. This organism could be used as a biological weapon, most likely by aerosol release. *F. tularensis* can enter the body via the skin, mucous membranes, gastrointestinal tract, or lungs.[42]

Onset of symptoms of tularemia is usually abrupt, with high fever, headache, chills and rigors, generalized body aches (often in the low back), runny nose, and sore throat. A variety of other symptoms can occur, including cough, shortness of breath, pleuritic pain, and production of sputum, which may be bloody. Nausea, vomiting, and diarrhea can occur, as can sweats, progressive weakness, loss of appetite, and weight loss. Skin ulcers can occur.

Where individual patient management is possible, parenteral therapy with streptomycin, the drug of choice, or gentamicin is recommended. In a mass casualty setting, doxycycline and ciprofloxacin are the preferred choices for both adults and children. A live attenuated vaccine has been available as an investigational new drug. It is now under review by the Food and Drug Administration.[42]

Botulism

Botulism is caused by the extremely potent neurotoxin that is produced by the bacterium *Clostridium botulinum*. Of the 174 cases of botulism in the United States reported to the CDC in 1999, there were 107 cases of infant botulism (due to spores germinating and producing toxin in the gastrointestinal tract), 41 cases of wound botulism (due to spores germinating in wounds, including those of injection-drug users), and 26 cases of foodborne botulism. Foodborne botulism is considered a public health emergency because there may be contaminated food remaining that could cause botulism in others.[42]

Clinically, botulism is characterized by symmetric, descending flaccid paralysis of motor and autonomic nerves, most often starting with the cranial nerves. Common symptoms are double vision, blurred vision, drooping eyelids, slurred speech, difficulty swallowing, dry mouth, and muscle weakness. Without treatment, botulism can progress to cause descending paralysis of the respiratory muscles and the muscles of the arms and legs. Botulinum antitoxin, which is supplied by the CDC, can, if administered early, prevent progression of the disease and shorten symptoms in severe cases. About 5 percent of those affected die of the disease, often from respiratory failure. Survivors may suffer from fatigue and shortness of breath for many years after recovery.[42] (See also Chapter 15.)

Smallpox

Smallpox is a highly contagious and deadly viral disease, for which human-to-human transmission is possible.[43-45] Smallpox was last diagnosed in humans in 1981, after an extraordinary international effort to eradicate the disease. Allegations of the weaponization of smallpox by the Russians and possibly others have raised concerns that smallpox may be used as a biological weapon, with potentially devastating consequences[12] because of the cessation of vaccination programs in the wake of the successful global effort to eradicate the disease. Once smallpox was "conquered," the only remaining stockpiles of the virus were to be safeguarded by the United States and Russia until their planned destruction—a goal that has been put on hold.[46,46a]

Smallpox can be transmitted by inhalation, through the fluid from the rash carried to the mucous membranes, and from handling clothing, bedding, or scabs of a person who has smallpox. The maculopapular rash of smallpox erupts quickly, rather than in stages as in chickenpox. It starts as small red macules, which become 2- to 3-mm papules within 1 to 2 days, then become 2- to 5-mm vesicles 1 to 2 days later. The rash first appears in the mouth and throat and then on the face and extremities, spreading slowly to the rest of the body. Then 4- to 6-mm pustules develop, remain present for 5 to 8 days, followed by crusting (Figure 10–2). Smallpox skin lesions are usually all at the same stage of development. In the past, drug eruptions, secondary syphilis, chickenpox, acne, insect bites, monkeypox, and generalized vaccinia and eczema vaccinatum were frequently confused with smallpox. Symptoms usually start between 10 and 12 days after exposure, but can begin as early as 7 days or as late as 17 days after exposure. High fever (often more than 40°C) occurs between 1 to 2 weeks after infection, often accompanied by malaise, prostration, headache, and backache; abdominal pain and delirium may also develop.[47]

Usually, smallpox is transmitted from person to person within families and among close contacts. The infected person is most contagious during the first week after the rash appears. A single person or small number of individuals infected with smallpox would probably be cared for at home, with close contacts identified and quarantined. After infection with smallpox begins, antibiotics for secondary infections and supportive therapy are indicated for treatment. No antiviral agents have been effective against the disease. Smallpox vaccine, however, can be administered within 4 days after exposure to lessen the severity of, or even prevent, illness.[47]

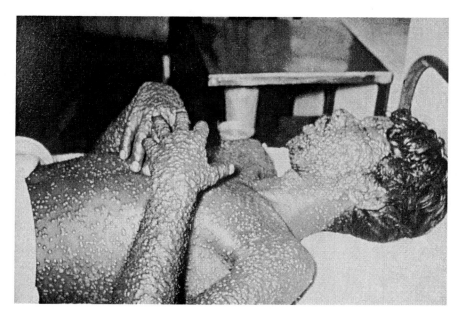

FIGURE 10–2. Man with smallpox lesions (Public Health Image Library/Centers for Disease Control and Prevention).

In the event smallpox is used as a biological weapon, hospitals must be prepared to isolate entire wards and to revaccinate hospital employees who had received vaccinations in childhood. Respiratory isolation (negative pressure ventilation) and contact precautions (using gloves, gowns, and masks) are necessary. Strict standard precautions must be followed in handling linen and clothing.

Vaccination for smallpox in the United States ceased after 1972. It is unknown whether those who had been vaccinated prior to 1972 remain immune. As a result of the discovery in March 2002 of approximately 75 million doses of previously stored smallpox vaccine, the stockpile of smallpox vaccine in the United States may be adequate for immunizing the entire population. Yet 250 out of every 1 million people vaccinated will probably have an adverse reaction, and an estimated 180 people will be likely to have fatal reactions if approximately 300 million Americans are vaccinated. It is not clear whether the best strategy will be to immunize everyone in the United States, or wait until an outbreak occurs and then attempt to quickly immunize contacts of those affected—the strategy that was used in the latter phases of the successful global program in the 1960s and early 1970s to eradicate smallpox (see Chapter 15 and Figures 15–1 and 15–2).[48,49] In June 2002, the CDC's Advisory Committee on Immunization Practices rejected a proposal to offer vaccine to everyone living in the United States. The Committee recommended immunizing only the estimated 15,000 health care and law enforcement workers who would likely respond to a biological agent attack and come in contact with victims.[50] In late 2002, President Bush ordered vaccination of 500,000 active-duty troops. Plans are being prepared to vaccinate selected health-care and emergency workers; there is considerable controversy about these plans.[50a]

Viral Hemorrhagic Fevers

These fevers are divided into several categories, including those caused by filoviruses, such as Ebola and Marburg viruses, and those caused by arenaviruses, such as Lassa virus. These viruses can be tramsmitted to humans when activities of infected reservoir hosts, or vectors, and humans overlap. The viruses carried in rodent reservoirs are transmitted when humans contact urine, fecal matter, saliva, or other body excretions from infected rodents. Viruses associated with arthropod vectors are spread most often when the vector mosquito or tick bites a human, or when a human crushes a tick. Some vectors may spread virus to animals, and humans can become infected when they care for or slaughter the animals. Ebola, Marburg, Lassa, and other viruses can spread from one person to another.[42]

Symptoms and signs vary, but initially they often include high fever, fatigue, dizziness, muscle aches, loss of strength, and exhaustion. With severe cases, there is bleeding under the skin, in internal organs, or from body orifices such as the mouth, eyes, and ears. Severe illness may also be accompanied by shock, nervous system malfunction, coma, delirium, and seizures.[42]

Treatment is supportive in nature. There is no established curative treatment. With the exception of yellow fever and Argentine hemorrhagic fever, for which vaccines exist, there are no vaccines that protect against these diseases.[42]

WHAT HEALTH PROFESSIONALS CAN DO

Health care providers should immediately report cases of possible bioterrorism to state health departments. They should not hesitate to request clinical and public-health consultation when they encounter patients with suspicious illnesses.

Overuse of antibiotics can create bacteria resistant to antibiotics that could pose a more substantive health threat than many hypothetical bioterrorist scenarios. Widespread public fear may lead to pressure on health care providers to prescribe antibiotics when it is not prudent to do so. Health care providers should resist this pressure and prescribe antibiotics only as they deem appropriate. Health care providers also need to warn patients that unnecessary use of antibiotics can also cause serious side effects. In addition, many antibiotics are contraindicated for children, teenagers, and pregnant or nursing women.

Health professionals can educate their patients, the general public, and other health professionals about biological weapons and about prudent measures that can be undertaken to address potential diseases that can be caused by bioterrorist action, as well as, more broadly, other infectious diseases of public health importance, including AIDS, tuberculosis, hepatitis B, and hepatitis C. They can assist epidemiologists in the investigation of disease outbreaks when they occur. Health professionals working in clinical or research laboratory settings can help restrict access to biological agents and equipment that could be used in producing biological weapons.[51]

A serious attempt to prevent bioterrorism must include the development of the controls and safeguards necessary to eliminate biological weapons— and all other weapons of mass destruction. Health professionals can advocate the United States' reversing its rejection of the international community's recent attempts to strengthen the BWC with strong inspection and verification protocols.[52–54] As with nuclear weapons, the best civil defense can never really offer protection from truly catastrophic scenarios. Real biological security can only come from merging the best global controls over weapons technologies with the commitment to finally eradicate specific diseases worldwide.

While addressing potential biological agents and the diseases they can cause, it is critically important that health professionals maintain—and strengthen—support for other public health priorities, many of which are related to infectious diseases. For example, there are an estimated 76 million cases of foodborne illness in the United States each year that are associated with 325,000 hospital admissions and 5,000 deaths.[55] Many of these cases of foodborne illness can be prevented with relatively inexpensive measures, such as training commercial food handlers and inspecting restaurants and other food service establishments.

Support for international control of infectious diseases, which is essential to reduce human misery and as a collateral benefit may help reduce international bioterrorism, may be even more urgent. For example, in India in 1999, there were two million new cases of tuberculosis (TB), causing approximately 450,000 deaths. Effective treatment of TB in India costs about US $15 per person treated.[56] The United Nations has estimated that about US $10 billion invested in safe water supplies could reduce by one-third the current four billion annual cases of diarrheal disease that result in 2.2 million deaths.[57] Yet the United States continues to spend far less in relation to its vast wealth on international development assistance than other industrialized countries. Health professionals have a special responsibility to call attention to these failures and to work to overcome them.

From a broad perspective, biological security in the 21st century must address bioterrorism, but it must also address other major issues, including: (a) control of emerging infectious diseases; (b) control of established major infectious diseases, such as HIV/AIDS, malaria, tuberculosis, diarrheal disease, and acute respiratory infection; (c) development by microorganisms of increasing resistance to antibiotics and other antimicrobials; (d) changing patterns of vectors and other biological consequences of climate change; (e) poverty, war, and various forms of social injustice that are important contributing causes of the transmission of much infectious disease; and (f) insufficient resources and insufficient political will to comprehensively address these problems globally.[58]

Acknowledgment

We acknowledge the contributions of Hillel W. Cohen and Robert M. Gould to some of the policy analyses in this chapter.

REFERENCES

1. Sidel VW, Goldwyn RM. Chemical and biological weapons. *N Engl J Med* 1966; 274:21–27.
2. *Health Aspects of Chemical and Biological Weapons: Report of a WHO Group of Consultants.* Geneva: World Health Organization, 1970.
3. Sidel VW, Cohen HW, Gould RM. Good intentions and the road to bioterrorism preparedness. *Am J Public Health* 2001; 91:716–718.
4. Geiger HJ. Terrorism, biological weapons, and bonanzas: assessing the real threat to public health. *Am J Public Health* 2001; 91:708–709.
5. Sidel VW, Gould RM, Cohen HW. Bioterrorism preparedness: Co-optation of public health. *Med Global Survival* 2002; 7:82–89.
6. Derbes VJ. DeMussis and the great plague of 1348: a forgotten episode of biological warfare. *JAMA* 1966; 196:59–62.
7. Tucker JB. *Scourge: The Once and Future Threat of Smallpox.* New York: Atlantic Monthly Press, 2001.
8. Harris R, Paxman J. *A Higher Form of Killing: The Secret Story of Chemical and Biological Warfare.* New York: Hill and Wang, 1982.
9. Williams P, Wallace D. *Unit 731: The Japanese Army's Secret of Secrets.* London: Hodder & Stoughton, 1989.
10. Wright S. Evolution of biological warfare policy: 1945–1990. In: Susan Wright (ed.), *Preventing a Biological Arms Race.* Cambridge, Mass.: MIT Press, 1990, pp. 26–68.
11. Cole LA. *Clouds of Secrecy: The Army's Germ Warfare Tests over Populated Areas.* Totowa, NJ: Rowman & Littlefield, 1988.
12. Alibek K with Handelman S. *Biohazard.* New York: Random House, 1999.
12a. Broad WJ, Miller J. Report provides new details of Soviet smallpox accident. *New York Times,* June 15, 2002, A1.
13. Miller J, Engelberg S, Broad W. *Germs: Biological Weapons and America's Secret War.* New York: Simon and Schuster, 2001.

13a. Garrett L. *Betrayal of Trust: The Global Collapse of Public Health.* New York: Hyperion, 2000.

14. Guillemin, J: *Anthrax: Immunization of a Deadly Outbreak.* Berkeley: University of California Press, 1999.

15. Török, TJ, Tauxe RV, Wise RP, et al. A large community outbreak of salmonellosis caused by intentional contamination of restaurant salad bars. *JAMA* 1997; 278: 389–395.

16. Piller C, Yamamoto KR. "The U.S. Biological Defense Research Program in the 1980s: A Critique," in S Wright (ed.), *Preventing a Biological Arms Race.* Cambridge, Mass.: MIT Press, 1990, pp. 133–168.

17. King J, Strauss H. "The Hazards of Defensive Biological Warfare Research," in Wright (ed.), *Preventing a Biological Arms Race,* pp. 120–132.

18. Wright S, Ketcham S. "The Problem of Interpreting the U.S. Biological Defense Research Program," in Wright (ed.), *Preventing a Biological Arms Race,* pp. 243–266.

19. Piller C, Yamamoto KR. *Gene Wars: Military Control over the New Genetic Technologies.* New York: William Morrow, 1988.

20. Preston R. The bioweaponeers. *The New Yorker.* March 9, 1998, pp. 52–65.

21. United Nations Special Commission (UNSCOM), Report to the Security Council, 25 January 1999. Available at http://www.fas.org/news/un/iraq/s/990125/index.html. Accessed April 20, 2002.

22. DiGiovanni C Jr. Domestic terrorism with chemical or biological agents: psychiatric aspects. *Am J Psychiatry* 1999; 156:1500–1505.

23. Norwood AE, Holloway HC, Ursano RJ. Psychological effects of biological warfare. *Mil Med* 2001; 166 (Suppl 2):27–28.

24. Romano JA Jr, King JM. Psychological casualties resulting from chemical and biological weapons. *Mil Med* 2001; 166(Suppl 2):21–22

25. Swartz MN. Recognition and management of anthrax—an update. *N Engl J Med* 2001; 345:1621–1626.

26. Cole LA. "Anthrax Hoaxes: Hot New Hobby?" *Bulletin of Atomic Scientists* 1999; 55:6–11.

27. Brachman PS, Gold H, Plotkin SA, et al. Field evaluation of a human anthrax vaccine. *Am J Public Health* 1962; 52:632–645.

28. Committee on Veterans' Affairs, United States Senate. Is Military Research Hazardous to Veterans' Health? Washington, D.C.: U.S. Government Printing Office, 1994.

29. Ivins BE, Pitt MLM, Fellows PF, et al. Comparative efficacy of experimental anthrax vaccine candidates against inhalation anthrax in rhesus macaques. *Vaccine* 1998; 16:1141–1148.

30. Friedlander PS, Pittman PR, Parker GW. Anthrax vaccine: evidence for safety and efficacy against inhalation anthrax. *JAMA* 1999; 282:2104–2106.

31. Stepanov AV, et al. Development of novel vaccines against anthrax in man. *Journal of Biotechnology* 1996; 44:155–160.

32. Wade N. Anthrax findings fuel worry on vaccine. *New York Times.* February 3, 1998, A6.

33. Broad WJ. Gene-engineered anthrax: is it a weapon? *New York Times.* Feb. 14, 1998.

34. Wade N. Tests with anthrax raise fears that American vaccine can be defeated. *New York Times,* March 26, 1998.

35. Sidel VW, Nass M, Ensign T. The anthrax dilemma. *Med Global Survival* 1998; 5:97–104.

36. Graham B. Military chiefs back anthrax inoculations. *Washington Post.* 2 Oct. 1996, A12.

37. Myers SL. U.S. armed forces to be vaccinated against anthrax. *New York Times*. December 16, 1997, A1, A22.

38. Anthrax Immunization. Policy Statement 9930, American Public Health Association, 1999. Available at http://www.apha.org. Accessed April 21, 2002.

39. Strong C. FDA cites 30 deficiencies in anthrax vaccine production. Associated Press, December 15, 1999.

40. Sciolino E. Shortage forces Pentagon to cut anthrax inoculations. *New York Times*, July 11, 2000, A14.

41. Sciolino E. Anthrax vaccination program is failing, Pentagon admits. *New York Times*, July 13, 2000.

41a. Stolberg SG, Miller J. Researchers call anthrax vaccine safe and likely to work. *New York Times*, March 7, 2002.

42. CDC website on bioterrorism: www.bt.cdc.gov.

43. Tucker JB. *Scourge: The Once and Future Threat of Smallpox*. New York: Atlantic Monthly Press, 2001.

44. Henderson DA, Inglesby TV, Bartlett JG, et al. Smallpox as a biological weapon. *JAMA* 1999; 281:2127–2137.

45. Facts About Smallpox at http://www.bt.cdc.gov/DocumentsApp/FactsAbout/Facts About.asp.

46. Miller J. U.S. set to retain smallpox stocks. *New York Times*, Nov. 16, 2001.

46a. W.H.O. delays end of smallpox virus. *New York Times*, May 19, 2002, A5.

47. Breman JG, Henderson DA. Diagnosis and management of smallpox. *N Engl J Med* 2002; 346:1300–1308.

48. Fauci AS. Smallpox vaccination policy—the need for dialogue. *N Engl J Med* 2002; 346:1319–1320.

49. Bicknell WJ. The case for voluntary smallpox vaccination. *N Engl J Med* 2002: 346:1323–1325; and correspondence. *N Engl J Med* 2002; 347:691–692.

50. Altman LK. Panel rules out smallpox shots for all. *New York Times*, June 21, 2002, A16.

50a. Sternberg S. Scientists call for smallpox revaccination campaign. *USA Today*, December 23, 2002, 39.

51. Sidel VW. Biological weapons research and physicians: historical and ethical analysis. *PSR Quarterly* 1991; 11:31–42.

52. Allen M, Mufson S. U.S. scuttles germ warfare conference; move to halt stuns European allies. *Washington Post*, Dec. 8, 2001, A1.

53. Falk R. Inhibiting reliance on biological weaponry: the role and relevance of international law." In: Wright S, ed. *Preventing a Biological Arms Race*. Cambridge, Mass.: MIT Press, 1990, pp. 241–266.

54. Call for the United States to Support a Strengthened Biological Weapons Convention. Policy Statement LB-01–07, American Public Health Association, 2001. Available at http://www.apha.org. Accessed April 21, 2002.

55. Mead PS, Slutsker L, Dietz V, et al. Food-related illness and death in the United States. *Emerg Infect Dis* 1999; 5(5):607–650.

56. Dugger CW. India wins battle in war on TB, but it has a long way to go. *New York Times*, March 25, 2000.

57. Price of safe water for all: $10 billion and the will to provide it. *New York Times*, Nov. 23, 2000.

58. Sidel VW, Levy BS. Security and public health. *Social Justice* 2002; 29:108–119.

11

Chemical weapons

HERMAN SPANJAARD AND OXANA KHABIB

A chemical weapon, according to the Chemical Weapons Convention (CWC), is "any chemical which, through its chemical effect on living processes, may cause death, temporary loss of performance, or permanent injury to people and animals." Chemicals are also present in explosives and incendiary weapons, but the destructive force of these weapons depends on blast and heat that chemicals can produce (Chapter 9); chemical weapons, by definition, depend on the direct toxic effects of chemicals.

HISTORY

As early as the Peloponnesian war in the 4th century B.C., the Spartans used fire and smoke in attacking the Athenians at Delium. Invented in the 7th century A.D., "Greek fire," which consists of sulphur, saltpeter, resin, lime, naphtha, and pitch, was used by naval forces to set wooden ships on fire because it floats on water and remains burning.[1] Fire and smoke are not today regarded as chemical weapons, however; neither are the more modern incendiary weapons such as napalm.

The development of chemical weapons coincided with major scientific and technological advances in chemistry. This science developed rapidly at the start of the 19th century, when Germany was becoming a leading world power. The German military recognized the importance of this development and began working on military uses of chemicals. In 1899, the First International World Peace Conference in The Hague, an international meeting addressing the effects of war, formally forbade the use of chemical weapons.

World War I

As World War I began, however, these weapons were further developed and used. Approximately 110,000 tons of toxic chemicals were disseminated during World War I, affecting 1.3 million individuals and causing 90,000 deaths.[1] A German chemical weapon attack on French troops on April 22, 1915, was described in great detail: Suddenly, at about 4 p.m., a strange opaque cloud of greenish-yellow fumes rose from the German trenches opposite the lines occupied by French colonial troops. A light breeze from the northwest wafted this cloud toward the French, who fell gasping in agony. Terror and panic spread through the ranks from the front to the rear lines. A French soldier wrote:

> We saw figures running wildly in confusion over the fields. Greenish clouds swept down upon them, turning yellow as they traveled over the country blasting everything they touched and shriveling up the vegetation. No human courage could face such a peril. Then there staggered into our midst French soldiers, blinded, coughing, chests heaving, faces an ugly purple color, lips speechless with agony, and behind them in the gas soaked trenches, we learned that they had left hundreds of dead and dying comrades. It was the most fiendish, wicked thing I have ever seen.[2]

From 6,000 cylinders, the Germans had released 150 tons of chlorine gas. Later in the war, phosgene was mixed with the chlorine. Its effect, though terrifying, did not change the trench mode of warfare common at that time, as some had expected.

Physicians and other health professionals became involved because the victims needed treatment. Preventive measures, in the form of gas masks (respirators) and other personal protective equipment, were developed. Many casualties occurred because people lacked the discipline to keep wearing their masks. Wearing masks affected people both physically, causing cardiac and respiratory effects; and psychologically, causing discomfort and fear that masks would be inadequate. Furthermore, when masks were used, troops had difficulty recognizing and communicating with each other.

In 1917, the United States entered World War I and started manufacturing chemical weapons. As masks improved, the impact of the use of chlorine and phosgene diminished, and new types of chemical weapons were invented. In 1917, the Germans introduced mustard gas (dichlorethyl sulfide), delivered by artillery shells. Because the gas is heavier than air, it settled on the surface and collected in low-lying areas. Because it is persistent, it remained active for days.

After World War I

The horror produced by the effects of chemical weapons led in 1925 to the negotiation of the Geneva Protocol outlawing the use of chemical weapons (see Box 11–1). During subsequent years, many new chemical weapons were nonetheless developed. In the 1920s and 1930s in Afghanistan, Morocco, and Ethiopia, colonial powers used mustard bombs against native populations. Many physicians and others were led to believe that chemical agents were more humane than bullets, shells, and shrapnel. This belief changed when the Germans, during World War II, developed and manufactured the lethal nerve gases tabun, sarin, and soman, but these gases were not fielded militarily. The Nazis used other gases in the concentration-camp gas chambers: carbon monoxide, pesticides, prussic acid, and hydrogen cyanide (Zyklon-B). The Allied powers also developed and stockpiled chemical weapons; the explosion of 100 tons of mustard gas, resulting from German bombing of a U.S. ship in the harbor of Bari, Italy, caused the deaths of more than 600 military personnel and many civilians.[3]

Since World War II, chemical weapons have been used in several parts of the world. In the 1980s, Iraq, in its war with Iran, used mustard gas and the nerve agent GA, as confirmed by a UN investigation, and possibly used the nerve agent GB. Later, the Iraqi government used hydrogen cyanide (Zyklon-B) against its own Kurdish population.[4] By the end of the Cold War, the Soviet Union had accumulated 40 metric tons of chemical weapons, and the United States, 29 metric tons.[5] In addition to the huge known stockpiles not yet destroyed in these two countries, stockpiles remain in other countries.

Qualities and Physicochemical Properties of Chemical Agents

Tens of thousands of toxic substances are known, but only a few are considered suitable for chemical warfare. About 70 different chemicals were used or stockpiled as chemical weapons during the 20th century. To be selected as a chemical weapon, a chemical must be "suitably highly toxic," but it must be possible to protect against it during manufacture. It must be storable for long periods without degradation or corrosion of the packaging. In addition, when used it should not lose its toxicity prematurely under normal atmospheric conditions. Finally, when dispersed by an exploding shell, it must be able to withstand heat. Combining these factors often leads to consideration of a spray attack as the most effective.

Box 11–1. International Control of Chemical Weapons.

The Geneva Protocol (the Protocol for the Prohibition of the Use in War of Asphyxiating, Poisonous or Other Gases, and of Bacteriological Methods of Warfare) was opened for signature in 1925 in response to widespread abhorrence of the use of chemical weapons in World War I. The Protocol entered into force for each state party (nation) individually at the time of its ratification. By 2002, a total of 132 states parties had ratified or acceded to it. Many of these nations reserved the right to use chemical weapons if such weapons were first used against them. The Protocol does not address possession or destruction of chemical weapons and does not include any implementation or verification provisions.

The Convention on the Prohibition of the Development, Production, Stockpiling and Use of Chemical Weapons and on Their Destruction (the "Chemical Weapons Convention," or CWC) was opened for signature in Paris in 1993 and entered into force in 1997, when the required number of states parties had ratified or acceded to it.

The CWC is the first disarmament agreement negotiated within a multilateral framework that provides for the elimination of an entire category of weapons of mass destruction. Its scope, the obligations assumed by states parties, and the system of verification envisaged for its implementation are unprecedented. The CWC prohibits all development, production, acquisition, stockpiling, transfer, and use of chemical weapons. It requires each state party to destroy its chemical weapons and chemical weapons production facilities, as well as any chemical weapons it may have abandoned on the territory of another state party. The verification provisions of the CWC affect not only the military sector but also the civilian chemical industry worldwide through certain restrictions and obligations regarding the production, processing, and consumption of chemicals that are considered relevant to the objectives of the convention. These provisions are to be verified through a combination of reporting requirements, routine onsite inspection of declared sites, and short-notice challenge inspections. The CWC also contains provisions on assistance in case a state party is attacked or threatened with attack by chemical weapons and on promotion of the trade in chemicals and related equipment among states parties.

The Organization for the Prohibition of Chemical Weapons (OPCW) was established in The Hague after the entry into force of the CWC. It is responsible for the implementation of the CWC. The OPCW is mandated to ensure the implementation of the provisions of the CWC, including those for international verification of compliance with it, and to provide a forum for consultation and cooperation among states parties.

—Merav Datan

Volatility Versus Persistence

Duration of the hazard reflects the degree to which the substance is persistent. Volatile substances are not persistent; they rapidly disperse or evaporate. Surfaces are usually not contaminated by volatile substances. The danger is primarily from inhalation and secondarily from skin exposure. Appropriate gas masks can often provide enough protection from these agents in the short term. Phosgene and hydrogen cyanide are examples of such non-persistent agents. On the other hand, persistent substances are not volatile and can cover surfaces; they can remain in an area for long periods—for example, up to a few weeks for the nerve agent VX. The danger is primarily from skin contact and secondarily from inhalation of vapors. Respiratory and dermal protection, including protective footwear, may be required.

Route of entry of a chemical agent can be via inhalation, absorption through the skin, or ingestion. The specific route is highly dependent on the relative volatility/persistence. Increasing ambient temperature increases volatility and decreases persistence. Increased temperature, therefore, increases the vapor and the inhalation hazard. There are relative distinctions between lethal and incapacitating agents and between lethal and incapacitating doses. For example, for nerve agents, the ratio of the incapacitating and lethal doses is approximately 1:10. On the other hand, tear gas, usually a harassing agent, can become lethal if a person is exposed to a high concentration in a confined space.

CLASSIFICATION OF CHEMICAL WEAPONS

The major way that chemical agents are classified is by the type of toxic effects that they have on the body (see Table 11–1). Table 11–2 contains more specific information on nerve agents, mustard, phosgene oxime, Lewisite, riot-control agents, cyanide, and pulmonary agents. (Note that different organizations use slightly different terms in categorizing these agents.) Five of the major groups are described in more detail below:

Nerve Agents.   Nerve agents are compounds that bind irreversibly to molecules of acetylcholinesterase (AChE), the enzyme that terminates the action of the neurotransmitter acetylcholine (ACh), leading to the accumulation of ACh and persistence of the cholinergic effect.[6] In addition, some nerve agents have a direct effect on the postsynaptic ACh receptor that mimics the effect of ACh. The effects of the excessive cholinergic stimulation can be summarized as muscarinic, nicotinic, and those affecting the central nervous system (CNS). The muscarinic effects may include miosis (decreased pupil size),

TABLE 11–1. Chemical Agents by Type of Effect.

VESICANTS OR BLISTERING AGENTS	INCAPACITATING AGENTS
Distilled mustard (HD)	Agent 15
Lewisite (L)	BZ
Mustard gas (H)	Cannabinoids
Nitrogen mustard (HN-2)	Fentanyls
Phosgene oxime (CX)	LSD
Ethyldichloroarsine (ED)	Phenothiazines
Lewisite 1 (L-1)	
Lewisite 2 (L-2)	NERVE AGENTS
Lewisite 3 (L-3)	Cyclohexyl sarin (GF)
Methyldichloroarsine (MD)	GE
Mustard/Lewisite (HL)	Sarin (GB)
Mustard/T	Soman (GD)
Nitrogen mustard (HN-1)	Tabun (GA)
Nitrogen mustard (HN-3)	VE
Phenodichloroarsine (PD)	VG
Sesqui mustard	V-Gas
	VM
BLOOD AGENTS	VX
Arsine (SA)	
Cyanogen chloride (CK)	RIOT-CONTROL/TEAR AGENTS
Hydrogen chloride	Bromobenzylcyanide (CA)
Hydrogen cyanide (AC)	Chloroacetophenone (CN)
	Chloropicrin (PS)
CHOKING/LUNG/PULMONARY-DAMAGING AGENTS	CNB—(CN in benzene and carbon tetrachloride)
Chlorine (CL)	CNC—(CN in chloroform)
Diphosgene (DP)	CNS—(CN and chloropicrin in chloroform)
Cyanide	CR
Nitrogen oxide (NO)	CS
Perfluoroisobutylene (PHIB)	
Phosgene (CG)	VOMITING AGENTS
Red phosphorous (RP)	Adamsite (DM).
Sulfur trioxide-chlorosulfonic acid (FS)	Diphenylchloroarsine (DA)
Teflon and perfluoroisobutylene (PHIB)	Diphenylcyanoarsine (DC)
Titanium tetrachloride (FM)	
Zinc oxide (HC)	

(Adapted from website of Centers for Disease Control and Prevention, www.bt.cdc.gov, accessed April 25, 2002.)

dim vision, smooth-muscle contraction, and copious hypersecretion from all exocrine glands (sweating, tearing, and runny nose), along with incontinence. The nicotinic effects may include skeletal muscle weakness and paralysis. The CNS effects may include changes in mood, decreased mental status, seizures, and coma. Deaths usually result from respiratory failure, with or without seizures and apnea, which cause hypoxia and, in turn, terminal ar-

TABLE 11–2. Chemical Agents: Symptoms and Treatment.

NERVE AGENTS (GA, GB, GD, GF, VX)	MUSTARD (HD, H)
Signs and Symptoms: Vapor: *Small exposure*—Miosis, rhinorrhea, and mild dyspnea. *Large exposures*—Sudden loss of consciousness, convulsions, apnea, flaccid paralysis, copious secretions, and miosis. Liquid on skin: *Small to moderate exposure*—Localized sweating, nausea, vomiting, and feeling of weakness. *Large exposure*—Sudden loss of consciousness, convulsions, apnea, flaccid paralysis, and copious secretions.	Signs and Symptoms: Asymptomatic latent period (hours). Erythema and blisters on the skin, irritation, conjunctivitis, corneal opacity, and damage in the eyes; mild upper respiratory signs, marked airway damage; also gastrointestinal effects and bone marrow stem cell suppression
Decontamination: Large amounts of water with a hypochlorite solution.	Decontamination: Large amounts of water with a hypochlorite solution.
Immediate Treatment/Management: Administration of atropine and pralidoxime chloride (2PAM); diazepam in addition if casualty is severe; ventilation and suction of airway for respiratory distress.	Immediate Treatment/Management: Decontamination immediately after exposure is the only way to prevent/limit injury/damage. Symptomatic management of lesions.

LEWISITE (L)	PHOSGENE OXIME (CX)
Signs and Symptoms: Lewisite causes immediate pain or irritation of skin and mucous membranes. Erythema and blisters on the skin and eyes and airway damage similar to those seen after mustard exposure develop later.	Signs and Symptoms: Immediate burning and irritation followed by wheal-like skin lesions and eye and airway damage.
Decontamination: Large amounts of water with a hypochlorite solution.	Decontamination: Large amounts of water.
Immediate Treatment/Management: Immediate decontamination; symptomatic management of lesions the same as for mustard lesions; a specific antidote British Anti-Lewisite (BAL) will decrease systemic effects.	Immediate Treatment/Management: Immediate decontamination; symptomatic management of lesions.

(continued)

TABLE 11–2. (*continued*)

CYANIDE (AC, CK)	PULMONARY AGENTS (CG)
Signs and Symptoms: Few. After exposure to high estimated dose (Ct): seizures, respiratory and cardiac arrest.	Signs and Symptoms: Eye and airway irritation, dyspnea, chest tightness, and delayed pulmonary edema.
Decontamination: Skin decontamination is usually not necessary because agents are highly volatile. Wet, contaminated clothing should be removed and the underlying skin decontaminated with water or other standard decontaminates.	Decontamination: Vapor: fresh air. Liquid: copious water irrigation.
Treatment: Antidote: intravenous sodium nitrite and then sodium thiosulfate. Supportive care: oxygen and correct acidosis.	Treatment: Termination of exposure, ABCs of resuscitation, enforced rest and observation, oxygen with or without positive airway pressure for signs of respiratory distress, other supportive therapy as needed.

RIOT-CONTROL AGENTS (CS, CN)

Signs and Symptoms:	Decontamination:
Burning and pain on exposed mucous membranes and skin, eye pain and tearing, burning nostrils, respiratory discomfort, and tingling of the exposed skin.	*Eyes*: thoroughly flush with water, saline or similar substance. *Skin*: flush with copious amounts of water, alkaline soap and water, or a mildly alkaline solution (sodium bicarbonate or sodium carbonate). Generally decontamination is not required if wind is brisk.
	Treatment: Usually none is necessary; effects are self-limiting.

(Adapted from: *Medical Management of Chemical Casualties Handbook*, 2nd edition, Chemical Casualty Care Office, United States Army Medical Research Institute of Chemical Defense, Aberdeen Proving Ground, Maryland, 1995.)

rhythmias. The effects on heart rate vary due to the mix of vagal and sympathetic stimulation of the heart.

Long after immediate life-threatening effects of anti-AChE agents clear, residual effects may possibly be observed. Follow-up studies of people exposed to sarin in the Tokyo subway attack in 1995 suggest that, in addition to post-traumatic stress disorder, acute sarin poisoning may cause a chronic decrement in psychomotor performance and a delayed adverse effect on the vestibulo-cerebellar system.[7,8]

Low-dose exposure to nerve gas may produce a variety of symptoms.[9] Up to one-third of all exposed subjects report one or more of the following symptoms: irritability, impaired memory, impaired concentration, depression, visual difficulties, or fatigue. It is difficult to determine whether these complaints were of pure psychic origin due to the stress associated with exposure or whether they were the consequence of disturbed cholinergic neurotransmission, an unmasking of one or more preexisting conditions, or some combination of these mechanisms. Regardless of what mechanism is responsible for the production of the symptoms, disabling symptoms may occur with some frequency.

Since relatively few people have been exposed to sublethal doses of nerve agents, it is possible that additional effects could occur. This is a difficult problem to approach experimentally because there appears to be much species-specific variation in the effects of the various anticholinergic agents, in spite of an apparently common mechanism of action. Thus, it is impossible to predict the effects of sublethal exposures of large populations that might be due to organic lesions in the nervous system.[10]

Vesicants.   Vesicants were used widely in World War I, and there is convincing evidence for their use—largely ignored by the world community—in conflicts between Iraq and Iran. These agents all act by producing chemical burns, typically affecting epithelial membranes of the skin and respiratory tract.[11] Severe exposure, particularly by inhalation, impairs gas exchange in the lungs, and victims die of hypoxia. Nonfatal inhalations may be followed by pneumonia. Severe skin burns may also be fatal due to loss of body fluids or secondary infections (Figure 11–1). Nonfatal exposures produce permanent disability due to damage to the epithelial surfaces of the lung, cornea, and other tissues.

Sulfur mustard is probably the only vesicant agent that has been used in war, and most likely to be used again. Mustard is a DNA alkylator and "radiomimetic" with triphasic effects: the skin and eyes affected early, then the lungs, and finally the bone marrow. Mustard is very insidious in its effects. It rapidly penetrates or fixes to tissue before producing any symptoms. Once symptoms have begun, decontamination is no longer effective. Mustard produces many incapacitating casualities due to skin and eye burns with low lethality; fatalities arise mainly from pulmonary complications. If treatment resources are not overwhelmed, modern burn and respiratory treatment, along with use of antibiotics, would likely reduce mortality. Increasing ambient temperature decreases the persistence of mustard, but increases the vapor hazard.

Many of these vesicants are mutagenic and carcinogenic. This property of these compounds has received less attention than the properties that cause death or long-term disability.[10]

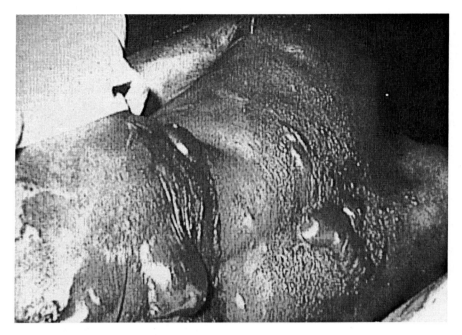

FIGURE 11–1. Victim of vesicant exposure with prominent skin blisters (Courtesy of the U.S. Army Office of the Surgeon General).

Pulmonary-Damaging Agents.   These include phosgene and chlorine. Phosgene, a colorless, but highly toxic gas, causes, after exposure to concentrations of 3 to 5 ppm, immediate irritant effects, including conjunctivitis, rhinitis, pharyngitis, bronchitis, tearing, spasm of the eyelids, conjunctival hyperemia, and upper respiratory tract irritation. After exposure to higher doses, severe pulmonary toxicity may occur. On rare occasions, pulmonary edema can be delayed for a period up to 48 hours. If the victim survives for 48 hours, prognosis is usually favorable. Treatment involves decontamination, including administration of 100 percent humidified supplemental oxygen, symptomatic and supportive treatment, and treating pulmonary edema if it occurs. Chlorine is also severely irritating to the eyes, skin, nose, throat, and mucous membranes. As with phosgene, respiratory symptoms may be immediate or delayed for several hours. Increased airway reactivity and decreased residual volume have occurred as sequelae, for up to 12 years following an acute exposure. Treatment is similar to that of phosgene exposure.[12]

Blood Agents, or Cyanides.   These chemicals include arsine, cyanogen chloride, and hydrogen cyanide. Cyanide, an example of these agents, can cause serious consequences and death within a few minutes. Cyanide is extremely volatile and tends to evaporate and be blown away; being lighter than air, it tends not to stay close to the ground. The dose needed to cause adverse health effects may be relatively large. Cyanide causes its adverse health effects by combining with a cellular enzyme and inhibiting its activity. Symptoms are often nonspecific, including rapid and deep breathing, feelings of anxiety and apprehension, agitation, dizziness, weakness, nausea, and muscle trembling. With higher doses, there is loss of consciousness, decreased respiration, seizures, and arrhythmias. Cyanogen chloride is very irritating and produces burning of the eyes, the nose, and the airways. Treatment of cyanide exposure may include administration of two antidotes, given sequentially: first, a nitrite, and the second, sodium thiosulfate. Oxygen (100% oxygen) should be given, even though the oxygen content of blood is normal.[13]

Riot-Control Agents: Tear Gas as an Example. In addition to widespread use of tear gas by civil authorities to control crowds and disable people, military forces have also used these compounds for similar reasons.[14] Tear gas, when correctly used, is purported to be safe because the effects are believed to be transient and free of long-term effects. Use of these compounds is alleged to be more humane than alternative, more violent measures. Deaths due to direct toxic effects of tear gas have been documented, however. Explosions of tear gas bombs or impacts by delivery vehicles may also cause injury or death. Because of these considerations, 80 countries voted that tear gas should be banned by the Geneva Protocol.

About 15 compounds have been used as tear gas. Of these, four have been used more extensively (omega-chloroacetophenone, or CN; o-chlorobenzylidenemalonitrile, or CS; 10-chlor-5, 10-dihydrophenarasazine; and α-bromo-α-tolunitril). These chemicals are potent lacrimators and irritants. Other populations, such as children and patients with asthma or obstructive or restrictive pulmonary disease, are likely to be more susceptible to these agents and are at greater risk. Studies in animals have shown that ingestion can cause gastroenteritis with perforation. CS is metabolized to form cyanide in peripheral tissues. It is not clear whether the amounts of cyanide formed under these circumstances are likely to have important biological effects. Long-term human studies are nearly impossible to perform because of the circumstances that surround use of these agents.[10]

Potential Risks of Treatment

Certain treatments for the effects of chemical weapons are not without risk. For example, temporary relief from the effects of nerve agents may be provided by the use of cholinergic drugs such as atropine (Table 11–2). In Israel during the Persian Gulf War, self-injecting syringes filled with atropine were provided to the population. Although there was no evidence that a nerve agent was used against Israel, a number of cases of atropine poisoning from self-injection were reported.[15,16] In addition, there were some deaths in Israel due to asphyxiation from incorrect use of respirators (gas masks), especially in young children.

CHEMICAL TERRORISM

It is difficult to predict which chemical weapons terrorists are likely to use.[17–19] Chemical agents, according to their presumed likelihood of use, are described in Table 11–3. Terrorist groups that have ideological motives and want public support may hesitate to use chemical weapons because these weapons have abhorrent effects and might harm the image of the user. Groups whose objective is to create chaos and fear may not hesitate to use chemicals as weapons. Given that terrorists used civilian aircraft as weapons of mass destruction, they may utilize commercial or industrial chemical substances or attack chemical production or storage sites.

The first documented use of chemical weapons by terrorists occurred in Matsumoto, Japan, in 1994, and a year later in the Tokyo metro. The Aum Shinrikyo group used sarin in both attacks, killing a total of 19 people and injuring more than 5,000.[20,21] These attacks made people worldwide realize that chemical weapons could be used in terrorist attacks (see Box 11–2 and Figure 11–2).

To terrorists, the use of chemical weapons would appear to have several advantages over other types of weapons: They are cheap to manufacture. Only simple technology is needed to produce them. They are difficult to detect. They are highly efficient. And, very important, they are extremely frightening.

Psychological effects can be associated either with actual or threatened use of chemical weapons. Chemically hazardous civilian environments can produce physical or psychological symptoms. Awareness of a chemical terrorist threat or living in an environment contaminated with chemicals may make people chemophobic—fearful of a "chemical catastrophe." For example, in Russia, there are more than 3,600 businesses that use hazardous chemicals and 146 cities situated in chemically endangered areas. According to the Russian Ministry of Disaster Resources, from 1992 to 1996, approximately 250 chemical incidents ("accidents") occurred, with discharges of extremely toxic chemicals affecting more than 800 people and killing 69.[22] In the United States each year, there are thousands of chemical spills, leaks, and explosions, many of which are classified as "serious," with hundreds affected. However, about three-fourths of all chemical accidents are controlled without any recognized adverse health effects in humans. A threatened attack can

TABLE 11-3. Characteristics of Selected Chemical Weapons of Potential Bioterrorist Use.

	EASE OF MANUFACTURE	ENVIRONMENTAL PERSISTENCE/STABILITY	LETHAL EFFECTS	OBSERVATIONS
NERVE AGENTS				
VX	Difficult to manufacture.	High	Very high	**Not likely weapon**, because of manufacturing problems.
Soman	Difficult.	Moderate	High	**Not likely**, because of manufacturing problems.
Sarin	Moderately difficult.	Not persistent	High	**Likely agent**, but restrictions on ingredients needed in intermediate steps could create difficulties for production.
Tabun	Relatively easy.	Moderate	High	**Likely agent**, because of ease of manufacture.
CHOKING AGENTS				
Chlorine	Industrial product.	Not persistent	Low	**Likely agent**, widely available commercially.
Phosgene	Industrial product.	Not persistent	Low	**Likely agent**, widely available commercially.

(General Accounting Office. *Risk Assessments: The Chemical Threat.* As reported in the *New York Times*, November 1, 2001, p. B7.)

Box 11–2. Sarin Attacks in Japan.

Although use of chemical weapons against civilian populations in the Iran-Iraq War was well documented,[1] it has received relatively little international attention. The more recent use of a nerve agent in two separate terrorist attacks in Japan, however, awakened considerable public concern.[2–5] The attacks are alleged to have been planned and executed by the Aum Shinrikyo sect. Since these attacks occurred in densely populated areas where excellent medical care and high media attention were instantly available, they are particularly well documented and publicized.

The first attack occurred in June 1994 in Matsumoto (population 200,000) in the central highlands of Honshu. The initial ambulance call was made by a man whose wife had lost consciousness and whose dog had died outside their home. Within the next three hours, three people were found dead, four died on their way to hospitals, 56 were admitted to hospitals, and 253 consulted physicians. Ten days later, police and governmental officials announced that they had found traces of sarin, which was identified by gas chromatography and mass spectrometry in samples taken from a pond.

The second attack occurred in the Tokyo subway system in March 1995. There were 12 deaths, and approximately 5,000 people were injured. Many of those hospitalized— 39 at one hospital alone—were emergency medical technicians who were exposed to sarin while conducting rescue operations (Figure 11–2).

These two attacks received extensive media coverage. Details of the clinical presentation, treatment, and long-term observation of exposed victims have been published in prominent medical journals. A number of points have emerged from this experience.

The first attack occurred at night with release of sarin in an open environment, with relatively calm winds (0.5 m/s). There has been speculation that this attack was conducted as an exercise to prepare for the subsequent attack. Even under these conditions, which were less than ideal for maximizing casualties from sarin, there were many casualties. The second attack, conducted in the Tokyo subway system, targeted highly vulnerable civilians and was seemingly designed to maximize casualties. Subways in Tokyo are densely populated, particularly during rush hour, and air exchange rates are low, confining the gas to a small volume of air occupied by many people.

In the wake of these attacks, questions were again raised about control of chemical weapons. Since many of the raw materials are common reagents, such as pyrophosphate and phosphoric acid, complete control of all of them is neither practical nor desirable in a free economy. An editorial in *Nature*, however, noted that "the treaty on chemical weapons signed last year is weaker than it should be because of the reluctance of legitimate chemical manufacturers to volunteer full disclosure of their use of raw materials."[2] Predictably, there were also suggestions that monitoring systems should be considered to detect the release of chemical agents so that corrective action might be taken sooner.

BOX REFERENCES
1. Hu H, Cook-Deegan R, Shukri A. The use of chemical weapons: conducting an investigation using survey epidemiology. *JAMA* 1989; 262:640–643.

(continued)

(continued)
2. Murder on the metro. *Nature* 1995; 374: 392.
3. Morita H, Yanagisawa N, Nakajima T, et al. Sarin poisoning in Matsumoto, Japan. *Lancet* 1995; 346: 290–293.
4. Suzuki T, Morita H, Ono K. Sarin poisoning in Tokyo subway (letter). *Lancet* 1995; 345:980.
5. Lifton RJ. *Destroying the World to Save It: Aum Shinrikyo, Apocalyptic Violence and the New Global Terrorism*. New York: Harry Holt and Company, 1999.

(Adapted from: Lockwood, AH. "The Public Health Effects of the Use of Chemical Weapons." In: BS Levy, VS Sidel, eds. *War and Public Health*. New York: Oxford University Press, 1997, pp. 93–94.)

influence the behavior of military personnel as well as civilians, and may cause adverse health effects from fear. "Expectancy" symptoms are nonspecific and may include shortness of breath, anxiety, irritability, disturbed vision, loss of the sense of time, poor concentration, confusion, disorientation, hallucinations, tremor, and nausea. Some of these symptoms may be due to wearing personal protective equipment, which can restrict vision and movement and increase body heat.

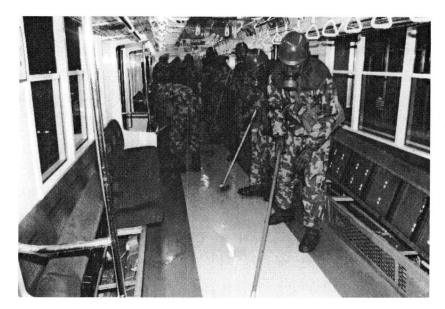

FIGURE 11–2. Workers with gas masks and full protective equipment decontaminate a subway car in Tokyo after the sarin attack in 1995 (Kyodo News International, Inc.).

Civilian Use of Chemicals

Problems related to the use of chemicals, from leaks and explosions in civilian production and use to military and terrorist use of chemicals, are intertwined. Since 2001, a World Health Organization (WHO) working group of chemical experts from around the world has been making an inventory of response mechanisms to chemical incidents.[23] The best mechanisms that were identified could serve as models for regional, national, and international responses to any chemical incident. Ideally, an early warning system would enable teams of standby health and safety professionals, police and firefighters, and, if need be, military personnel, to respond quickly to treat those affected and prevent further adverse health consequences. Internet and mobile communication mechanisms could help activate other responders. Where there are existing response mechanisms, local community workers and health and safety professionals would be involved in the response, as would military personnel in response to a suspected terrorist incident due to chemical weapons. In addition, on a global scale, teams of the OPCW will also respond to such an incident.[24,25] Hazardous materials (hazmat) teams and local emergency planning committees (LEPCs) have become well-established in the United States over the last decade, and also prepare and train for terror contingencies. The United States Chemical Safety and Hazard Investigation Board, which began operations in 1998, was established to promote the prevention of major chemical accidents at fixed facilities.

Many countries, especially the less-developed countries, lack adequate response mechanisms for chemical incidents. Many industrial and agricultural chemical incidents have occurred, including:

- Release of methyl isocyanate (MIC) from a pesticide factory in Bhopal, India, in 1984, causing 4,035 deaths and seriously affecting 50,000 others;[26] and
- Release of dioxin (2,3,7,8-tetrachlorodibenzo-p-dioxin, or simply TCDD) from a chemical plant in Seveso, Italy, in 1976, exposing as many as 300,000 people in 11 municipalities.

Personal Protective Equipment

Personal protective equipment will be important to military and emergency personnel, but will not be a viable means of protecting the public at large. Since the primitive masks worn during World War I, the development of new types of personal protective equipment has kept pace with the development of new types of chemical weapons. Currently available masks, each consisting of an aerosol filter and an activated-carbon gas filter, can protect against inhalation of chemicals. The skin also requires protection against liquid and solid chemical agents.

The level of protection depends on a number of considerations, such as: How much time is needed to put on the equipment? Will there be any advance warning? What is the absorbent capacity of the respiratory filter? What is the likely degree of leakage? For protective clothing, both penetration (passage through hole or seams) and permeation (diffusion through material) must be considered. In the past, protective clothing was impermeable, creating problems in heat regulation and fluid balance, especially in warm climates and during exercise. Modern clothing is permeable and has a layer of activated carbon; when designed in one piece, penetration is minimal. If heavy exposure is possible, an impermeable suit can be worn for a short period of time.

Over the years, demand for comfortable protective clothing and equipment has increased, in part because of the need for long-term use. (When there is uncertainty if chemical weapons will be used, as was the case during the Persian Gulf War, protective equipment may be required continuously.) For masks, inhalation and exhalation have been made easier, the visual field has been enlarged, and communication has been improved by installing speech devices.

Decontamination

When early warning and avoidance of contamination fail, decontamination of both personnel and equipment is necessary. Because chemicals can penetrate surfaces and thus cause prolonged release of toxic gases, decontamination becomes more difficult. Decontamination can be achieved by physical or chemical destruction of the agent, isolating it, washing it off, absorbing it, or evaporating it. Some decontaminants, although very effective, may not be suitable for all surfaces. The better the identification of the agent, the more closely the decontaminating process can be matched to it (see Table 11–2). In decontaminating a person, the most important consideration is time: the longer the exposure has been, the greater the damage. In removing clothes of a contaminated person, care must be taken to avoid transferring the chemical to the skin. Good results may be achieved with water and soap, talc, or flour. Personal decontaminants—such as chloramines in alcohol for mustard agents and either sodium phenolate or sodium cresolate in alcohol or bentonite as an absorbent powder for nerve agents—may be useful.

If decontamination is not possible, contact with the chemical must be avoided until the chemical has lost its toxicity. The time needed varies according to the characteristics of the chemical used and the surface on which it is located. For example, on metal surfaces, soman disappears within 5 hours, but the nerve agent VX may last as long as 1 week.

Improving Preparedness

There are other measures that are likely to be more effective in strengthening systems and protecting people. These include stockpiling of appropriate antidotes against chemical agents (see Table 11–2), developing decontamination facilities that could quickly be made operational as needed, and better preparing hospitals and other medical-care facilities. A survey published in 2001 found that fewer than 20 percent of respondent hospitals had plans for biological or chemical weapons incidents. Only 6 percent had the minimum recommended physical resources for a hypothetical sarin incident. It concluded that hospital emergency departments generally are not prepared in an organized fashion to treat victims of chemical or biological terrorism, and that substantial additional resources at the local level will be required to improve domestic preparedness.[27]

CONTROL OF CHEMICAL WEAPONS AND THEIR HEALTH CONSEQUENCES

The Chemical Weapons Convention (CWC)

More than 10 years of negotiations resulted in the CWC, which came into force in 1997. An independent international institution, the Organization for the Prohibition of Chemical Weapons (OPCW), was established in The Hague to provide verification and other services to the member states, including assistance in case of an alleged attack (see Box 11–1).

Member states have been required under the CWC to declare their relevant chemical substances within 30 days of active participation in the Convention. Chemical weapons under government control are easily declarable. Through inspections, chemical weapons are monitored and will be destroyed, as required by the CWC, in special facilities by the end of 2012.

The civilian chemical industry does not reveal much information, however, in part because of patent laws and fears of industrial espionage. Industry has new concerns about publicly disclosing chemical inventories because they might become targets of an attack to steal chemicals that could be misused or become targets of attacks designed to provoke catastrophic hazardous materials releases. These concerns must be balanced against the public's right to know and emergency planners' need to prepare.

The OPCW has inspection teams with experts in different fields of chemistry. These teams perform onsite inspections in the following three categories:

1. *Inspection of chemical weapons and related facilities*
   Following the declaration by a member state of its chemical weapons, its stockpiles of these weapons are sealed and regularly reinspected until all of them have been destroyed. Because of previous experience with similar inspection teams for other weapon reduction treaties, such as the START I Treaty (see Chapter 12), there has been almost no resistance from political or military leaders.

2. *Industry inspections*
   Because civilian chemical industry facilities are geographically diffuse and quite variable in nature and magnitude, it is not easy to monitor them. Managers of these companies, however, have understood that willingness to cooperate would be wise for public-relations reasons. For confidentiality purposes, a facility agreement is made for every inspection, in which the mode of inspection and degree of access are agreed upon. Previous experience with similar inspections, such as by the International Atomic Energy Agency (IAEA; see Chapter 12), have been helpful in facilitating these inspections.

3. *Challenge inspections*
   Every member state has the right to request an onsite challenge inspection, if there is a good reason to do so. Such requests are carefully evaluated by the executive council of the OPCW because they have consequences for possible noncompliance with the treaty and possible financial implications for the requesting party.

Based on the requirements of the CWC, facilities to destroy chemical weapons have been built in the United States and planned in Russia. Destruction of chemical weapons can be accomplished by chemical detoxification or by burning, which may cause environmental problems if not performed safely. Seven destruction facilities for chemical weapons are planned to be built in Russia; at Shchuchye, the largest and most important of these facilities; 5,400 tons of VX are slated for destruction.[28] The financial situation in Russia makes it unable to meet its obligations to destroy all of its chemical weapons in the short term, even though the European Union and the United States have provided financial support for the destruction of these weapons.

In the United States, destruction facilities have been built, often despite community objections, in several states in which chemical weapons are stockpiled. This has been done in order to minimize the risk of transporting these weapons. U.S. chemical weapons were transferred from Europe to an island in the Pacific Ocean for destruction, and destruction of them is reported to be completed.

POTENTIAL CHEMICAL WEAPONS OF THE FUTURE

The line between biological weapons (Chapter 10) and chemical weapons is being blurred by rapid developments in biotechnology and the emergence of a new generation of toxins and bioregulators. Many of them exceed the toxicity of nerve agents by several orders of magnitude.

Modern biotechnological weapons can be based on sophisticated application of the structure-activity relationships of toxins and substances produced within the body, and targeted at particular cell receptors in selected organs. Although these new weapons are mainly in research and developmental stages today, their potential threat includes: activity in very low concentrations; a pattern of toxicity that is difficult to diagnose and treat; the ability to be completely broken down within the body; lack of antidotes for medical protection and treatment; and lack of detection techniques and devices.[4]

Acknowledgment

We acknowledge the assistance of Stefanos Kales, M.D., M.P.H., who reviewed an earlier draft of this chapter and made many helpful comments and suggestions.

Editors' Update

There is recent evidence that both Russia and the United States are developing new forms of "non-lethal" chemical weapons. On October 26, 2002, Russian special forces reportedly used a gas that was based on the opiate fentanyl to incapacitate approximately 50 heavily-armed Chechen insurgents who were holding hundreds of civilians hostage in a Moscow theater. The Russian health minister later estimated that more than 100 hostages had died from the effects of the drug. The minister declared that chemical compounds that could fall under the authority of the CWC were not used during the course of the special forces operation. The use of this agent reignited debate about the use of "non-lethal" chemical weapons and their status under the CWC. In the course of this debate, it was revealed that the U.S. Department of Defense had in the year 2000 sought corporate bids to perform research on the development of "non-lethal" chemical compounds for military or law-enforcement use. Analysts are concerned that the Moscow episode could be a harbinger of future events, and that modern advances in the life sciences could be applied to the development of new types of chemical weapons.

REFERENCES

1. Medical aspects of chemical and biological weapons. *Textbook of Military Medicine.* Office of the Surgeon General, Department of the Army, USA, 1997.

2. Watkins OS. Methodist report. In: Fries AA, *Chemical Warfare*. New York: McGraw-Hill, 1921.

3. Infield GB. *Disaster at Bari*. New York: Macmillan Company, 1991.

4. Defence Research Establishment (FOA), Sweden. *A FOA Briefing Book on Chemical Weapons*. Stockholm: FOA, 1992.

5. www.sbccom.army.mil/programs/stockpile.htm

6. Lockwood AH. Nerve gases. *PSR Quarterly* 1991; 1:69–76.

7. Yokoyama K, Araki S, Murata K, et al. Chronic neurobehavioral effects of Tokyo subway sarin poisoning in relation to posttraumatic stress disorder. *Arch Environ Health* 1998; 53:249–256.

8. Yokoyama K, Araki S, Murata K, et al. A preliminary study on delayed vestibulo-cerebellar effects of Tokyo subway sarin poisoning in relation to gender difference: frequency analysis of postural sway. *J Occup Environ Med* 1998; 40:17–21.

9. Fullerton CS, Ursano RJ. Behavioral and psychological responses to chemical and biological warfare. *Mil Med.* 1990; 155:54–59.

10. Lockwood AH. The public health effects of the use of chemical weapons. In: BS Levy, VW Sidel, eds. *War and Public Health*. New York: Oxford University Press, 1997, pp. 84–97.

11. Carnes SA, Watson AP. Disposing of the U.S. chemical weapons stockpile: an approaching reality. *JAMA* 1989; 262:653–659.

12. Sifton DW (ed.). *PDR Guide to Biological and Chemical Warfare Response*. Montvale, NJ: Thomson/Physicians' Desk Reference, 2002.

13. Maniscalco PM, Christen HT (eds.). *Understanding Terrorism and Managing the Consequences*. Upper Saddle River, NJ: Prentice Hall, 2002.

14. Hu H, Fine J, Epstein P, et al. Tear gas: Harassing agents or toxic chemical weapon? *JAMA* 1989; 262:660–663.

15. Amitai Y, Almog S, Singer R, et al. Atropine poisoning in children during the Persian Gulf crisis. A national survey in Israel. *JAMA* 1992; 268:630–632.

16. Almog S, Winkler E, Amitia Y, et al. Acute pyridostigmine overdose: a report of nine cases. *Isr J Med Sci* 1991; 27:659–663.

17. www.terrorismfiles.org

18. http://web.nps.navy.mil/~library/tgp/tgpndx.htm (Centre for Non-Proliferation Studies).

19. http://cns.miis.edu/research/cbw/index.htm (Monterey Institute of International Studies).

20. OPCW. Synthesis, summer 2001.

21. http://rcmp-learning.org/docs/

22. Chimitcheskoye Razoruzheniye (Chemical Disarmament; http://pfo.metod.ru/data/issue/otrasli/ho/index.html)

23. WHO expert working group on chemical incidents, internal report, 2001.

24. www.opcw.org

25. ISIS Briefing Paper No. 75, January 2000.

26. Centre for European Disaster Medicine (CEMEC).

27. Wetter DC, Daniell WE, Treser CD. Hospital preparedness for victims of chemical or biological terrorism. *Amer J Pub Health* 2001; 91:710–716.

28. http://www.nandotimes.com, February 9, 2001, Health & Science.

12

Nuclear, radiological, and related weapons

PATRICE M. SUTTON AND ROBERT M. GOULD

The potential use by terrorists of nuclear, radiological, and related weapons expands the nuclear weapons threat to new actors with links to the global complex of nuclear weapons and nuclear power facilities. Measures to address this enhanced threat need to move well beyond law enforcement and military action, to the strengthening of stable, long-term global mechanisms in order to safeguard nuclear weapons and nuclear materials. At the same time, specific plans need to be developed to eliminate all nuclear weapons.

TYPES OF WEAPONS

Nuclear Weapons

A nuclear weapon suddenly releases vast quantities of energy by splitting the nuclei of atoms (fission) and/or by fusing the nuclei of pairs of atoms (fusion) (Figure 12–1). It is estimated that even a crude nuclear weapon has potential explosive force at least 1,000 times higher than the most powerful conventional explosive ever deployed.[1]

The essential ingredients of every nuclear weapon are fissile material compressed into a "supercritical mass" so that the number of fissions will esca-

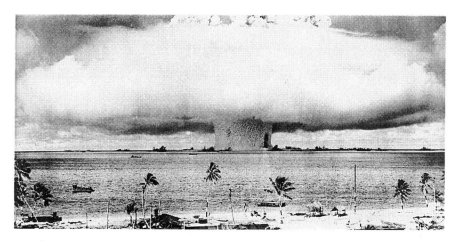

Figure 12–1. United States atomic-bomb test at Bikini atoll in the Pacific in 1946 (Library of Congress, Negative LC-USZ 62-66049).

late very rapidly and create a nuclear explosion.[2,3] The two principal fissile materials used in making nuclear weapons are uranium-235 and plutonium-239. Uranium found in nature contains less than 1 percent uranium-235.[3] To produce the supercritical mass required for nuclear weapons, uranium must be "enriched" chemically to increase the percentage of uranium-235 to 90 percent or more. Uranium enriched to more than 90 percent is considered weapons-grade, highly enriched uranium (HEU), but uranium enriched to significantly lower percentages is also weapons-usable.[4] Virtually all plutonium-239 is produced by bombarding uranium-238 with neutrons in nuclear reactors.[5]

Radiological Weapons ("Dirty Bombs")

A radiological weapon ("dirty bomb") disperses radioactive materials with a conventional device, rather than with a nuclear explosion. During World War II, the United States initiated a research program to determine the feasibility of dispersing radioactive material with the use of conventional weapons.[6] More recently, Iraq has acknowledged to the United Nations that it explored the use of radiological weapons against Iran.[7] Iraq reportedly tested a radiological bomb meant to weaken enemy forces by inducing radiation sickness, but abandoned this type of weapon because radiation levels created were not sufficiently high.[8] In 1995, alleged Islamic rebels from Chechnya were reported to have buried—but not to have detonated—a 30-pound box of cesium-137 and dynamite near the entrance of a busy Moscow park.[9] Radioactive materials in wide use in the United States, such as certain isotopes

of cesium and cobalt rods used for food irradiation, have also been identified as possible source materials for radiological weapons.[10] In early 2002,
the U.S. government was reported to be interested in developing the ability
to use radiological weapons to destroy stockpiles of chemical or biological
agents.[11] In March 2002, the *Washington Post* published an analysis of the
ways radioactive cesium and strontium in radiothermal generators that had
been abandoned in, or stolen from, the former Soviet Union could be used
in radiological weapons.[11a]

Although characterized as "conventional" weapons by the United States
and the North Atlantic Treaty Organization (NATO) and not strictly intended
as radiological weapons, the use of depleted-uranium weapons, according to
the World Health Organization (WHO), may pose a radiation and chemical
exposure hazard for military personnel, children, and others who may be exposed if the depleted uranium enters the body through inhalation, ingestion,
or through wounds.[12] Depleted uranium is the material remaining after enriched uranium (containing a higher percentage of the uranium-235 isotope)
is removed for use in nuclear power plants. Depleted-uranium weapons were
used by the United States in 1991 during the Persian Gulf War and in 1999
in the war in the Balkans.[13]

Targets as Weapons: Nuclear Power Facilities and Transportation Routes

Nuclear power plants, as technologically complex repositories of vast quantities of radioactive materials, are potential targets of terrorist attacks. Statements by the International Atomic Energy Agency (IAEA) and research studies conducted by the U.S. Department of Energy have demonstrated that the
containment structures around nuclear reactors may be breached by attacks
such as those that occurred at the World Trade Center in 2001.[14,15] In addition, areas outside the containment structure are equally, if not more, vulnerable to terrorist attacks.

Normally, after nuclear material used as fuel in power production is depleted through irradiation, the "spent fuel" is placed underwater in pools
outside of the reactor containment structure in order to shield the radiation and dissipate the heat that continues to emanate from the fuel.[16] Spent
fuel pools contain more long-lived radioactivity than reactor cores.[17] If the
pools sustain structural damage so that the water boils or drains away, the
spent-fuel assemblies will overheat and either melt or catch on fire.[16,17]
Control rooms are also vulnerable, as they are located outside of containment structures, in far less robust structures.[18] Highly radioactive fuel is
also stored at nuclear power facilities outdoors in large dry casks. At some
plants, casks are surrounded by chain-link fences, but stored in areas that

are unguarded. In other instances, the casks are visible from places of open access.[16]

Transporting highly radioactive materials away from nuclear power plants presents additional opportunities for the intentional or unintentional release of radioactive materials into the environment. If implemented, recently authorized plans for the transport of highly radioactive waste from nuclear power plants across the United States to a proposed long-term storage site at Yucca Mountain, Nevada, would involve the transport of tens of thousands of shipments of highly radioactive waste by train and truck across 43 states over the next 30 years; 50 million people would be living within one-half mile of the projected routes.[19,20] Two experiments conducted in cooperation with the U.S. Army at the Aberdeen Proving Ground in 1998 demonstrate that the containers used to transport radioactive materials are vulnerable to attack.[21]

USE OF NUCLEAR AND RELATED WEAPONS

To date, the use of nuclear and related weapons has been the sole purview of nation-states. A nuclear weapon was first used in warfare on August 6, 1945, at 8:15 a.m., when the United States exploded a nuclear weapon over Hiroshima. The bomb had an explosive force equivalent to 15,000 tons of TNT. Three days later, the United States exploded a bomb equivalent to 21,000 tons of TNT over Nagasaki (Figure 12–2).[22]

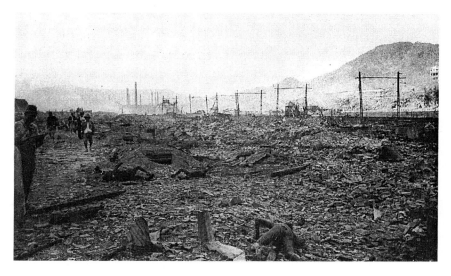

FIGURE 12–2. Nagasaki, August 10, 1945 (the day after the bombing), near the Matsuyan–Machi intersection close to the hypocenter (Photograph by Yosuke Yamahata; used with the permission of Shogo Yamahata).

Non-state actors could acquire a nuclear weapon by: (1) stealing or gaining control of a weapon already made by a nation with nuclear weapons; or (2) stealing, or otherwise illegally acquiring, military or civilian weapons-usable fissile material and fabricating an explosive device for detonating it.[4] According to U.S. Energy Secretary Spencer Abraham, "The theft of only a very small quantity of highly enriched uranium or plutonium . . . would be enough for a crude but potentially devastating nuclear weapon."[23] Since 1993, the IAEA has recorded 16 cases involving illicit trafficking of plutonium or enriched uranium.[24]

In order to achieve their putative political objectives, *non-state* actors would not necessarily require weapons that possess the yield, "safety," reliability, and technical sophistication that are desired in *state* weapons programs.[1] A non-state actor could construct a crude, highly enriched uranium bomb, with the explosive power of several hundred to a few thousand tons of TNT, that could be transported by and detonated in an ordinary van.[4] Other potential terrorist scenarios involve the holding of a nuclear weapon, nuclear power facility, or nuclear plant personnel for political or economic blackmail.[4,25]

PROLIFERATION OF NUCLEAR AND RELATED WEAPONS

The proliferation of nuclear weapons and related technologies over the past half-century has resulted in the wide distribution of vast quantities of nuclear weapons and fissile and other radioactive materials throughout the world (Table 12–1). The numbers of nuclear weapons in the U.S. and Russian stockpiles have been decreasing over the past decade. Yet recent U.S. government decisions—to abrogate the Anti-Ballistic Missile Treaty, to deploy a national missile defense system (which would be ineffective against most scenarios of nuclear terrorism), and to develop a new generation of nuclear weapons— may stimulate additional global proliferation (see Box 12–1).[29,30]

Plutonium from civilian nuclear reactors can be used to make nuclear and radiological weapons.[4,31] The relationship between nuclear power and nuclear weapons has been described as a form of "latent proliferation"—short of the actual possession of nuclear weapons, but accounting for a supply of raw materials and intellectual know-how that are capable of producing nuclear weapons.[31] The proliferation potential from civilian nuclear power programs has been illustrated by: (a) reactor-grade plutonium being used to fabricate a nuclear weapon exploded by the U.S. military in 1962; and (b) civilian nuclear power and research programs being integrally involved with the nuclear weapons programs of both India and Pakistan.[4,32]

Civilian plutonium is contained in an irradiated form (spent fuel) or in a separated, non-irradiated form. In order to be used in nuclear weapons, plu-

TABLE 12–1. Proliferation of Nuclear Weapons and Radioactive Materials.

SOURCE	QUANTITY
Nuclear Weapons*	Global nuclear weapons stockpile of approximately 25,000 to 33,000 weapons is distributed among eight countries: United States, 10,500–12,000; Russia, 13,000–20,000; France, 400–482; China, 400–410; Great Britain, 200; India, enough separated weapons-grade plutonium to make 85–90; Israel, enough weapons-grade fissile material for 100 weapons; and Pakistan, 15–25. Iran, Iraq, North Korea, and Libya are believed to be attempting now, or have in the past attempted, to develop nuclear weapons.[26]
Plutonium and Highly-Enriched Uranium (HEU) Stockpiles	Global plutonium stockpile, as of 1999, was 1,520 tons. Of the 1,270 tons in civilian stores, 205 tons (16 percent) are in separated form; of the 250 tons in military stores, more than 90 percent is in separated form. Separated form is more usable in weapons. Global highly enriched uranium (HEU) stockpile, as of 1999, was 1,690 tons (1,670 tons military, 20 tons civilian).[27]
Nuclear-Power Plants	In the United States: 103 licensed nuclear-power reactors, located at 65 plant sites in 31 states;[28] 14 decommissioned plants, some of which still contain radioactive material;[14] 40,000 metric tons of spent nuclear fuel are stored in pools at 110 operating and closed reactor sites, with over two billion curies of long-lived radioactivity;[17] globally: 433 nuclear-power plants are operating in 44 countries.[26]

*Estimates include strategic and non-strategic weapons. Estimates for U.S. and Russian warheads include those in active, operational forces as well as retired, non-deployed warheads awaiting dismantlement and weapons in reserve.

tonium must be chemically extracted from the spent fuel at "reprocessing" plants.[33] Worldwide, there is about five times more total plutonium in civilian stores than in military stockpiles.[27] Because the overwhelming amount of civilian plutonium is in the form of irradiated fuel, however, civilian stockpiles (205 tons) and military stockpiles (225 tons) of separated plutonium are almost equal.[27] The amount of separated plutonium from civilian nuclear power plants will rapidly increase as more reprocessing capacity becomes operational.[4]

ADVERSE CONSEQUENCES OF PRODUCTION AND USE

Detonation of a nuclear weapon results in blast, heat, and the release of radiation. Radiological weapons result in the release of radiation and, depending on the scenario of use, the much lower blast force of a conventional weapon or explosive.

There is no comprehensive treaty banning the use or mandating the destruction of nuclear weapons. Instead, a series of overlapping incomplete treaties has been negotiated:

The Partial Test Ban Treaty (PTBT) of 1963, promoted, in part, by public health concerns, banned nuclear tests in the atmosphere, underwater, and in outer space.

The expansion of the PTBT, the Comprehensive Nuclear-Test-Ban Treaty (CTBT), a key step towards nuclear disarmament and preventing proliferation, was opened for signature in 1996 and has not yet entered into force. It bans nuclear explosions, for either military or civilian purposes, but does not ban computer simulations and subcritical tests (tests involving chain reactions that do not reach criticality), which some nations rely on to maintain the option of developing new nuclear weapons. As of early 2002, the CTBT had been signed by 165 nations and ratified by 89. Entry into force requires ratification by the 44 nuclear-capable nations, of which 31 had ratified the CTBT by early 2002.

The Treaty on the Non-Proliferation of Nuclear Weapons (the "Non-Proliferation Treaty," or NPT) was opened for signature in 1968 and entered into force in 1970. By early 2002, a total of 187 states parties (nations) had ratified the treaty. The five nuclear-weapon states recognized under the NPT—China, France, Russia, the United Kingdom, and the United States—are parties to the treaty. The NPT attempts to prevent the spread of nuclear weapons by restricting transfer of certain technologies. It relies on safeguards, such as inspections carried out by the International Atomic Energy Agency (IAEA), which also promotes nuclear energy. In exchange for the non-nuclear weapons states' commitment not to develop or otherwise acquire nuclear weapons, the NPT commits the nuclear-weapon states to good-faith negotiations on nuclear disarmament. Every five years since 1970 the states parties have held a review conference to assess implementation of the treaty. The review conference in 2000 identified and approved 13 practical steps towards the total elimination of nuclear arsenals. The next NPT Review Conference is scheduled for 2005.

Another part of the patchwork quilt of anti-nuclear war treaties was the establishment of Nuclear Weapons Free Zones. These zones are to be kept free of nuclear weapons; they are enforced with varying degrees of rigor, the newer ones tending to have more developed implementation provisions. They include the Treaty on the Southeast Asia Nuclear Weapon-Free Zone (Bangkok Treaty), the African Nuclear-Weapon-Free-Zone Treaty (Pelindaba Treaty, which is not yet in force), the South Pacific Nuclear Free Zone Treaty (Treaty of Raratonga), and the Treaty for the Prohibition of Nuclear Weapons in Latin America and the Caribbean (Treaty of Tlatelolco).

The Anti-Ballistic Missile (ABM) Treaty between the United States and the Soviet Union was signed and entered into force in 1972. The treaty was amended in 1974. It was modified in 1997 to include successor states of the Soviet Union: Russia, Ukraine, Kazakhstan, and Belarus.

(continued)

(continued)

The ABM Treaty, by limiting defensive systems that would otherwise spur an offensive arms race, has been seen as the foundation for the Strategic Arms Reduction Treaties (START) process. In late 2001, President George W. Bush announced that the United States would withdraw from the ABM Treaty within six months and gave formal notice, stating that it "hinders our government's ability to develop ways to protect our people from future terrorist or rogue-state missile attacks."

The ABM Treaty, START I and II, and the pending framework for START III have been regarded as the framework for strategic arms control and nuclear reductions between the United States and the Soviet Union, and now Russia. When the U.S. government announced its intention to withdraw from the ABM Treaty, it said it would replace the START process with unilateral mutual reductions—with less accountability and transparency than provided by the START process. Following Russian pressure and public criticism, the United States later agreed to codify these reductions in a treaty. Unlike the START proposals, however, this treaty will not include destruction of weapons removed from deployment and its verification provisions are likely to be less comprehensive than under START.

START I, signed in 1991 by the United States and the Soviet Union, required the reduction of U.S. and Soviet arsenals by 50 percent. START II, signed in 1993 by the United States and Russia, was ratified in 1996 by the United States and in 2000 by Russia (conditional on the United States' not deploying a national missile defense). START II would reduce, by the year 2007, the strategic nuclear arsenals of each country to between 3,000 and 3,500, and eliminate multiple independently targeted warheads (MIRVs) on land-based strategic missiles. Given President Bush's late-2001 announcement of strategic reductions outside the START framework, START II appears, as of March 2002, unlikely to enter into force. But some aspects of the treaty, including its verification provisions and the ban on multiple-warhead ICBMs, may be maintained in the new treaty between the United States and Russia on codifying future strategic reductions.

In 1997, U.S. President Bill Clinton and Russian President Boris Yeltsin had agreed on a framework for START III negotiations, building on START II provisions. Under the START III framework, by 2007 the United States and Russia would have had no more than 2,500 deployed strategic nuclear warheads on intercontinental ballistic missiles, submarine-launched ballistic missiles, and heavy bombers. As of early 2002, START III appeared unlikely to be further negotiated.

—Merav Datan

Use of a nuclear or radiological weapon, or an attack on a nuclear power facility that results in the release of radiation, would lead to exposure to ionizing radiation. How ionizing radiation enters the body depends on its form. Beta particles and gamma rays penetrate the human body; in contrast, alpha particles do not penetrate human skin. Radiation also enters the body through inhalation and ingestion of contaminated food and water, and through wounds.[34]

The adverse health effects associated with the use of nuclear weapons, radiological weapons, and radiation releases from nuclear power facilities are summarized in Table 12–2. Many of the tens of thousands of deaths at Hiroshima and Nagasaki were caused by ionizing radiation.[22] Individuals exposed to radiation at levels sufficient to cause acute radiation sickness may die within a few hours, days, or weeks.[34]

For individuals who do not receive doses high enough to cause acute illness, the primary health impacts of radiation exposure are cancer and inheritable genetic damage.[34] Most of these health impacts will appear years later, making causal inferences difficult.[35] For populations acutely exposed to high doses of ionizing radiation, it is well established that the risk of cancer is

TABLE 12–2. Adverse Health Effects Associated with the Use of Nuclear Weapons, Radiological Weapons, and Radiation Releases from Nuclear Power Facilities, Many of Which Can Be Fatal or Lead to Long-Term Disabilities.

- Acute radiation sickness (nausea, vomiting, diarrhea, fever, hemorrhage, and other symptoms)
- Burns
- Other types of injuries
- Psychological disorders
- Respiratory disorders
- Cancer
- Immunological disorders
- Chromosomal aberrations, birth defects (congenital malformations), and inheritable genetic damage
- Sterility and impaired fertility
- Cataracts
- Premature aging
- Hair loss

IPPNW Global Health Watch Report Number 1: Crude Nuclear Weapons. Proliferation and the Terrorist Threat. Cambridge, Mass.: International Physicians for the Prevention of Nuclear War, 1996.

Yokoro K, Kamada N. The public health effects of the use of nuclear weapons. In: *War and Public Health.* Updated edition. Washington, D.C.: American Public Health Association, 2000, pp. 65–83.

Sumner D, Hu H, Woodward A. Health hazards of nuclear weapons production. In: *Nuclear Wastelands: A Global Guide to Nuclear Weapons Production and Its Health and Environmental Effects.* Cambridge, Mass.: MIT Press, 1995, pp. 65–104.

Last JM. *Public Health and Human Ecology.* Stamford, Conn.: Appleton and Lange, 1998, pp. 185–186.

Forrow L, Blair B, Helfand I, et al. Accidental nuclear war—A post–Cold War assessment. *N Engl J Med.* 1998, 338:1326–31.

Lamb M, Resnikoff M. *Radiological Consequences of Severe Rail Accident Involving Spent Nuclear Fuel Shipments to Yucca Mountain: Hypothetical Baltimore Rail Tunnel Fire Involving SNF,* prepared on behalf of Pacific World History Institute, September 2001.

proportionate to the dose, and no threshold of exposure exists below which there is no cancer risk.[36,37] However, there is considerable controversy concerning the risk of cancer in populations exposed over longer periods of time to lower levels of ionizing radiation. It is generally accepted that the same linear dose–response relationship applies to lower doses,[36] so that the release of even low levels of radiation over a large, densely populated area will, over time, result in many additional cases of cancer. Studies of adult and child community residents near, or workers at, nuclear power facilities indicate that these low-level exposures may result in increased rates of malignancies, including leukemia, non-Hodgkin's lymphoma, thyroid cancer, and multiple myeloma.[38]

Moreover, the long-term health impacts of exposure to radiation from nuclear or radiological weapons are not limited to cancer. They may also include psychological and stress-related disorders, and illnesses related to economic and social disruption. As with other environmental hazards, the risk of harm will not be evenly distributed in the exposed population, given local weather patterns, variations in individual susceptibility, and other factors.

The potential magnitude of health consequences from use of nuclear or radiological weapons, and other radiation releases by non-state actors, are presented in Table 12–3. The scenarios presented identify reasonable estimates of the scale of consequences related to each type of incident. The explosive yields of crude nuclear devices produced or used by terrorists are more unpredictable than the expected yields of weapons developed through rigorous testing protocols in nation-state weapons programs.[1,4] All of the estimates involve additional large uncertainties due to factors that will significantly influence the scope of damage, including: the size of the radiation release, types and chemical form of the isotopes involved, explosive device used, heat generated, weather conditions, population density and location, estimated health risk of exposure to radiation, risk of other non-cancer health impacts related to exposure to ionizing radiation, and transport of radioactive substances in the food chain and the environment.

Some models of consequences may provide a sense of the potential toll from terrorist attacks. Ira Helfand and colleagues estimated that the detonation of a 12.5-kiloton nuclear weapon in New York City by a terrorist would cause more than 250,000 deaths from blast, heat, and exposure to radiation directly and through fallout.[39] Another study, by Lachlan Forrow and colleagues, indicates the potential toll of a terrorist takeover of a nuclear submarine, with the launch of its missiles bearing nuclear weapons, could result in approximately seven million fatalities.[40]

Peter Taylor and David Sumner have estimated the consequences of the use of a radiological weapon to disperse plutonium in a large city. According to their model, such a weapon is unlikely to result in short-term doses

TABLE 12–3. Estimated Magnitude of Health Consequences of the Use of a Nuclear or Radiological Weapon or Other Radioactive Releases by a Non-State Actor.

TYPE OF WEAPON	SCENARIO	MAGNITUDE OF HEALTH CONSEQUENCES
Nuclear	1. 12.5-kiloton nuclear weapon brought into port in New York City on a ship.[39]	• 52,000 people killed immediately from blast and heat; • 238,000 people exposed to direct radiation from the blast—44,000 would suffer radiation sickness and 10,000 would receive a lethal dose; • 1.5 million people exposed to fallout—200,000 fatalities from 24-hour cumulative dose and another 300,000 cases of radiation sickness; and • Thousands of people with thermal and mechanical injuries.
	2. Takeover of a Russian nuclear submarine and intermediate-sized missile launch (based on estimates of an unintentional nuclear detonation).[40]*	• Approximately seven million deaths from firestorms in eight U.S. cities; and • Millions of other people exposed to potentially lethal doses of radiation in fallout.
"Dirty bombs"	3. Use of a crude dispersal mechanism, such as an incendiary device, to disperse 35 kg of bomb-grade plutonium in London.[4]	• 2,805 to 10,337 cases of cancer, with approximately 80 percent overall mortality; the vast majority lung cancer, with the remainder mostly neoplasms of bone, bone marrow, and liver.
Nuclear power reactor	4. Unintentional release of large amounts of radiation into atmosphere from a nuclear power plant of various possible sizes.[41]**	• 700 to 100,000 early fatalities, depending on the size of the reactor; • 3,000 to 40,000 deaths from cancer; and • 4,000 to 610,000 injuries.
	5. Spent-fuel pool fire.[17]***	• 28,000 cancer deaths; • $59 billion in damage; and • 188 square miles uninhabitable.
	6. Release of radioactive material from a single cask of spent nuclear fuel during a transportation accident followed by a fire in a tunnel in Baltimore.[42]	• 4,401 to 28,164 latent cancer deaths from 50-year dose; and • 10 km² with moderate contamination and 10 km² with heavy contamination.

*Russian nuclear experts have raised concerns that terrorists could gain control of a Russian nuclear missile facility and initiate an attack against the United States using strategic nuclear missiles.[39]

**Based on a study by Sandia National Laboratory, conducted subsequent to the partial meltdown at Three Mile Island in 1979, of the consequences of an unintentional release of large amounts of radiation at reactors that were operational or nearing completion at the time.

***Estimate based on studies of consequences of unintended release.

sufficient to cause radiation sickness or other acute effects of plutonium exposure. Fear and other social impacts would probably be large, however, and cancer risk would be increased, although delayed for many years.[4]

Hundreds to tens of thousands of casualties could result from a terrorist attack on a nuclear power reactor, depending on the size of the reactor, as suggested by government assessments of unintentional large releases from nuclear power plants.[41] A study by Matthew Lamb and Marvin Resnikoff of an unintentional release of radiation during the transport of spent fuel demonstrates that, if such an incident were initiated by terrorists, it could result in thousands of fatalities from cancer and widespread environmental contamination.[42]

Together, these examples indicate that the magnitude of the health consequences of the intentional release of radiation by a non-state actor, beyond large-scale fear and panic, could range in scale from a few thousand deaths from cancer to millions of immediate and long-term fatalities due to the detonation of a nuclear weapon. Depending on the isotopes released, vast areas of land could become contaminated for thousands of years.

RESPONDING TO ATTACKS AND MITIGATING HEALTH CONSEQUENCES

Evaluation of the sequelae to the 1986 releases of radiation from the Chernobyl nuclear power reactor in Ukraine indicates that a plan for mitigation measures in the event of an intentional or unintentional release of radiation from a nuclear power plant should include:

1. *Keeping populations indoors prior to subsequent evacuation*:[43] Initial restriction of populations to indoor areas may reduce exposure to radioactive hazards. Yet even with thoughtful preparation, mass evacuation of a large urban area affected by any variety of larger-scale nuclear terrorist scenarios would be a daunting challenge. As underscored by testimony given during public hearings regarding the potential evacuation of the densely populated area around the Indian Point nuclear reactor located 30 miles north of New York City (Figure 12–3), the local roads—jammed at rush hour even on ordinary days—would be clogged with panicking families.[44]
2. *Restricting consumption of locally produced milk and foodstuffs*:[43] The absorbed dose from *inhalation* of external exposure to radioiodines is negligible compared to that from *ingestion* of milk or dairy products.[45] For example, the individuals receiving the highest doses of radioactive iodine-131 from Nevada Test Site fallout during open-air tests of nu-

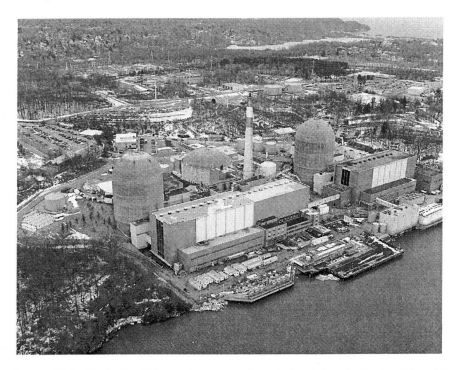

FIGURE 12–3. The Indian Point nuclear power plant site located on the Hudson River 30 miles north of New York City (AP/Wide World Photos).

clear weapons by the U.S. government between 1951 and 1962 were young children who consumed large amounts of milk from backyard goats and cows after the tests. The National Academy of Sciences has estimated that exposure of the public in the United States to radioactive iodine-131 through this and other pathways from U.S. nuclear-weapons testing in Nevada will ultimately result in a total of 11,300 to 212,000 excess cases of thyroid cancer.[46]

3. *Providing potassium iodide prophylaxis*: In the event of a radiological emergency at a nuclear power plant, federal and international agencies recommend rapid iodine prophylaxis of at-risk populations in order to reduce the radiation dose to the thyroid.[47,48] After September 11, 2001, the U.S. government purchased one million adult-strength tablets and 600,000 children's doses of potassium iodide for $180,000, with plans to spend $1 million to buy another five to ten million doses in 2002.[49] As of March 2002, at least four bills had been introduced in Congress that would require potassium iodide to be stockpiled at distances ranging up to 200 miles from all U.S. commercial nuclear power plants.[50,51] Despite universal acceptance of potassium iodide as an effective thyroid-

protective agent,[43] the proper implementation of such a policy is a matter of significant debate.[52–56]

4. *Worker protection, medical treatment, environmental sampling, and illness tracking*: Planning must also include protection of emergency responders; identification of treatment facilities where highly contaminated patients can receive definitive medical treatment, with safeguards for attending medical personnel; and environmental sampling and radiological monitoring.[45] An additional public-health challenge would be the follow-up surveillance, diagnosis, and management of chronic adverse health effects of radiation, including cancer, in survivors of the exposure as well as among emergency responders and other occupationally exposed individuals.

When considering attacks with nuclear weapons, a number of previously published assessments have provided extensive documentation of the inability to provide care for injured survivors.[57–60] Ira Helfand and colleagues have noted that casualties on the scale estimated by the terrorist use of a nuclear weapon would immediately overwhelm medical facilities, leading to a high mortality rate among those injured, but not killed, by the initial blast and thermal effects.[39] It is instructive in this regard to compare the Japanese experience after the Kobe earthquake of 1995, which resulted in fewer casualties than those posed by more than a minor hypothetical nuclear attack: 6,500 dead and 34,900 injured. While the situation in Kobe was not complicated by factors such as extensive radioactive contamination, there were long delays before outside medical assistance arrived.[39]

While preparedness measures are important, they have inherent limitations, especially if nuclear weapons are used. Hence, while health care providers and public health professionals should initiate and implement plans for mitigation measures (secondary and tertiary prevention), they should also support measures to limit the likelihood of a nuclear terrorist attack (primary prevention).

PREVENTION OF NUCLEAR TERRORISM

Since September 11, 2001, extensive resources have been dedicated to combining law enforcement and military action against the individuals and networks that would presumably carry out terrorist actions.[61,62] In addition, the U.S. government has advocated an expansion of anti-terrorist responses, including the possible use of nuclear weapons, towards a number of states, including those described by President George W. Bush in January 2002 as constituting an "axis of evil" that allegedly would directly carry out or support a terrorist action employing nuclear weapons or other weapons of mass destruction.[11,63] Notwithstanding the morbidity, mortality, and social, political, and economic costs of aggressive military solutions in a volatile, nuclear-armed world, exclusive focus on short-term suppression of the putative agents of nuclear terrorism can overlook the deeper, long-term threat posed by the persistence of the materials and methods of the global nuclear-weapons and nuclear-power infrastructure.

The threat of nuclear terrorism is related to the combined existence of nuclear weapons and a surfeit of weapons-usable material available to states and non-state actors who may be willing to use them for their own political agendas.[4] In order to address this threat, there is a need to develop a comprehensive, primary prevention approach that includes: (a) concerted international safeguarding of nuclear weapons and their constituent materials that are already dispersed throughout the world in nuclear power facilities and nuclear weapons stockpiles; (b) utilizing and strengthening existing treaties aimed at curbing proliferation and promoting nuclear disarmament; and (c) moving beyond current treaty obligations to develop even stronger global agreements to drastically reduce and ultimately eliminate materials and weapons that could have catastrophic consequences for humankind (see Box 12–1).

SAFEGUARDING NUCLEAR POWER FACILITIES AND NUCLEAR WEAPONS STOCKPILES

"Mock intruder" tests conducted by the Nuclear Regulatory Commission between 1991 and 1998 demonstrated that security regulations at nuclear-power facilities are inadequate and need to be strengthened.[64,65] Various short- to moderate-range measures have been proposed to address the vulnerabilities of nuclear-power facilities, including, but not limited to: increasing and strengthening the security regulations and security-force capabilities at these facilities; increasing Coast Guard patrols around coastal nuclear reactors; establishing no-fly zones around nuclear power facilities; placing caps on the amount of spent fuel produced at nuclear power plants; and moving spent fuel into dry-cask storage onsite.[14,17,64–69]

While important deterrents, the most sophisticated safeguards on materials and facilities can never be fully protective. For example, even under optimal conditions, current safeguards on plutonium in bulk-handling facilities, such as reprocessing plants, are ineffective. With the large amount of plutonium being processed, measurement uncertainties hamper accurate accounting, so that diversion of plutonium to weapons pathways can occur undetected.[4]

Global procedures and practices used to safeguard state-owned and stored fissile material are chaotic and ineffective, and permit leakage, theft, and smuggling on the nuclear black market, as exemplified by the situation in Russia and the former Soviet republics.[4] Currently, 603 metric tons of weapons-usable nuclear material are stored at 53 different sites in Russia—enough to make 41,000 additional nuclear bombs.[39]

The United States is spending between $900 million and $1 billion annually on a number of related nuclear-threat-reduction programs in Russia and the former Soviet republics.[70] The purpose of these programs includes securing these stockpiles and ensuring employment of weapons scientists who might otherwise provide scientific and technical know-how for would-be nuclear terrorists or states.[70] However, current funding, comprising less than 1 percent of U.S. defense spending, is inadequate to meet this challenge.[70]

Paradoxically, while many aspects of current U.S.–Russia initiatives could have a positive impact on reducing terrorist threats, some agreements, such as those providing for the disposition of excess weapons-grade plutonium at mixed-oxide (MOX) fuel plants, create their own terrorist risk. This risk is due to vulnerabilities of increased transport and storage of weapons-capable materials, and the subsequent generation of additional fissile materials in the reactors.[71] These U.S.–Russia agreements would compound the proliferation risks posed by current commercial reprocessing, which is the main contributor to the growth of nuclear weapons-usable materials in the world.[72]

In conclusion, without explicit linkage to move simultaneously towards elimination of new sources of weapons-grade materials flowing from continued nuclear weapons and nuclear power programs, the long-term efficacy of programs to safeguard nuclear materials and nuclear facilities is self-limited. Simply put, the more that weapons-usable and weapons-grade materials are available, the greater the risk will be that some of these materials will be acquired illegally and used to produce nuclear explosives.[4]

ENDING PROLIFERATION OF FISSILE MATERIALS AND NUCLEAR WEAPONS WHILE PROMOTING DISARMAMENT

International concerns about the proliferation potential inherent in all nuclear facilities were a key stimulus to the signing, ratification, and unlimited extension of the Non-Proliferation Treaty (NPT) (see Box 12–1). Towards this end, the IAEA is responsible for monitoring more than 900 facilities throughout the world in order to ensure that no nuclear materials at these facilities are diverted to military use.[24]

Unfortunately, the NPT, even if stringently enforced, is inadequate to cope with the persistence of highly concentrated sources of nuclear fuel and nuclear waste in nuclear reactors that are globally distributed and may serve as targets and sites of unintentional releases. Moreover, by virtue of the NPT's support for the development of nuclear power, the IAEA simultaneously plays two apparently conflicting roles—discouraging active proliferation, while encouraging "latent" proliferation.[31]

Examining the relationship between nuclear power and the proliferation of nuclear and radiological weapons could logically lead to support of phasing out nuclear power as a key element in the prevention of nuclear terrorism.

However long the global nuclear economy persists, there will be a continued need for vigorous enforcement of the NPT in order to stem the diversion of materials and technical knowledge from civilian nuclear programs to military programs of state or non-state actors. The necessary global political will to apply the force of the NPT steadfastly is, however, itself contingent on the need for the nuclear weapons states to uphold their clear obligations, under Article VI of the NPT, to formulate concrete steps towards global disarmament.

A key demonstration of support by the nuclear powers for carrying out their disarmament obligations would be for all of them to ratify the Comprehensive Test Ban Treaty (CTBT) (see Box 12–1). But in 1999, the U.S. Senate rejected ratification, and in 2002, the Bush administration announced that it might resume nuclear testing.[73] Renewed testing would facilitate U.S. plans, as reflected in its recent Nuclear Posture Review, that call for developing and deploying new nuclear weapons—steps that could well unravel the entire treaty-based nonproliferation system.[11,74,75] Even U.S. proposals to reduce the number of deployed strategic warheads—from the current level of approximately 6,000 to a level between 1,700 and 2,200 within 10 years—involve placing the warheads in storage, from which they could be reactivated, instead of destroying them.[76] Under the Department of Energy "Stockpile Stewardship" program, the U.S. government is currently spending $5.3 billion a year on nuclear weapons research, development, testing, and production.[29,77] The explicit discussion in the Nuclear Posture Review of contingencies for U.S. use of its proposed improved "nuclear strike capabilities"[11,75] constitutes a significant legitimization of the utility of nuclear weapons. This policy inevitably undermines global disarmament efforts and will therefore facilitate a new era of weapons proliferation by states and by terrorist groups.

In summary, current U.S. policy embraces the potential use of nuclear weapons against states that allegedly either (a) pose a threat of attack, or (b) support terrorists who would attack the United States with nuclear, chemical, or biological weapons.[11,75] To this end, the United States is also actively pursuing the development of so-called mini-nukes ("low-yield" nuclear weapons) for use against hardened targets, such as caves and deep underground command centers.[74,78] In addition to undermining internationally sanctioned nonproliferation efforts, American plans to integrate nuclear weapons into a broad spectrum of war-fighting capabilities increase the likelihood of their use, with consequent potential catastrophic morbidity and mortality.

NUCLEAR ABOLITION

Real primary prevention of the entwined threats of nuclear weapons proliferation and terrorism can ultimately be achieved only by universally sanctioned and verifiable programs that move towards the complete elimination of nuclear weapons. Nuclear abolition has been supported by numerous global political and military leaders and has been endorsed by leading medical and public health organizations, including the American Medical Association, the American College of Physicians, the American Public Health Association, and International Physicians for the Prevention of Nuclear War and its U.S. affiliate, Physicians for Social Responsibility.[79–84] By integrating strong support for the abolition of nuclear weapons—and all other weapons of mass destruction—with other concerted measures to reduce the availability of deadly nuclear materials and technologies, health professionals can help significantly reduce the dangers of nuclear terrorism well beyond what individual and collective preparedness efforts can accomplish.

REFERENCES

1. Maerli MB. *The Threat of Nuclear Terrorism: Nuclear Weapons or Other Nuclear Explosives Devices.* Symposium on International Safeguards: Verification and Nuclear Material Security. International Atomic Energy Agency: Vienna, Austria, October 10, 2001. Available at: http://www.iaea.org/worldatom/Press/Focus/Nuclear_Terrorism/maerli.pdf.
2. U.S. Department of Energy, Office of Environmental Management. *Linking Legacies. Connecting the Cold War Nuclear Weapons Production Processes to Their Environmental Consequences.* DOE/EM-0319. January 1997, p.12.
3. Mahkijani A, Saleska S. The production of nuclear weapons and environmental hazards. In: Makhijani A, Hu H, Yih K. *Nuclear Wastelands. A Global Guide to Nuclear Weapons Production and Its Health and Environmental Effects.* Cambridge, Mass.: MIT Press, 1995.
4. *IPPNW Global Health Watch Report Number 1: Crude Nuclear Weapons. Proliferation and the Terrorist Threat.* Cambridge, Mass.: International Physicians for the Prevention of Nuclear War, 1996.

5. U.S. Department of Health and Human Services, Agency for Toxic Substances and Disease Registry. *Toxicological Profile for Plutonium*. TP-90-21. December 1990, p. 85.

6. Report by Col. James P. Cooney, Medical Corps. General indoctrination. 24 February 1950, p.1. As quoted in U.S. Department of Defense, *Report on Search for Human Radiation Experiment Records 1944–1994*, Vol. 1. Assistant to the Secretary of Defense for Nuclear and Chemical and Biological Defense Programs.

7. Lynch C. Iraq worked on radiation bomb to use against Iran. *Washington Post*. May 12, 2001, A19.

8. Iraq's no-go dirty nukes. *Bulletin of the Atomic Scientists*. May 3, 2001. Available at: http://www.thebulletin.org/bulletinwirearchive/BulletinWire010503.html. Accessed March 17, 2002.

9. Verrengia JB. Experts fear crude radioactive device as potential terror weapon. *News and Observer*. Raleigh, N.C. December 18, 2001.

10. Glanz J, Revkin AC. Some see panic as main effect of dirty bombs. *New York Times*. March 7, 2002.

11. Gordon MR. U.S. nuclear plan sees new targets and new weapons. *New York Times*. March 10, 2002, A1.

11a. Warrick J. Nuclear litter of Soviet days raises fears of "dirty bombs." *Washington Post*, March 19, 2002.

12. World Health Organization, Department of Protection of the Human Environment. Depleted uranium: sources, exposures and health effects. WHO/SDE/PHE/01.1. Geneva: April 2001. Available at: http://www.who.int/environmental_information/radiation/Depluraniumintro.pdf.

13. Wozniak C. *Depleted Uranium Weapons*. Issue Brief. Washington, D.C.: Physicians for Social Responsibility. July, 1999. Available at: http://www.psr.org/duissuebrief.html Accessed March 17, 2002.

14. Physicians for Social Responsibility, Center for Global Health and Security. Issue Brief: *Vulnerability of U.S. Nuclear Power Plants to Terrorist Attack and Internal Sabotage*. Available at: http://www.psr.org/s11/plants.html#notes. Accessed January 6, 2002.

15. Details of nuclear power left open. *The Guardian*, October 24, 2001. Available at: http://www.guardian.co.uk/uslatest/story/0,1282,-1260475,00.html.

16. Union of Concerned Scientists. Issue Brief. *Spent Fuel Security*. October 16, 2001.

17. Alvarez R. What about the spent fuel? *Bulletin of the Atomic Scientists* 2002; 58:45–47.

18. Lochbaum D. Union of Concerned Scientists. Letter to Anthony Roisman. December 4, 2001.

19. Nuclear Information and Resource Service & World Information Service on Energy. Available at: http://www.nirs.org/factsheets/whywecallitmobilechernobyl.htm. Accessed March 30, 2001.

20. Nevada Agency for Nuclear Projects, Office of the Governor. *A Mountain of Trouble: A Nation At Risk. Report on the Impacts of the Proposed Yucca Mountain High-Level Nuclear Waste Program*, Volume 1. February 2002. Available at: http://www.state.nv.us/nucwaste/yucca/impactreport.pdf Accessed April 1, 2002.

21. Grove B. Nuclear casks can be damaged. *Las Vegas Sun*. February 11, 2002.

22. Yokoro K, Kamada N. The public health effects of the use of nuclear weapons. In: Levy BS, Sidel VW (eds.), *War and Public Health*. Updated edition. Washington, D.C.: American Public Health Association, 2000, pp. 65–83.

23. Smith G. U.S., Russia in arms-to-fuel deal. *Copley News Service.* February 9, 2002.

24. Curtis C. *Reducing Nuclear Threats in the 21ˢᵗ Century.* Symposium on International Safeguards: Verification and Nuclear Material Security. Vienna, Austria: International Atomic Energy Agency. October 29, 2001. Available at: http://www.iaea.org/worldatom/Press/News/curtis.pdf. Accessed March 17, 2002.

25. U.S. Congress, Office of Technology Assessment. *Technology Against Terrorism, The Federal Effort.* OTA-ISC-481. Washington, D.C.: U.S. Government Printing Office, July, 1991, p. 20.

26. Ong C. *Nuclear Weapons States, Who They Are and How Many Weapons Each Possesses.* Abolition 2000. A Global Network to Eliminate Nuclear Weapons. Available at: http://www.abolition2000.org/issues/indecent-explosives.html.

27. Albright D, Gorwitz M. Tracking civilian plutonium inventories: end of 1999. *Plutonium Watch.* October 2000. Available at: http://www.isis-online.org/publications/puwatch/puwatch2000.html.

28. Holt M, Behrens CE. *Congressional Research Brief IB88090: Nuclear Energy Policy.* The National Council for Science and the Environment. March 22, 2001.

29. Lichterman A, Cabasso J. *U.S. Nuclear Weapons Policies, Ballistic Missile Defense, and the Quest for Weapons in Space: Military Research and Development and the New Arms Race.* Western States Legal Foundation. July, 2000. Available at: http://www.wslfweb.org/docs/spabull1.pdf. Accessed March 17, 2002.

30. Tauscher E. Missile defense system is not ready for prime time. *San Francisco Chronicle.* March 24, 2002.

31. Taylor TB. *Nuclear Weapons and Nuclear Power.* Santa Barbara, Calif.: Nuclear Age Peace Foundation. July 1996.

32. Dolley S. *Indian and Pakistani Nuclear Tests.* Nuclear Control Institute. June 9, 1998. Available at: http://www.nci.org. Accessed January 7, 2002.

33. Institute for Energy and Environmental Research. *Fissile Material Basics.* Available at http://www.ieer.org/fctsheet/fm_basic.html. Accessed April 1, 2002.

34. Sumner D, Hu H, Woodward A. Health hazards of nuclear weapons production. In *Nuclear Wastelands: A Global Guide to Nuclear Weapons Production and Its Health and Environmental Effects.* Cambridge, Mass.: MIT Press, 1995, pp. 65–104.

35. International Physicians for the Prevention of Nuclear War. *Radioactive Heaven and Earth: The Health and Environmental Effects of Nuclear Weapons Testing In, On and Above the Earth.* New York, N.Y.: Apex Press, 1991.

36. Geiger HJ, Rush D, et al. *Dead Reckoning. A Critical Review of the Department of Energy's Epidemiologic Research.* The Physicians Task Force on the Health Risks of Nuclear Weapons Production. Washington, D.C.: Physicians for Social Responsibility, 1992.

37. Last JM. *Public Health and Human Ecology.* Stamford, Conn.: Appleton and Lange, 1998, pp. 185–186.

38. Childhood Cancer Research Institute. Health risks of low-level ionizing radiation in adults and children: overview of epidemiologic studies. Worcester, Mass.: Childhood Cancer Research Institute, 1999.

39. Helfand I, Forrow L, Tiwari J. Medical effects of a nuclear terrorist attack. *BMJ.* 324:356–359, 2002.

40. Forrow L, Blair B, Helfand I, et al. Accidental nuclear war—A post–cold war assessment. *N Engl J Med* 1998; 338:1326–1331.

41. Lochbaum D. Nuclear Plant Risk Studies: Dismal *Quality.* In: *Science for Democratic Action.* Institute for Energy and Environmental Research. 9(1), 2000.

42. Lamb M, Resnikoff M. *Radiological Consequences of Severe Rail Accident Involving Spent Nuclear Fuel Shipments to Yucca Mountain: Hypothetical Baltimore Rail Tunnel Fire Involving SNF*, prepared on behalf of Pacific World History Institute, September 2001. Available at: http://www.state.nv.us/nucwaste/news2001/nn11459.pdf. Accessed April 2, 2002.

43. Becker DV, Zanzonico P. Potassium iodide for thyroid blockade in a reactor accident: administrative policies that govern its use. *Thyroid*. 1997; 7(2):193–7.

44. Worth RF. Hard questions for movement to shut Indian Point. *New York Times*. December 27, 2001.

45. Porter SW. Planning for management of radiation accidents. In Stellman JM, ed., *International Labour Office: Encyclopaedia of Occupational Health and Safety*, 4th edition. Geneva: International Labour Office. 1998; pp. 48.31–48.48.

46. *Exposure of the American People to Iodine-131 from Nevada Nuclear Tests: Review of the National Cancer Institute Report and Public Health Implications*. Institute of Medicine and National Research Council. Washington, D.C.: National Academy Press, 1999, p.6.

47. Federal Emergency Management Agency. Federal Policy on Use of Potassium Iodide (KI). *Federal Register*: January 10, 2002 (Vol. 67, no. 7). Available at: http://www.fema.gov/library/not02367.html. Accessed March 17, 2002.

48. World Health Organization. *Guidelines for Iodine Prophylaxis Following Nuclear Accidents*. WHO/SDE/PHE 99.6. Geneva. 1999. Available at: http://www.who.int/environmental_information/Information_resources/documents/Iodine/guide.pdf. Accessed March 17, 2002.

49. Government buys drug as safeguard. Associated Press, January 3, 2002.

50. Congressman wants anti-radiation drug near nukes. Reuters, November 15, 2001.

51. HR 3382, HR 3279, HR 3448, S 1746.

52. Nuclear Regulatory Commission. 10 CFR Part 50: *Consideration of Potassium Iodide in Emergency Plans*. Washington, D.C.: January 9, 2001. Available at: http://www.nrc.gov/reading-rm/doc-collections/cfr/fr/20010119part2.html. Accessed March 17, 2002.

53. Crane P. *The NRC's "Fighter Jet" Rule on KI*. September 13, 1999. Available at: http://www.ki4u.com/crane.htm. Accessed March 17, 2002.

54. Public Citizen Critical Mass Energy Project. *Potassium Iodide*. Washington, D.C.: March 25, 2001. Available at: http://users.rcn.com/agnews/PotassiumIodideKI-CMEP.htm. Accessed March 17, 2002.

55. Toner M. Feds stockpiling anti-radiation pills. *The Barre Montpelier Times Argus*. January 13, 2002. Available at: http://timesargus.nybor.com/Search/Categories/Article/40610. Accessed March 17, 2002.

56. Archibald RC. In shadow of reactors, parents seek peace of mind in a pill. *New York Times*. January 21, 2002. Available at: http://www.prop1.org/nucnews/2002nn/0201nn/020121nn.htm#110. Accessed March 17, 2002.

57. Ervin FR, Glazier JR, Arnow S, et al. Human and ecological effects in Massachusetts of an assumed thermonuclear attack on the United States. *N Engl J Med* 1962; 266:1127–37.

58. Sidel VW, Geiger HJ, Lown B. The physician's role in the post-attack period. *N Engl J Med*. 1962; 266:1137–45.

59. Abrams HL. Medical resources after nuclear war: availability vs. need. *JAMA*. 1984; 252:653–658.

60. *Effects of Nuclear War on Health and Health Services*, 2nd ed. Geneva: World Health Organization, 1987.
61. Gov't to spend $22B on security. Associated Press, January 31, 2002.
62. Bush's budget adds $48B for defense. Associated Press, February 4, 2002.
63. Bush calls for support against rogue nations. Associated Press. January 31, 2002.
64. Hirsch D. The NRC: what, me worry? *Bulletin of the Atomic Scientists* 2002; 58:38–44.
65. Union of Concerned Scientists. *Briefing: Nuclear Reactor Safety*. 2001. Available at: http://www.ucsusa.org/energy/br_safenplants.html. Accessed April 1, 2002.
66. Federal guards for nuke plants sought. Associated Press, November 16, 2001.
67. Gunboats, other security at waterways. Associated Press, October 5, 2001.
68. France surface-to-air missiles pulled from nuclear plants. *Agence France-Presse.* March 8, 2002.
69. Rattner R. Pacific Gas and Electric Shareholder's Proposal. Radioactive wastes: risk reduction policy. San Francisco, Calif. 2002.
70. Tiwari J. Issue Brief: *U.S. Non-Proliferation Initiatives in Russia and the Former Soviet Union States: Essential for National and Global Security*. Washington, D.C.: Physicians for Social Responsibility, 2001. Available at: http://www.psr.org/s11/ctr-full.html. Accessed March 17, 2002.
71. Makhijani A. *Plutonium End Game. Managing Global Stocks of Separated Weapons-Usable Commercial and Surplus Nuclear Weapons Plutonium*. Chapter 4: Disposition of U.S.-Russian surplus military plutonium. Institute for Energy and Environmental Research. Takoma Park, Md.: January 2001. Available at: http://www.ieer.org/reports/pu/ch4.html. Accessed March 17, 2002.
72. Makhijani A, Saleska S. *The Nuclear Power Deception. U.S. Nuclear Mythology from Electricity "Too Cheap to Meter" to "Inherently Safe" Reactors*. Institute for Energy and Environmental Research. New York: Apex Press, 1999. pp. 121–126.
73. Pincus W. U.S. to seek options on new nuclear tests. White House worries about arsenal's reliability. *Washington Post*, January 8, 2002, A04.
74. Physicians for Social Responsibility. *Nuclear Weapons in Counterproliferation: Responding to the Chemical and Biological Weapons Threat*. Washington, D.C., 2001. Available at: http://www.psr.org/s11/chembionucthreat.html. Accessed March 17, 2002.
75. Cushman J Jr. Rattling new sabers. *New York Times*, March 10, 2002, A1.
76. U.S. nuke proposal called shell game. *Associated Press,* January 10, 2002.
77. Schwartz SI. The new-nuke chorus tunes up. *Bulletin of the Atomic Scientists*. 57:30–35, 2001. Available at: http://www.thebulletin.org/issues/2001/ja01/ja01schwartz.html. Accessed March 17, 2002.
78. Lichterman A. *Looking for New Ways to Use Nuclear Weapons: U.S. Counterproliferation Programs, Weapons Effects Research, and "Mini-Nuke" Development*. Oakland, Calif.: Western States Legal Foundation, 2001. Available at: http://www.wslfweb.org/docs/mininuke.pdf Accessed March 17, 2002.
79. International Physicians for the Prevention of Nuclear War. *Vital Signs* 1995; 8:1.
80. American College of Physicians. Resolution from the Board of Governors, approved by the Board of Regents. Presented at: Meeting of the American College of Physicians, October 1996; Philadelphia, Pa.
81. American Public Health Association. Cessation of nuclear testing and abolition of nuclear weapons: policy statement No. 9605 (adopted by the Governing Council, November 20, 1996). *Am. J. Public Health* 1997; 87:500.

82. American Medical Association. House of Delegates Resolution 617 (I-96). Presented at: Meeting of the House of Delegates, American Medical Association, December 1996, Chicago, IL.
83. The Canberra Commission on the Elimination of Nuclear Weapons. Available at: http://www.dfat.gov.au/cc/cc_report1.html. Accessed March 17, 2002.
84. *Statement on Nuclear Weapons by International Admirals and Generals.* Available at: http://www.cornnet.nl/~akmalten/search.html. Accessed March 17, 2002.

BACKGROUND READING

Mettler FA, Voelz GL. Major radiation exposure—what to expect and how to respond. *N Engl J Med* 2002; 346:1554–1561.

III

Challenges and opportunities

13

Strengthening the public health system

C. WILLIAM KECK AND MARGUERITE A. ERME

The mission of public health is assuring the conditions in which people can be healthy. Terrorism is anathema to public health. This chapter reviews the evolution of the public health system in the United States, describes the strengths and deficiencies in the system that were revealed by the terrorist attacks in 2001, and provides recommendations for strengthening the public health system so that it can be more effective—in responding not only to the health consequences of terrorism but also to other major challenges as well.

BACKGROUND

The public health "system" in the United States is intended to protect the country's population from disease and injury. By some measures, it has been remarkably successful in doing so. It has been estimated that approximately 25 years of the 30-year gain in life expectancy during the 20th century was due to public health interventions, compared to 3.7 years for medical treatment and 1.5 years for clinical preventive services.[1] Yet, at the end of the 20th century, many people doubted that the public health system had the resources to meet ongoing public health needs, let alone respond to purposeful acts intended to injure or to spread disease.

Public health in the United States was inaugurated at the end of the 18th century to help control the spread of infectious diseases in Eastern seaboard port cities. The threat of great epidemics and the continual mortality caused by common infections created incentives to improve cleanliness and diminish crowding in cities during the 19th century. In many ways, however, public health came into its own during the first half of the 20th century. The focus on control of infectious diseases, fueled by rapid increases in the knowledge of bacteria, was balanced by attention paid to community-based health activities and health education of the public. States formed boards of health, and the federal government began to provide funding support and expertise to states for public health programs. After World War II, much attention was given to public health, but efforts focused more on medical care needs than on prevention, and health departments began a slow but steady decline. From the 1950s to the present, the prevalent assumption that health depended on medical care, coupled with an anti-government attitude in the United States, contributed to a failure of real expenditures on public health to keep pace with population growth.[2]

The Institute of Medicine Report

Concern about the status of public health led the Institute of Medicine (IOM) to convene a study committee to examine the nature of the discipline in the United States. Its report, *The Future of Public Health (1988)*, noted that:

> The current state of our abilities for effective public health action . . . is cause for national concern and for the development of a plan of action for needed improvements. . . . [W]e have slackened our public health vigilance nationally, and the health of the public is unnecessarily threatened as a result.[3]

Indeed, while cognizant and respectful of the significant contributions made by an underfunded and underappreciated public health system, the IOM declared that the public health system in the United States was a "system in disarray."[3] To be sure, the IOM report galvanized the public health community into action. Since its publication, considerable progress has been made in defining and organizing the discipline of public health, characterizing the needs of its practitioners, and redeveloping its ties with academia. Little or no progress has been made, however, in de-politicizing local and state health departments, in repairing a very frayed public health infrastructure, and in addressing the great differences in sophistication and capacity among health departments across the country.

Challenges Facing Local Health Departments

The National Association of County and City Health Officials (NACCHO) periodically surveys its local health department members in an effort to characterize them. Its latest survey, done in 1997, showed that local health departments nationally employ an average of 72 full-time equivalent personnel (FTEs) and a median of 16 FTEs.[4] More recent data showing an average of 67 FTEs and a median of 13 FTEs suggest a trend toward declining staff size in local health departments.[5] The difference in numbers of staff members among health departments serving populations of different sizes is dramatic. Departments serving fewer than 25,000 people employ an average of 13.9 and a median of 8.5 FTEs. Those serving populations in excess of 500,000 employ an average of 612 and a median of 437 FTEs. Half of local health departments serve jurisdictions with fewer than 25,000 people.[5]

This is the mosaic of the public health system that provides the first line of defense for public health threats in American communities. It is a system hampered by neglect of its infrastructure needs, by strong vestiges of home rule that hinder collaboration across geopolitical boundaries, by shortages of trained professionals, by politicization of its activities, and by an ever-expanding agenda that is not matched with expanding resources.

Concerns about Terrorism

At the end of the 20th century, concerns about terrorism and the potential use of biological warfare agents increased awareness of the need to improve public health infrastructure (see Chapters 10 and 15). The Centers for Disease Control and Prevention (CDC) report *Preventing Emerging Infectious Diseases: A Strategy for the 21st Century* outlined goals and objectives for protecting the United States from the threat of infectious diseases.[6] This plan did not specifically focus on bioterrorism, but the 1996 Presidential Decision Directive on emerging diseases and the growing threat of bioterrorism stimulated revision of the original 1994 plan. Nearly all the improvements recommended for the plan could be used to assess and react to a potential bioterrorism incident.

In 2000, the CDC published *Biological and Chemical Terrorism: Strategic Plan for Preparedness and Response*,[7] which highlighted the vulnerability of the United States to biological and chemical attacks and listed implementation priorities and specific recommendations for terrorism preparedness. In 2000, the CDC prepared *Public Health Infrastructure: A Status Report*[8] for the Appropriations Committee of the U.S. Senate. It emphasized three areas of the public health infrastructure necessary to handle the threats of the 21st century, including bioterrorism: a skilled public health workforce, robust information and data systems, and effective health departments and laboratories. The terrorist incidents of September and October 2001 highlighted how important these elements are and how much more work will be required to bring them to an acceptable level of capacity and competence.

DEFICIENCIES HIGHLIGHTED BY THE TERRORIST ATTACKS OF 2001

The terrorist attacks in the United States in September and October of 2001 and the resulting public concern were a major test of the capacity of local safety and public health agencies to respond appropriately. The purposeful airplane crashes into the World Trade Center in New York and the Pentagon in Virginia on September 11 required first response from community safety forces (fire and police) and supporting roles from local and state health departments (Chapter 2). The magnitude and viciousness of those events awakened health departments in other parts of the country to the need to review, confirm, modify, or develop disaster plans in their own communities, and to assure the health department's role in disaster response.

The Response to Anthrax

The first report, on October 4, 2001, of a human case of inhalational anthrax triggered a series of events that quickly led to the direct involvement of most local and state health departments (Chapter 6). When the number of cases of anthrax grew and several infected people died, public concern mushroomed. As it became clear that the anthrax had been spread through letters laced with powder containing anthrax spores to news-media outlets in Florida and New York City and to members of Congress and U.S. Senators in Washington, D.C., fear about the safety of the postal system spread rapidly.

Medical care providers and health departments in Florida, New York, New Jersey, Washington, D.C., Pennsylvania, and eventually Connecticut became first-responders to a terrorist act. Bioterrorism attacks tend not to begin with a "bang"; rather, they become noticed only when infected individuals develop symptoms and present themselves for diagnosis and treatment. Medical care providers are responsible for diagnosing and reporting cases of infectious disease to health departments, which are charged with tracking patterns of disease, identifying patterns consistent with an unexpected event, and enacting control measures. The presence of multiple cases of anthrax 3 weeks after September 11 raised concerns about bioterrorism, given the terrorists' threats of more attacks to come. The local health departments involved in communities where infection was demonstrated played their appropriate roles in strong partnership with state health departments and the CDC.

The intense publicity given to anthrax and "white powder," coupled with expectations that additional terrorist attacks were likely, fueled public anxiety and stimulated copycat anthrax hoax letters. In this atmosphere, people were encouraged to report suspicious packages and envelopes, and some sought medical attention for symptoms they thought might indicate anthrax. For their part, national medical and public health organizations and the federal government quickly developed and distributed information to the public and health professionals about potential bioterrorism agents, procedures for defining and handling suspicious packages, communication guidelines for safety and public health workers, and anthrax sampling and testing techniques.

For most of the country, the anthrax scare became a giant field exercise. In most areas, there were no anthrax spores in the environment, no one became infected, and there were no illnesses or deaths, but frightened people on high alert flooded public health and safety agencies with calls for information and assistance with suspicious packages and envelopes as well as powdery substances, 24 hours a day, 7 days a week. The only health risk was to mental health, yet the capacity of many agencies to respond was severely taxed (see Chapter 3 and Figure 1–3).

Public health, medical, emergency management, fire, and police officials had to communicate and cooperate, not only within their own communities, but also with their colleagues in neighboring communities. Working relationships had to be established with the Federal Bureau of Investigation (FBI) and the U.S. Postal Service. Rules of engagement were formulated to determine which agency's representatives should respond, based on the nature of the problem presented by each request for assistance. Respondents had to distinguish between credible and non-credible threats, determine the likelihood of exposure to a potential disease agent, and learn how to work in an environment that might be considered a crime scene as well as a health threat. Decisions had to be made about who would respond to questions from the news media. At the same time, all involved had to maintain their usual range of public services and other responsibilities. Without doubt, communication mechanisms between involved agencies and professionals were improved and response protocols were adjusted where experience dictated the need. A more important issue involved problems that were discovered not to be amenable to simple adjustment, such as shortages of communicable disease epidemiologists, insufficient laboratory capacity, inadequate communication technology, and uncertainty over how to meet community mental health needs.

Surveys of Local Health Departments

In December 2001 and January 2002, NACCHO assessed local health departments' response to anthrax concerns, the state of their response planning, and training needs for bioterrorism threats. A two-page survey was sent via blast-fax to a random, stratified sample of 1,024 local public health departments across the nation: about one-third of the nation's 3,000 local agencies. The response rate was 61 percent. Eighty percent of the survey respondents reported that since early October 2001 their health departments had responded to calls about suspicious powders. The average number of calls received was 97; the median was six. The number of calls varied widely depending on the population size of the jurisdiction served. In answer to a question about development of a written plan for emergency preparedness, only 26 percent of respondents reported having a completed plan in place, while 55 percent reported they had a plan at least 80 percent complete. Agencies were less prepared specifically for bioterrorism. Of those working on a plan, only 12 percent of respondents indicated that the bioterrorism portion of their plan was complete, although approximately 30 percent of respondents indicated that their bioterrorism plans were at least 80 percent complete. Eleven percent had not yet begun development of a bioterrorism component. Training needs identified included the role of public health in emergency response, operations and management of bioterrorism-related systems, use of emergency communication equipment, and understanding individual roles in emergency response.[9]

The National Association of Counties (NACo) also surveyed local health departments in the aftermath of the country's experience with anthrax. Its study revealed that fewer than 10 percent of respondents felt "fully prepared" to handle a bioterrorism attack, and fewer than 5 percent felt prepared enough to address the fallout from a chemical attack. Of the counties with populations above 250,000, none said that they were fully prepared. NACo estimated that 15,000 more public health workers are needed nationwide to bolster the public health system.[10]

In Ohio, based on our experience, the major challenges faced were: the inadequacy of our staffing for such an all-consuming event; the inadequacy of our laboratory support systems; the difficulty of managing adequate communication links among public health agencies, the medical community, safety forces, the news media, the community at large, and other interested or involved parties such as the U.S. Postal Service; providing necessary staff training; meeting community mental health needs; and maintaining day-to-day service requirements during an episode.

Staffing of Public Health Departments

Most public health departments do not have staff members with communicable-disease-control training that includes bioweapon agents. When unusual pathogens are identified, difficulties may therefore arise in understanding and implementing timely control measures, and in working closely with medical care providers in the community. In addition, public health departments tend to be staffed at levels that allow for timely response to communicable-disease problems anticipated from previous experience. Most public health responses are managed during the typical workday with some staff on call for occasional after-hours work. Unlike public safety agencies, health departments do not have several shifts of professionals. As a result, during the anthrax scares of 2001, front-line staff members were in danger of "burning out" after several weeks of calls for assistance around the clock. Marshalling additional resources to assist with the high workload provided only partial relief, because the special skills possessed by front-line staff members were not duplicated in other employees.

Laboratory Support

Most local health departments do not have their own laboratories, and some of the larger local health departments with laboratory facilities are limited in their ability to perform microbiology tests (see Chapter 14). The result is that most local health departments rely on state health department laboratories to provide the support necessary to diagnose and control infectious-disease outbreaks. At the height of anthrax control efforts in late 2001, state health department laboratories were inundated with requests to test suspicious substances and objects for the presence of anthrax. In Ohio, these requests forced the state laboratory to close for any other microbiological testing for several days until it could make arrangements for other laboratories to assist. Unfortunately, other disease processes did not stop just because the state laboratory was preoccupied with anthrax. In Akron, Ohio, for example, in the midst of a shigellosis outbreak in day-care centers, public health officials had to turn to local hospital laboratories for assistance (see Chapter 14).

Communication

In Akron, communication links were quickly formed, out of necessity, with the state health department, county emergency management agency, police department, fire department, the FBI, and the U.S. Postal Service. After some initial difficulty, roles were defined, communication was established, and good working relationships were developed among these agencies. Communication with neighboring public health agencies was also reasonably good. There was not enough time for personnel knowledgeable about anthrax to communicate effectively with other groups. Responding to requests for information and assistance from concerned individuals consumed the time of those involved, so there were few formal information or press releases prepared for the news media, the medical community, or the public at large. Local public health officials responded to calls from the news media in the course of other work, and relied on both national and local media reporting to keep the general public and medical community informed about events. Medical professional associations and the CDC ably provided information of interest to medical care providers, the news media, and the general public (see Box 13–1).

Staff Training

There had been little to no preparation of noncommunicable disease staff members for their role in dealing with a bioterrorism event. Clerical staff members were relatively unprepared to handle a large volume of calls about this problem or to deal with their own concerns about safety when opening packages or envelopes. Environmental staff members were not prepared to assist with environmental decontamination efforts, if they were required. Health education staff members, in the short run, were not prepared to help provide information on anthrax to the media, medical personnel, or the general public. They had had no training on bioterrorism agents and have little background in microbiology or the epidemiology of infectious diseases. Mental health counselors did not know if they had a role to play in the absence of infection or injury.

Mental Health

In most of the country, the major mental health problem was widespread personal anxiety, rather than the grief that would have accompanied loss of life or physical health (see Chapter 3). Although a number of agencies can provide mental health workers if needed, there are few, if any, mechanisms in place to coordinate their participation in disaster response. There has been little preparation for critical incident debriefing, particularly outside of the public safety agencies. In addition, it is not clear how many communities could deal with the long-term mental health impact of a major disaster.

Maintaining Usual Workload

The anthrax events were so consuming that some staff responsibilities had to be shifted in order to provide support for ongoing control of other commu-

Box 13–1. Communicating about Anthrax: Some Lessons Learned at the CDC.

Numbers are not the whole story, but they can tell us something about the magnitude of the communication challenge of the anthrax outbreak that began in October 2001 (see Chapter 6). From October 1, 2001, through January 19, 2002, the Centers for Disease Control and Prevention (CDC) Office of Communication managed what in normal times is a year's worth of media-relations work: 23 press briefings with an average of 80 journalists at each, 44 press releases, 7,737 telephone calls from the media, 306 television interviews, and 17,986 telephone calls from the public. The CDC bioterrorism website, www.bt.cdc.gov, hosted 5 million visitors who downloaded 12 million items from the site.

Audience research has shown that providing information that people can count on is a CDC attribute valued by public health professionals, decision-makers, the public, and the media. Communication staff members worked hard during the anthrax crisis to be sure we met these expectations. In the process, we validated much that we knew already and learned a number of lessons: Most important, stick to communication basics when dealing with the media and the public. Balance the timeliness and accuracy of the information being given—it has to be as exact as the current science will allow, but delivered in a way that meets the media's deadlines so that coverage will be both prompt and as accurate as possible. Respond to media calls. Plan ahead for the extra hands it will take to staff phone, e-mail, and fax lines seven days a week. Stay in constant touch with the experts. Learn the issues—especially the complicated ones—and help craft articulate messages to explain them. Work in partnership—state and local leaders are rightly "out front" in notifying the public and confirming situations in their areas, even when they are based on CDC confirmation. Even in a time of crisis, look for opportunities to promote public health and how the system works. Build the public's confidence that those in government working on the problem know what they are doing and can be trusted to protect lives.

CDC's communication response was from a national level, but sharing experiences with state and local public health colleagues through discussions and joint field assignments led to identifying lessons that can apply to any level of response: Communication professionals are an integral part of any response team. Include them as the team is being deployed, and plan to have them on site until the work is completed. Get the news out quickly but do not speculate. Silence or saying "we don't know" is better than giving the wrong information. Always be aware of the balance between the deadlines of the media and accuracy of the science. Find (and train) trusted spokespersons to talk with the media. Try to balance scientific expertise on the health problem with an understanding of the need for the media and the public to be reassured that they are getting sound advice on actions they need to take to reduce their own risks. Work with partners to define the niche the organization needs to fill during the outbreak—if it is public health, then try to stay in that role and not get into law-enforcement, political, state or local, or other roles. Do daily media updates—they help organize the response team's time and assure reporters of regular access to spokesper-

(continued)

Box 13-1. *(continued)*

sons and current information. If a critical piece of information is received between briefings, weigh with the team whether the importance of the information justifies an immediate release.

In individual and group conversations with public-information professionals at state and local levels, there was general agreement that it is important for those who may be involved in a response to plan ahead. Build partnerships with local media and with intermediaries who may be involved in a response effort, such as local hospitals, physicians in the community, and emergency management agencies. Have simple things, such as current lists of contact information, for immediately getting in touch with critical personnel no matter when or under what circumstances an incident occurs. Pull together basic information about the potential bioterrorism agents, such as fact sheets or treatment recommendations, and have it assembled for easy access by the first team members called into action. Train potential responders about appropriate management of persons exposed to a specific agent, and how the public health and emergency systems can be accessed during an event.

In short, tried-and-true techniques for public information and media relations will well serve the public's need to know and are an integral part of any crisis response.

—Kay S. Golan and Cheryl Lackey

BOX REFERENCES

Kirby S, Taylor M, Freimuth V, et al. Identity building and branding at CDC: a case study. *Social Marketing Quarterly* 2001; 3:16–35.

Emergency Risk Communication: NPHIC Communication Planning Checklist, from "Managing the Media and Public Health Communications," teleconference 11/15/01 (available at www.bt.cdc.gov), accessed 3/15/02.

CDC Responds: "Risk Communication and Bioterrorism." *December 6, 2001 satellite video conference.* Available at http://www.phppo.cdc.gov/phtn/bio1206.asp, accessed 3/15/02.

nicable diseases. Nurses and sanitarians, even those with minimal or no training in infectious disease control, had to assume routine tasks for controlling outbreaks. Removing staff members from other areas of work adversely impacted the level of service delivery in those areas, but this impact was manageable in the short run.

What If There Had Been a Chemical or Nuclear Attack?

Most local health departments have the capacity to deal with issues related to microbial infection on a regular basis. The dissemination of anthrax in late 2001 strained that capacity, but anthrax fits the models developed for communicable-disease control. If a chemical or nuclear attack had occurred, local health departments would have been much more limited in their capacity to respond. Very few local public health departments have staff members knowledgeable about chemical and nuclear weapons. Most departments are not prepared to implement the immediate and long-term measures that would be required to protect populations from exposure, respond to those who had been exposed, and provide the surveillance needed to assess the long-term health impacts (see Chapters 11 and 12).

IMPROVING CAPACITY OF LOCAL HEALTH DEPARTMENTS TO RESPOND TO TERRORISM

Many of the deficiencies in the U.S. public health system were highlighted by the terrorist acts of 2001. Shortcomings were identified in (a) disaster planning; (b) linkages with other agencies and institutions involved in disaster response; (c) capacity to communicate with special groups (such as federal and state government public agencies, safety agencies, and medical care providers) and the general public; (d) capacity to detect microbiological threats to health; and (e) capacity to detect other threats to health and respond to them. Contributing to the shortcomings were the large number of local health departments, varying widely in size and sophistication, operating in a politicized home-rule atmosphere, with a history of minimal funding. Many people believe that it is remarkable that the system responded as well as it did to these terrorist acts.

Long-term improvement of local public health capacity, in many locations, will require significant increases in the size and sophistication of state and local public health agencies. In recent years, progress has been made in unifying the public health profession and better describing its purpose and activities. Further depoliticization of state and local health departments, coupled with increases in funding and capacity, will need to come next. In addition, a number of specific issues need to be addressed, as described below. Along with strengthening the public health system, the medical care system will need to be strengthened as well (see Box 13–2).

Disaster Planning

The previously cited NACCHO data make it clear that many health departments are not engaged, or at least not *fully* engaged, in preparing for their appropriate roles should disaster occur in their communities. The terrorist-related events of 2001 caused many local health departments that did have emergency operations plans to scramble to find and activate them. In most disasters involving property damage or mass casualties, local health departments are secondary responders, responsible for post-disaster disease and in-

Box 13–2. Strengthening the Medical Care System.

The U.S. medical care system, while far better funded and very much larger than the U.S. public health system, must be considered part of the U.S. public health system when responses to terrorism are planned or implemented.

The medical care system responded very well to the WTC and Pentagon attacks. First-responders provided onsite emergency medical services to the injured and transported those seriously injured to nearby acute-care hospitals. In both the New York and Washington metropolitan areas, the capacity of medical care facilities was far more than sufficient for treating injured survivors, although some burn treatment units in New York hospitals were stretched to their limits (see Chapter 2).

The medical care system also responded reasonably well to the anthrax dissemination (see Chapter 6). Many medical care providers were not knowledgeable about the signs and symptoms of cutaneous and inhalation anthrax at the time that the dissemination occurred. In addition, public health officials, including those at the Centers for Disease Control and Prevention (CDC), had a relatively small base of scientific and medical knowledge on which to base their recommendations for diagnosis and treatment for anthrax cases and for prophylaxis for those who may have been exposed to anthrax spores. As medical care providers became better informed about the diagnosis, treatment, and prevention of anthrax, they responded effectively—in educating their patients and others, in evaluating suspected cases and treating them, and in participating in and promoting efforts to provide prophylaxis to those who may have been exposed. In some instances, inaccurate or inadequate information was provided and antimicrobials were inappropriately used.

We propose the following recommendations for strengthening the U.S. medical care system. Most of these recommendations include a closer working relationship between medical care and public health. And most focus on what needs to be done at the community level—before a terrorist attack or threat may occur. Strengthening the medical care system to better deal with terrorist acts and threats will also improve its ability to better respond to other unforeseen human-made and natural disasters and diseases caused by biological and chemical agents.

1. *Improving diagnostic capabilities*: Concerning diseases possibly caused by biological and chemical agents, medical care providers need to heighten their clinical suspicion and continually improve their diagnostic knowledge and skills. They need to learn where they can turn for expert information, including specific government agencies and academic institutions. Knowledge and skills concerning terrorism need to be incorporated into continuing education programs for health professionals and curricula for students in the health professions.

2. *Improving clinical surveillance*: Effective surveillance greatly depends, in part, on accurate clinical and laboratory-based diagnoses by medical care providers. Sur-

(continued)

(continued)

veillance systems need to be improved to facilitate reporting by clinicians and laboratories (see Chapter 14).

3. *Improving therapeutic and preventive capabilities*: Medical care providers will need to improve their ability to treat and prevent health problems caused by biological and chemical agents, including accessing large quantities of relevant antimicrobials, antitoxins, and vaccines, and learning decontamination procedures.

4. *Improving staffing of health care facilities*: There have been disturbing trends of increasingly inadequate staffing by nurses and other medical care professionals at medical care facilities in the United States. Inadequate staffing reduces the quality of medical care on an ongoing basis. A terrorist attack could further compromise the availability and quality of care. Policies and programs need to be established to ensure adequate staffing.

5. *Developing surge capacity*: Major terrorist attacks pose the likelihood of many injured people arriving at emergency departments and other acute-care facilities over a short period of time without warning. Medical care facilities need to develop surge capacity to provide appropriate care to all who need it in these situations, including establishing regional networks to draw on medical care personnel in neighboring communities or areas.

6. *Improving capabilities to diagnose and treat mental disorders*: Major consequences of terrorist attacks and threats are anxiety, depression, post-traumatic stress disorder (PTSD), and other mental-health disorders (see Chapter 3). There may be increased substance abuse among populations affected by terrorist attacks and threats. Availability and quality of mental health services and related resources need to be improved.

7. *Improving dissemination of information and communication with individuals and communities*: Medical care providers need to improve their ability to acquire information from their patients and impart information to them. Effective communication in an emergency situation is best achieved when trust has been previously established between medical care providers and their patients. The role of the news media is critically important in both acquiring and transmitting information. Medical care providers should develop ongoing working relationships with journalists and other news-media representatives.

8. *Improving insurance coverage*: Forty million Americans are without medical care insurance of any kind, and most other Americans have inadequate insurance coverage. Many people with no or inadequate medical insurance would not seek medical care if they had initially mild, nonspecific symptoms from a bioterrorist attack—potentially a situation of major public health significance.

9. *Engaging in preparedness planning*: Health professionals need to develop preparedness plans for terrorist attacks, and undertake drills and exercises to rehearse implementation of these plans. These plans need to be updated regularly, and should not inappropriately divert personnel and resources from other necessary tasks and services.

(continued)

> **Box 13–2.** *(continued)*
>
> 10. *Advocating prevention*: A large-scale biological or chemical weapon attack or even
>   a small-scale nuclear weapon attack would overwhelm medical care facilities. The
>   numbers of patients would far exceed the capacity of medical care personnel and
>   facilities. Medical care providers can advocate policies and programs that will help
>   prevent terrorist attacks and threats and that will lead to the reduction or elimina-
>   tion of weapons of mass destruction.
>
> —Barry S. Levy and Victor W. Sidel

jury prevention. Their roles include inspection and certification of emergency shelters, assurance of safe food and water, assurance of appropriate waste disposal, immunization of at-risk populations, and mitigation of environmental threats. Typically, practice of these functions during disaster drills has been minimal. Health departments will need to be active participants in planning and preparation for possible disasters. Public health workers will need to develop and improve their competencies for emergency preparedness (see Box 13–3).

Health departments are front-line responders to bioterrorist attacks (see Chapter 10). Their disease surveillance and response systems and communication links with the medical community are key components for the recognition of and response to bioterrorist attacks. Future attacks will most likely be discovered in physicians' offices, emergency departments, and public health agencies. Chemical and nuclear attacks would probably create needs for long-term disease surveillance of affected populations and for environmental assessment and hazard mitigation (see Chapters 11 and 12). Communities should be adding annexes on weapons of mass destruction to their emergency operations plans, and local health departments should be directly involved in planning and preparedness exercises.

Mutual Aid Agreements

Communities commonly have formal mutual aid agreements with neighboring safety agencies, asserting that assistance will be forthcoming should any particular department be faced with a situation that overwhelms its capacity to respond. These arrangements are especially common among fire departments. We suggest that public health departments consider similar arrangements with neighbor agencies.

Box 13–3. Emergency Preparedness Competencies for Public Health Workers.

In order for the public health system to meet performance standards in emergency preparedness, all public health workers must be competent to:

- Describe the public health role in emergency response in a range of emergencies that might arise. (For example: "This department provides surveillance, investigation, and public information in disease outbreaks, and collaborates with other agencies in biological, environmental, and weather emergencies.")
- Describe the agency chain of command in emergency response.
- Identify and locate the agency's emergency response plan (or in large agencies, the pertinent portion of the plan).
- Describe his/her functional role(s) and responsibilities in emergency response and demonstrate his/her role(s) in regular drills.
- Demonstrate correct use of all communication equipment used for emergency communication.
- Describe his/her communication role(s) in emergency response within the agency, with the media, with the general public, and personally (with family and neighbors).
- Identify limits to his/her own knowledge, skills, and authority, and identify key system resources for referring matters that exceed these limits.
- Apply creative problem-solving and flexible thinking to unusual challenges within his/her functional responsibilities, and evaluate the effectiveness of all actions taken.
- Recognize deviations from the norm that might indicate an emergency and describe appropriate action (such as communicating clearly within the chain of command).

Public health leaders and administrators must also be competent to:

- Describe the chain of command and management system ("incident command system" or similar protocol) for emergency response in the jurisdiction.
- Communicate the public health information, roles, capacities, and legal authority to all emergency response partners—such as other public health agencies, and other health agencies, other government agencies—during planning, drills, and actual emergencies. (This includes contributing to effective community-wide response through leadership, team building, negotiation, and conflict resolution.)
- Maintain regular communication with emergency-response partners. (This includes maintaining a current directory of partners and identifying appropriate methods for contacting them in emergencies.)
- Assure that the agency (or agency unit) has a written, regularly updated plan for major categories of emergencies that respects the culture of the community.
- Assure that the agency (or agency unit) regularly practices all parts of emergency response.

(continued)

Box 13–3. *(continued)*

- Evaluate every emergency response drill (or actual response) to identify needed internal and external improvements.
- Assure that knowledge and skill gaps identified through emergency response planning, drills, and evaluation are addressed.

Leader/administrative occupations involve the exercise of analytical ability, judgment, discretion, personal responsibility, and the application of a substantial body of knowledge of principles, concepts, and practices applicable to one or more fields of administration or management. (Adapted from the U.S. Office of Personnel Management.)

Public health professionals must also be competent to:

- Demonstrate readiness to apply professional skills to a range of emergency situations during regular drills. (For example: access, use, and interpret surveillance data; access and use lab resources; access and use science-based investigation and risk-assessment protocols; identify and use appropriate personal protective equipment.)
- Maintain regular communication with partner professionals in other agencies involved in emergency response. (This includes contributing to effective community-wide response through leadership, team building, negotiation, and conflict resolution.)
- Participate in continuing education to maintain up-to-date knowledge in areas relevant to emergency response. (For example: emerging infectious diseases, hazardous materials, and diagnostic tests.)

Professional occupations require knowledge acquired through education or training equivalent to a bachelor's degree or higher; require the exercise of discretion, judgment, and personal responsibility for the application of an organized body of knowledge that is constantly studied. (Adapted from the U.S. Office of Personnel Management.)

Public health technical and support staff must also be competent to:

- Demonstrate the use of equipment (including personal protective equipment) and skills associated with his/her functional role in emergency response during regular drills.
- Describe at least one resource for backup support in key areas of responsibility.

Technical occupations involve non-routine work and are typically supportive of a professional or administrative field; involve extensive practical knowledge gained through job training, though less than that represented by college graduation; and in-

(continued)

(continued)
volve elements of the work of the professional or administrative field, but at less than full competence.

Clerical/support occupations involve structured work in support of office, business, or fiscal operations; duties are performed according to established policies or techniques and require training, experience, or working knowledge related to the tasks. (Adapted from the U.S. Office of Personnel Management.)

—Centers for Disease Control and Prevention

Incident Command

An important element of disaster planning is an incident command system, which provides a clear delineation of roles, functions, and duties for those involved in responding to large public incidents. Incident command is an important element of the response by public safety professionals to community threats, but it is a new concept to most public health professionals. The inclusion of public health departments as responders (in partnership with fire, police, and hazmat teams, as well as the FBI) to any future terrorism threat mandates training in incident command for public health professionals.

Staff Capacity

Improving staff capacity will require: (a) clarification of the roles of health department staff members who will interact with the public at the time of a disaster; (b) cross-training of staff members to improve the depth of capacity; and (c) collaboration with other community agencies, including other health departments, in order to share personnel and expertise.

In any local or state health department, one of the best indicators of a publicized threat to the public's health is an increase—sometimes a dramatic increase—in the number of telephone inquiries. Most telephone calls are answered by clerical staff members who either deal with them or transfer them to others who can appropriately respond. It is very important that these initial public contacts be handled well. All staff members involved in responding to public inquiries should be provided with information on the threat and related information that will enable them to respond well and minimize the need to involve others who may be dealing with the threat more directly.

Most local public health departments are limited in the number of highly trained individuals available to respond to terrorist acts. During and after the anthrax dissemination in 2001, for example, available staff members were quickly overwhelmed by the number of telephone calls and the demands for service that continued around the clock. One way to improve the effectiveness of "experts" is to cross-train, in advance, public health nurses, environmental health specialists, health educators, and others to handle the routine activities of communicable-disease control so they can be quickly called upon to do so when necessary.

Collaboration with others, particularly other health departments, can be very helpful for most agencies, but it is especially critical for local public health agencies that are limited in size and sophistication. State health department backup is very important, but county or regional (multi-county) communicable-disease reporting and response systems, bringing hospitals, health departments, and other agencies and organizations together into a co-ordinated system, can simplify the task of reporting and assure a competent, coordinated response.

Disease Surveillance

The capacity to identify and track the occurrence of both communicable and non-communicable chronic diseases at the local level in the United States has expanded significantly with the general improvement in electronic technology, but the presence of this technology and the personnel needed to utilize it effectively are quite variable across the country (see Chapter 14). Communicable-disease reporting has always been limited by the common reluctance of physicians and other health care providers and the occasional reluctance of laboratories to report their findings. This reluctance is often heightened by the multiplicity of reporting authorities that may exist in a region, and the perception that the public health response will be less than adequate. In order to provide an effective communicable-disease surveillance system for every community in this country, the following four objectives will need to be achieved: (1) epidemiological expertise in communicable-disease control available for every jurisdiction; (2) centralized communicable-disease reporting and response systems in regions with multiple reporting agencies; (3) disease surveillance systems to identify disease early in its course; and (4) electronic technology to track, evaluate, and communicate the results of disease surveillance.

In addition, chronic-disease surveillance, which also could benefit from this kind of attention, has importance for potential terrorist events. A chemical or nuclear attack, for example, could increase the risk of future onset of chronic diseases, which might not become manifest for years or even decades.

Local public health agencies will need to have the capacity to track the health status of populations exposed to chemical or nuclear agents over long periods of time. A growing body of evidence about post-traumatic stress disorder (PTSD) suggests that mental health disorders resulting from involvement in a disaster may be common and may take a long time before becoming apparent (see Chapter 3).[11] Surveillance systems for mental health, currently primitive or nonexistent, also need to be developed.

Communication

Reliable communication networks and processes are essential to successfully manage a response to a major public health threat or incident. Communication must occur vertically among local health departments and state and federal public health agencies, as well as horizontally among local health departments, local health care providers and institutions, safety agencies, emergency management agencies, and the general public. Local health departments should have radios, pagers, cell phones, electronic mail, fax machines, and other equipment required to assure that communication links remain functional, even when unforeseen communication disruptions occur. Local health departments should be included in safety agency communication grids, as appropriate, and participate in exercises designed to teach communication protocols, use of available technology, and preparedness for communication disruptions.

Local jurisdictions should also have access to personnel skilled in communicating to the public. Knowledge helps forestall or minimize panic. Public safety and public health professionals are often too involved in assessment and control of an emergency situation to write press releases for the media or information alerts for the health care community (see Chapter 7).

Laboratory Capacity

Most local health departments depend on state health department laboratories to provide microbiological testing for recognizing, tracking, and controlling outbreaks of infectious disease. The anthrax dissemination in the fall of 2001 resulted in state laboratories being flooded with requests to test substances for anthrax, reduced the capacity of some laboratories to support other local communicable-disease activities, and demonstrated the need for greater laboratory redundancy. Some states may be able to address this problem by agreements to become partners with other laboratories in time of special need. Local capacity may also need to be increased, however. This recommendation is not to suggest that local laboratories should be organized to support the investigation of bioterrorist attacks—a specialized capacity that should not necessarily be duplicated. Rather, local capacity may need to be expanded to perform more routine testing for the investigation and control of commonly encountered infectious diseases (see Chapter 14).

Laboratories should also be included as an important component of surveillance systems. For example, if a laboratory received a request to test a sample for anthrax or plague bacteria or another agent known to be a potential biological weapon, it should automatically notify the communicable-disease control office of its local health department.

Public Health Law

Many people believe that public health statutes at the state and local level will need to be strengthened to address possible bioterrorist threats. A Model State Emergency Health Powers Act has been proposed (see Box 13–4).

Education of Public Health Professionals

Schools of public health, schools with community health and preventive medicine programs, health education programs, and other academic programs in public health need to include in their curricula many aspects of terrorism as they apply to public health, in order to ensure that future public health professionals are prepared to address these challenges. A variety of continuing-education activities has already been developed to improve the knowledge and awareness of the public health workers who are currently grappling with terrorist threats. The subject of anthrax has been covered quite well, and there have been some initial efforts to help people understand smallpox as a weapon of terror. Information has come through satellite video conferences, later made available on videotape; faxes; electronic mail distributed by the Health Alert Network; articles printed in newsletters and journals; grand rounds in hospitals; and a variety of professional conferences. Material has been both general and oriented toward the needs of specialized groups, such as administrators and clinicians. The CDC has produced and distributed most of the information, and professional associations have assisted in giving it wide distribution.

The continued development and distribution of such information is very important. There should be a careful evaluation of the education and training needs of the public health workforce. Attention should be focused on agents that might be used as weapons but have so far received little notice, including not only infectious organisms, but also chemical and nuclear weapons. In addition, it will be important to continue to offer educational materials in a wide variety of formats. There are still, after all, some local health departments that do not have electronic mail and that may be open less than five days a week.

Box 13–4. The Model State Emergency Health Powers Act.

In the aftermath of the September 11 attacks and the intentional dissemination of anthrax through the mail, it became clear that the public health system was ill-prepared for a potential bioterrorism attack. The Center for Law and the Public's Health at Georgetown University and Johns Hopkins University drafted the Model State Emergency Health Powers Act (MSEHPA, available at www.publichealthlaw.net) at the request of Centers for Disease Control and Prevention and in collaboration with members of national organizations representing governors, legislators, attorneys general, and health commissioners.

State public health statutes are frequently outdated, having been built up in layers during the 20th century. Consequently, these laws often do not reflect contemporary scientific understandings of disease, in terms of surveillance, prevention, and response; or legal norms for protection of constitutional rights, such as equal protection and due process; and statutory rights, such as protection against discrimination on the basis of disability.

The purpose of the MSEHPA is to facilitate the detection, management, and containment of public health emergencies, while appropriately safeguarding personal and proprietary interests. The scope of the Act includes major events of bioterrorism or naturally occurring infectious diseases affecting large portions of the population. The Act is structured to reflect five basic public health functions to be facilitated by law. The first two functions (planning and surveillance) would go into effect immediately, and the other three functions (management of property, protection of persons, and communications) would go into effect only after a declaration of a public health emergency by the governor of a state. These five functions are:

Preparedness and planning: The Public Health Emergency Planning Commission (appointed by the Governor) must prepare a plan that includes coordination of services; procurement of necessary material and supplies; housing, feeding, and caring for affected populations (with appropriate regard for their physical and cultural/social needs); the proper vaccination and treatment of individuals in the event of a public health emergency; and ethical criteria for rationing scarce resources.

Surveillance: The Act contains detailed provisions for surveillance, including prompt reporting of all critical agents of bioterrorism, interviewing persons infected, and tracing persons potentially exposed. It facilitates the exchange of health information among public health, emergency management, law enforcement, and other relevant agencies, as well as private-sector entities, including pharmacies, hospitals, and managed-care organizations. This surveillance allows for rapid detection and monitoring of health hazards.

Management of property: The state's designated public health authority may close, decontaminate, or procure facilities and materials to respond to a public health emer-
(continued)

265

Box 13–4. *(continued)*

gency; destroy dangerous goods and materials; dispose of infectious waste safely; perform appropriate burials; and obtain and deploy health care supplies, such as needed medicines and vaccines. The public health authority must compensate owners for public use of private property, but it need not compensate them for closure or destruction of dangerous facilities. This distinction conforms with modern constitutional law.

Protection of persons: The Act permits the public health authority to physically examine and test individuals as necessary to diagnose or to treat illness; vaccinate or treat to prevent or ameliorate an infectious condition; and isolate or quarantine individuals to prevent or limit the transmission of an infectious disease. The public health authority also may waive licensing requirements for health care professionals and direct them to assist in vaccination, testing, examination, and treatment of patients. To ensure an appropriate sphere of liberty and justice, the Act contains a modernized, extensive set of conditions and principles to safeguard human rights, including procedural due process, respect for religious and cultural beliefs, and care of persons in isolation and quarantine.

Communication and public information: The Act provides for a set of powers and duties to ensure appropriate public information and communication. The public health authority must provide information to the public regarding the emergency, including protective measures to be taken and information regarding access to care for physical and mental illness. An authoritative spokesperson for public health should be designated.

The Act facilitates the exercise of critical public health functions within a framework of personal rights and freedoms protected by law. As Justice John Harlan wrote in the seminal United States Supreme Court case of *Jacobson v. Massachusetts*, "The whole people covenants with each citizen, and each citizen with the whole people, that all shall be governed by certain laws for the common good." The Act strikes such a balance.

—Lawrence O. Gostin

(Editors' note: A critique of the Act appears in Box 17–1 in Chapter 17.)

Coordination and Funding of Research

The threat and reality of bioterrorism have stimulated a significant amount of research aimed at developing approaches that can protect the U.S. population. In 1999, the IOM published a report entitled, *Chemical and Biological Terrorism Research and Development to Improve Civilian Medical Response*, which analyzed preparedness at four levels of intervention: (a) local emergency response personnel, (b) initial treatment facilities, (c) state departments of emergency services, and (d) state departments of public health.[12] In its discussion of public health, the report emphasized the importance of surveillance for microbial agents, chemicals, and toxins, and also noted: "No research effort, no matter how important or sophisticated, will be productive until the nation rebuilds the public health infrastructure to a level at which the results of appropriate research can be properly applied. This infrastructure improvement would have enormous value to the average citizen on a day-to-day basis and would generate significant health benefits beyond readiness for terrorist events."[12]

The committee offered some specific research suggestions: (a) determine the benefits and drawbacks to using Internet and electronic-mail technologies to improve reporting and access to expertise during a biological or chemical release; (b) develop quick and accurate nucleic-acid "fingerprinting" techniques for microbes that may be used by terrorists, and make these techniques available for general use; and (c) develop symptom-based, automated decision aids to assist physicians in the early recognition of unusual diseases, and test these aids for validity and accuracy.

The Department of Defense, the National Institutes of Health (NIH), and the CDC have developed bioterrorism research agendas. NIH work emphasizes detecting microbes, developing antimicrobial therapeutic agents and vaccines, and performing basic microbial research.[13] (See also Chapter 15.)

The anthrax dissemination in 2001 raised many potential research questions (Chapter 6). Our understanding of the transmission, treatment, and prognosis of inhalational anthrax had been based on limited and dated information. The recent "real world" experience with anthrax demonstrated that some parts of this understanding need to be changed. That experience, coupled with concern about other agents that might be deliberately released, raised some additional questions that need to be answered, such as: How long must chemoprophylaxis be continued after exposure to anthrax spores? Is it reasonable to offer people post-exposure anthrax vaccine? Should patients exposed to smallpox virus be treated with an antiviral agent?

Research projects addressing bioterrorism questions are difficult to design because of the ethical issues inherent when working with dangerous organisms that occur rarely in human hosts. Nevertheless, it is important to learn what we can so that use of untried and unexamined treatments can be minimized in exposed or ill victims of a terrorist attack. It would also be helpful to find a way to coordinate research funding concerning terrorism to ensure that the most important questions are addressed, that duplication of effort is minimized, and that competition for research support takes place in a constructive manner.

CONCLUSION

The public health system in the United States, entrusted with promoting health and preventing disease and injury in the population, is troubled. In recent years, many of its shortcomings have been identified, and the profession has made significant progress in addressing some of them. Nevertheless, serious problems still hamper the capacity of the system to respond to large and complex threats to public health.

Improvements in the ability of this system to respond to terrorist threats will depend on progress in three areas: improving organization and structure, developing collaborative partnerships, and increasing funding for infrastructure. There are too many very-small local health departments that cannot begin to meet the obligations a terrorist event would thrust upon them. For some, the best option for their constituents would be to merge with a larger neighboring health department. Others might be able to improve their capacity by developing strategic partnerships or by sharing resources in other ways. Certainly, all local health departments need to establish good working relationships with the medical care community, safety agencies, neighboring health departments, the state health department, emergency management agencies, professional associations, and other relevant agencies, institutions, and organizations.

The issue of paramount importance, however, is that the 50-year decline in support for public health infrastructure in the United States must be reversed. Funding must be provided for obtaining communication equipment and expertise, for improving the epidemiological capacity at the local level for both infectious and chronic noninfectious diseases, and for expanding laboratory capacity. The good news is that investments in public health infrastructure will improve the capacity of local health departments to accomplish their usual tasks of health promotion and disease prevention. This will result in improvements in health status across the United States, even if there never is another major episode of terrorism in this country.

REFERENCES

1. Bunker JP, Frazier HS, Mosteller F. Improving health: measuring effects of medical care. *The Milbank Quarterly* 1994; 72:225–258.
2. Fee E. "History and Development of Public Health." In: D Scutchfield, CW Keck (eds.) *Principles of Public Health Practice.* Albany, New York: Delmar Publishers, 1997; pp. 10–30.
3. Institute of Medicine, Committee for the Study of the Future of Public Health. *The Future of Public Health.* Washington, D.C.: National Academy Press, 1988; pp. 1–2.

4. Milne T. "The Local Health Department." In Scutchfield D, Keck CW (eds.) *Principles of Public Health Practice* (2nd edition). Albany, New York: Delmar Publishers, 2002; Chap. 8.

5. National Association of County and City Health Officials. *Local Public Health Agency Infrastructure: A Chartbook.* Washington, D.C.: NAACHO, 2001.

6. Centers for Disease Control and Prevention. Preventing emerging infectious diseases: a strategy for the 21st century. *MMWR*, 47(No. RR-15), 1998.

7. Centers for Disease Control and Prevention. Biological and chemical terrorism: strategic plan for preparedness and response, *MMWR*, 49(no. RR-4), 2000.

8. Centers for Disease Control and Prevention. Public health's infrastructure: a status report. Prepared for the Appropriations Committee of the United States Senate, 2000.

9. National Association of County and City Health Officials. *Research Brief: NACCHO Emergency Response Survey, #6.* Washington, D.C.: NACCHO, February 2002.

10. Gonzales J. *A Report from the Front Lines: Safeguarding America's Communities from Terrorism.* National Association of Counties, January 2002. Available at http://www.naco.org, accessed January 31, 2002.

11. McFarlane AC. "The Prevalence and Longitudinal Course of PTSD." In: Yehuda R, McFarlane AC (eds.) *Psychobiology of Posttraumatic Stress Disorder.* New York: New York Academy of Sciences, 1997; Vol. 821, pp. 10–23.

12. Institute of Medicine, Committee on R&D needs for improving civilian medical response to chemical and biological terrorism incidents. In: *Chemical and Biological Terrorism Research and Development to Improve Civilian Medical Response.* Washington, D.C.: National Academy Press, 1999.

13. Portfolio Summary of NIAID-Supported Research on Bioterrorism, October 2001. http://www.niaid.nih.gov/factsheets/btrsch.htm, accessed December 27, 2001.

14

Improving epidemiology, surveillance, and laboratory capabilities

J. LYLE CONRAD AND JAMES L. PEARSON

In the United States, the first health responder to disease outbreaks, terrorist threats, or terrorist attacks is the local public health authority—and if indicated, the local law authority. This local public health response is based on constitutional law that was first established in 1791. Health and welfare became the responsibility of state governments, which passed laws governing the practice of medicine, the reporting of disease, and the licensing of laboratories and hospitals. By 1925, all states reported some diseases to the U.S. Public Health Service (PHS) in Washington, D.C. In 1961, this reporting and response function was transferred to the then–Center for Disease Control.[1] All states and territories have a laboratory designated as the state (or territorial) public health laboratory (PHL). Originally formed to test milk, drinking water, and specimens from patients with suspected venereal diseases or tuberculosis, these laboratories continue to be a vital component of public health surveillance and prevention.

CURRENT STATUS

Reporting and investigating disease outbreaks are state functions. Each state health department has delegated these functions to the "state epidemiologist," although he or she may not be an epidemiologist by training, job title, or experience. Today, each state and territory has at least one person designated as the state epidemiologist, and most major cities have a senior epidemiologist as well. The state epidemiologists' national organization, the Council of State and Territorial Epidemiologists (CSTE),[2] establishes guidelines for the national surveillance of disease and standardized case definitions. State epidemiologists are often directly involved in the administration of disease-control grants from the Centers for Disease Control and Prevention (CDC) and other federal agencies, and the preparation of state budget requests. By tradition and necessity, state epidemiologists coordinate control efforts with state public health laboratories, and share information on disease occurrence in their jurisdictions with neighboring states and the CDC.

Depending on the size of its population, a state may have one to 50 staff epidemiologists working in specialty areas, such as acute communicable-disease epidemiology, chronic-disease epidemiology, injury epidemiology, and environmental-disease epidemiology. These epidemiologists may have had previous education and training as physicians, dentists, veterinarians, nurses, and statisticians or in other health professions. In times of emergency, they all can assist on any type of problem.

Disease surveillance and control are the primary functions of the epidemiologist. Primary-care-physician practices, emergency departments, public health department clinics, and laboratories provide most disease reports. These reports are sent to the local health department, the state health department, or both, depending on the process defined by the state. The state compiles all of the reports received, collates and analyzes them, and, on a weekly basis, provides reports to medical care providers in the state and to the CDC. The CDC collates and analyzes data for the entire nation and reports national disease and injury data and other information on its website and in the Morbidity and Mortality Weekly Report (*MMWR*).[3]

Over the past 100 years, the disease surveillance system has evolved from weekly postcards to telephonic and facsimile reports, to computer-based reporting by medical care providers to health departments. The most recent development in reporting, the National Electronic Disease Surveillance System (NEDSS), captures electronic reports from medical care providers, augmented by direct entry of reports received by telephone or other means. City, county, district, and state health departments across the country are adding computers, enabling more rapid reporting, analysis, and distribution of population-based disease data to medical care providers and community-based prevention programs. Medical care providers, hospital emergency departments, and clinical laboratories are also moving toward electronic reporting, providing the opportunity for the next step: daily incident, or real-time, reporting. The CDC and some states have used active daily surveillance in special situations or for special events, such as the Olympics, the Goodwill Games, and the presidential inauguration, with good results. But such a system is very labor-intensive and cannot be maintained routinely or nationally without an enormous infusion of human and financial resources.

Public health laboratories are integral to the surveillance and epidemiological investigation of disease. Some states have one PHL, while others have several laboratories in cities, counties, or local health districts. The specific testing that they provide for public health and clinical diagnosis varies. Many PHLs offer direct services to local medical care providers and public health clients in local health departments. Some have courier services, while others depend on mail, commercial delivery services, and customer drop-off. Each state and territory has a person designated as the state public health laboratory director. The Association of Public Health Laboratories (APHL) provides advocacy and support for laboratory science, presents training programs for laboratory staff members, and sponsors conferences as fora for discussing issues.

Public health laboratories are a neglected treasure. For too long, we have been lulled into complacency by the quiet success of public health interventions that have decreased morbidity and mortality in our communities. Because government officials who make funding decisions seldom see graphic reminders of the need for public health, there has been a steady erosion of funding for vital infrastructure such as PHLs. Ideally, today's PHL has sophisticated tools to analyze specimens from people, food, water, and the environment that provide valuable data for surveillance, case finding, patient diagnosis, intervention, and prevention. In reality, however, PHL tools are aging, the workforce is dwindling in number, facilities are deteriorating, and budgets are usually declining, while the workload and the cost of providing essential laboratory services continue to rise. Today's mantra is: "Do more with less."

Surveillance depends on several resources, among which laboratory-based reporting of significant disease is a vital component. With declining resources, PHLs must either reduce services or charge for them. Today, several state PHLs are partially or completely supported by fees. Without substantial financial support from government, PHLs are severely limited when needs for emergency services arise.

CHALLENGES POSED BY TERRORISM

Terrorism has brought new challenges to the public health system. In 1984, when the first modern-day bioterrorist attack in the United States occurred, the Oregon state health department was inundated by more than 700 cases of salmonellosis and requested help from the CDC (see Box 10–2 in Chapter 10). This outbreak demonstrated that basic services were in place and operating, but it also gave warning that the public health system was inadequately prepared for bioterrorism.

Concerns about the use of biological and chemical agents of terrorism had been discussed for years in public health and academic circles. With heightened awareness of the potential for terrorist attacks on the United States during the Persian Gulf War, Congress began to consider the risk. In 1998, the CDC received initial funding from Congress for bioterrorism preparedness. Part of these funds was designated for competitive grants to state health departments and state public health laboratories to begin preparation at the state level. While the funding was insufficient to provide start-up funding for every state, territory, and major city, it did allow for a modest beginning.

The CDC began training of health department staff members. States offered training to physicians and nurses on signs and symptoms of diseases most likely to be spread by terrorists. PHLs began training staff of clinical and commercial laboratories to be alert for "select agents" in clinical specimens, and giving instruction on shipping suspicious isolates to the PHL. The CDC, the American Society for Microbiology, the United States Army Medical Research Institute of Infectious Diseases (USAMRIID), the Federal Bureau of Investigation (FBI), and the APHL teamed up to prepare standardized procedures to rule out the presence of these organisms in clinical specimens. They were instructed to immediately refer an isolate to a PHL and contact the local health department if a potential bioterrorist agent was identified.

The Laboratory Response Network (LRN) was established by the CDC, the APHL, and other agencies and organizations to provide clear guidance on which laboratories could provide reliable and timely services. The CDC prepared and distributed reagents and laboratory diagnostic materials to LRN members, according to the levels of service that laboratories were prepared to deliver. Readiness improved slowly, but steadily.

The almost simultaneous appearance of anthrax infections in October 2001 ushered in a new era (Chapter 6). A physician in Florida suspected anthrax in a patient, and the local branch of the state public health laboratory confirmed *Bacillus anthracis* from clinical specimens from this patient. Surveillance, disease reporting, and epidemiological investigation by the Florida Department of Health and the CDC proceeded rapidly. During the next several weeks, additional cases were reported in New York City; Virginia; Maryland; Washington, D.C.; and Connecticut. The CDC dispatched more than 100 epidemiologists to assist cities and states. Public health professionals demonstrated that letters containing anthrax spores that had been sent through U.S. Postal Service mail were the source of the infections.

In retrospect, it was clear that our local and national public health services had been stretched to the limit.[5] Epidemiologists employed by public health agencies were in short supply locally and nationally; few were available for other problems during this three-month period. Laboratory services were overwhelmed at the local, state, and national levels. Several CDC specialty laboratories were pressed into service to test for anthrax in human and environmental samples. Regular services were delayed.

State PHLs were inundated with environmental samples to test for anthrax. "White powder" flooded the system. Some initial reports of positive anthrax samples were later rescinded. PHLs in some jurisdictions did not have timely access to the materials necessary to perform standard laboratory protocols for anthrax testing. Protocols for testing specimens from humans were available for some of the select agents, but had not been validated and distributed for all organisms likely to be used by bioterrorists. Methods of testing environmental samples, including dust and powders, for anthrax had not been completely validated and needed immediate revisions. State and local PHLs responded admirably, but they did not have the necessary material resources and number of staff members to provide the testing needed to satisfy the insatiable demand for information. As of late February 2002, LRN laboratories had processed over 150,000 samples for suspected anthrax, and specimens were still being received.

The news media were often the first to report significant information; unfortunately, these reports were not always accurate (see also Chapter 7). Another facet of communication was also found wanting. Fact sheets were prepared and distributed by city, county, district, state, and federal government agencies; but often the information contained in these sheets conflicted with information distributed by other entities. Public health agencies were slow to provide knowledgeable and respected spokespersons to supply accurate scientific information to the media.

While anthrax has not been unknown in the United States, the public health profession had little recent experience with the disease. Studies on transmission were either very old or of limited scope. Science was vague on several issues, including the infectious dose by the airborne route, the incubation period, and effective treatment. Political involvement also kept the public health system in turmoil. Initially, top political leaders and their appointees showed a lack of understanding of infectious disease and the role of public health in control and prevention. As these leaders learned the complexity of disease control, public health officials took over responsibility for public communication, which helped reduce public anxiety. Gradually, public understanding of the problems led to more reasonable public expectations that these problems could not be instantly solved, despite political demands.

An impressive array of infectious agents and chemicals may be used in terrorist attacks (Chapters 10 and 11). Explosives as well as nuclear and radioactive weapons expand the possibilities (Chapters 9 and 12). Physicians, nurses, epidemiologists, and laboratory specialists have been challenged to learn new skills necessary to quickly identify disease that may be linked to an intentional act. Demand for epidemiologists with general training will be high, for these "epi-generalists" will be the first to investigate suspected terrorist incidents. If the initial investigation suggests a terrorist attack, epidemiologists and laboratory scientists with special training and skills will need to be available to advise on how to proceed.

The shortage of PHL scientists and epidemiologists in the United States is not new. For a variety of reasons, including salaries that lag behind the private sector, many of these positions go unfilled. The United States will need far more epidemiologists and laboratory scientists with additional skills and training to perform the investigations and analyses in order to provide early warning of an attack. These professionals will need to be distributed throughout the United States.

Surveillance systems must be modernized. Data collection and analysis must be more rapid, and distribution to those who need to know, more timely. Most important, data sources will need to be expanded. Since a terrorist attack may involve explosives, or biological, chemical, or nuclear or radioactive weapons, or a combination of those weapons, data must be collected from a wide variety of sources. These sources could include various groups of workers, and people of all ages and population groups. The laboratory must be able to identify agents that previously were not considered in the differential diagnosis—not only from human or animal specimens, but also from food, water, air, or other environmental sources. Surveillance must extend throughout the medical care system. Clinicians must have low thresholds of suspicion and promptly report suspected cases of terrorism to public health authorities and provide appropriate specimens to competent laboratories for identification or referral.

Epidemiologists must be available to promptly visit sites involved to consult and to evaluate the risk of the spread of disease to others. If potential for spreading is suspected, teams of properly trained and equipped professionals must be organized and engaged so that the problem is competently, safely, and completely investigated. If a terrorist attack is extensive, the resources required may need to be increased several-fold. Rapid response is critical to minimize disease, disability, and death.

Laboratory services will also need to be expanded due to the complexity of the challenge. But questions abound: Should each state have a full-service PHL, or should those services be consolidated? Should the system have many very competent and complex laboratories to meet national needs, or a few larger laboratories that are complete in every aspect of microbiology, chemistry, and physics, with links to the surrounding area by rapid, on-demand couriers? Solutions to long-neglected problems will be very expensive.

DEFICIENCIES IDENTIFIED IN EPIDEMIOLOGY, SURVEILLANCE, AND LABORATORY CAPABILITIES

Since the formation of the CSTE in 1951 and the establishment of the Epidemic Intelligence Service (EIS) at the then–Communicable Disease Center in 1951, the shortage of epidemiologists has been recognized, publicized, and acknowledged. This shortage exists at all levels—local, state, and national—and in academia as well. Several studies during the past 15 years have addressed the need for more epidemiologists in the public sector.[4] The distribution of epidemiologists in the United States is also a major concern. When the nation called on CDC epidemiologists for help to investigate the anthrax dissemination in 2001, it meant that many other services at the CDC had to be temporarily discontinued. Epidemiologists from the CDC were sent to states and cities affected by anthrax that did not have enough trained staff members to conduct the necessary investigations. Some states have only one epidemiologist and little funding for additional staff.

Gunn and colleagues (1989) reviewed the number of public-sector epidemiologists in the United States and offered a formula for the distribution of epidemiologists to each state according to its population.[4] They recommended a minimum of four doctoral-level epidemiologists in the public section per state, supported by an equal number of non-doctoral epidemiologists with training for specific diseases, and an additional senior epidemiologist and supporting epidemiologist for each one million people—a goal to be realized within 15 years. These recommendations were made before the need for terrorism surveillance was recognized. Georgia, with 50 epidemiologists and a state population of eight million, meets these goals. North Dakota, South Dakota, Montana, Arizona, Maine, Idaho, Pennsylvania, Virginia, North Carolina, South Carolina, and many other states do not. With the added responsibilities of investigating suspected terrorism, the shortage is profound.

The anthrax attack also demonstrated deficiencies in surveillance (see Chapter 6). Several patients were in the hospital and near death before reports were distributed through the system, resulting in a substantial delay in case investigation. A weekly surveillance report with a medical practitioner as the principal source of information is not enough in today's world. Reporting must occur at least daily, with a goal of real-time reporting if the nation is serious about reducing the impact of a terrorist attack. Surveillance should be expanded to include occupational groups, such as postal workers and airline employees, public health clinics, health maintenance organizations, insurance companies, and emergency departments. Computer-based reporting must be enhanced nationally. Every county and local health department should have at least one computer and the necessary number of qualified staff members dedicated to compiling and sending reports to, and receiving reports from, the national disease reporting system—on a daily basis. This system will require enough epidemiologists to analyze data as they are received, to recognize clusters, and to assure that local epidemiologists are notified and that investigations are completed promptly enough to prevent additional exposures. A comprehensive national surveillance system has yet to be designed, but it will be needed if the residents of the United States are to be protected from another exposure to anthrax or other microorganisms in a terrorist attack.

Deficiencies in PHL services were also notable. The anthrax laboratory at the CDC was overrun with environmental and human specimens. Other CDC laboratories with proper containment were converted to support anthrax studies, and personnel from other areas who had training and experience working in a containment laboratory were reassigned to work on the influx of anthrax samples. States like Virginia, Maryland, and New York had similar problems. States without adequate or available laboratory containment facilities had extreme difficulty finding other laboratories with the capacity and capability to test the huge volume of samples generated by public fear. PHLs across the country were called on to analyze unusual dust and powder samples for anthrax spores.

Testing protocols developed by APHL and the CDC were modified to allow rapid screening of environmental samples. APHL provided consultation and testing services to the U.S. Postal Service. PHLs also accepted the additional burden of receiving samples collected as evidence by law enforcement, fire, and hazardous materials officers, and maintaining these samples under strict chains of custody.

Pending results of laboratory analyses, airports, public facilities, and businesses were closed when unexpected packages or letters without return addresses were received, or when people found powder on the floor. PHLs became highly visible for the first time in decades. In order to ensure that the public's health was protected, emergency procedures were implemented, facility security was enhanced, and staff members provided 24-hour, 7-day-a-week coverage. Routine work was delayed or not performed. Scientists were reassigned from other areas to provide relief for those who had worked for excessively long periods.

The deficiencies in the laboratory system became clear. Equipment was old and in short supply. Reagents were difficult to obtain. Supplies dwindled. Containment facilities were too small to handle the volume of work. There were not enough facilities. Many were not designed to meet current safety standards. And most important, there was a major shortage of trained laboratory scientists to perform analyses.

The anthrax outbreak of 2001, initiated by sending letters containing anthrax spores through the mail, showed our vulnerability. Previously, some experts had challenged the possibility of a biological agent's being effectively used by a terrorist, claiming that delivery devices were not available or not reliable. Delivery devices used in the 2001 anthrax dissemination were readily available and, in retrospect, highly efficient. They could easily have resulted in millions of exposures had letters been sent—and anthrax dispersed—more broadly.

IMPROVING EPIDEMIOLOGY

The current shortage of epidemiologists and laboratory scientists is acute. Training additional people for these vital public service careers must begin immediately. At the CDC, the incoming class of EIS officers should be doubled or tripled, at latest by July 2003, recognizing that it takes at least five years to develop fully competent epidemiologists (Figures 14–1 and 14–2).

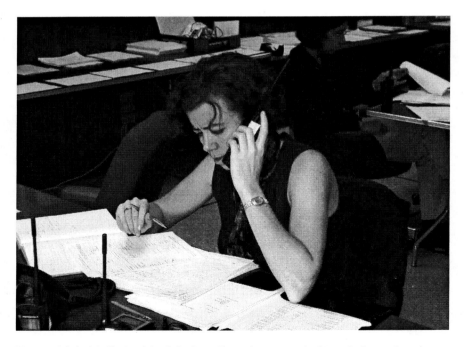

FIGURE 14–1. Medical epidemiologist collects data over telephone during anthrax investigation in New York City in the fall of 2001 (Photograph by John Redd).

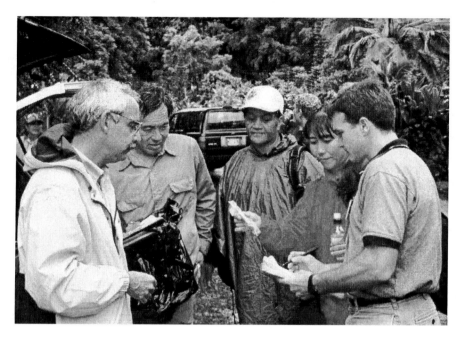

Figure 14–2. Medical epidemiologists and other investigators collect field specimens during an outbreak of dengue fever in Hawaii (Photograph by John Mosely Hayes).

Skilled supervision of these officers, so critical to their success, will require a significant commitment of time from already hard-pressed professionals at the CDC and state and local health departments. Schools of public health are another important source of epidemiologists. If funding were made available, graduates of two-year public health graduate programs could move into supervised three-year field assignments with the EIS. After five years of training, these epidemiologists would be able to assume major responsibilities in health departments. But where would they end up?

The distribution of trained epidemiologists is not uniform in the United States. DeKalb County, Georgia, with a population of 700,000, is home to the CDC headquarters. County residents include approximately 1,000 active and retired epidemiologists, perhaps the greatest concentration on earth. North Dakota, with a population of 635,000, two Strategic Air Command (SAC) bases, missile sites, Garrison Dam on the Missouri River, and an over-the-horizon radar station, has just one epidemiologist. In order to improve the distribution of trained epidemiologists, recruitment, retention, and support must be addressed. Successful recruitment of trained professionals for the sparsely populated or remote areas of the United States will require a different strategy. Candidates from those areas will be more likely to return to those areas to practice upon completion of their training. In order to retain people in those areas, positive working environments must be established, with good support staff, necessary equipment, competitive salaries, and strong public health laboratories. Even more important are strong, well-trained, and highly motivated local supervisors who understand what public health is and is not, and who have access to skilled consultants to provide guidance for unusual situations. Support of the local political leadership is also vital to sustaining public health epidemiology. If such an environment cannot be provided by the political jurisdiction, federal epidemiology officers could perform the necessary surveillance and epidemiology functions for the population. Supervision of these officers would present another challenge, although the CDC or nearby academic centers with trained epidemiologists could provide guidance. Action is needed now to address these difficult challenges.

As of early 2002, the magnitude of the current shortage of epidemiologists is unknown, but the CSTE is studying the problem, and answers should be available in the near future. We roughly estimate that there are now approximately 1,000 public-sector epidemiologists. In the absence of hard data, a reasonable goal is to have at least one practicing public health epidemiologist working in the public sector per 100,000 people nationwide by 2004—a total of approximately 2,000 additional epidemiologists. These new epidemiologists will need high-quality supervision and practical experiences to expand their skills, putting additional pressure on experienced epidemiologists who will be expected to provide supervision and guidance.

Continuity is also a challenge. About 100 senior epidemiologists retire every year after, on average, a career of about 30 years; another 100 leave public-sector positions every year, often because of frustration with political leadership, inadequate salaries, or lack of local support. Over the past several years, the annual demand for experienced senior epidemiologists has exceeded 200.[6]

The attacks on the World Trade Center and the Pentagon, followed by the anthrax dissemination, demonstrated yet another problem. In late 2001, when the CDC reassigned 100 or more EIS officers to the East Coast to respond to these terrorist attacks, their original assignments were neglected until the end of the crisis. These EIS officers provide the nation's "surge capacity" of epidemiologists. Unfortunately, with a disaster of this magnitude, the need far outstripped the supply. Other vital public health services were not performed at the CDC and in state and local health departments. Trained personnel were not available to fill in the gaps left by those who were reassigned.

In order to meet the shortfall, about three times as many EIS officers are needed—about half of these for assignment to states and major cities for training. Once trained, these additional officers could provide the necessary surge capacity when terrorist attacks or natural disasters occur, with other services vital to the public's health being provided with only minimal disruption. The needs can seem overwhelming. Enhanced recruitment for the next generation of epidemiologists and establishment of more training programs should begin immediately.

IMPROVING SURVEILLANCE

Public health surveillance has made enormous strides in the past generation. Early in the 20th century, diseases were reported by postcard from the medical care provider to the county health department, then these reports were forwarded to the state health department. The process took months to complete. Once a year, totals were summed and a report prepared and distributed to the U.S. Public Health Service in Washington, D.C. Immediate problems, such as disease outbreaks, were investigated locally, with an occasional assist from the state health department if it could respond. By 1961, states were sending weekly reports to the CDC; if they did not arrive, follow-up phone calls were initiated to collect the data. During the 1970s and 1980s, states began to encourage reporters to call in reports weekly, with modest success. Reporting was still delayed. With the acceptance of computers by health departments, and the development of electronic reporting programs, timeliness began to improve. The National Electronic Telecommunications System for Surveillance (NETSS) began to take shape. By the end of the 1980s, all states were reporting weekly to the CDC by computer, and the CDC was compiling and placing those reports on its the website, making data available much faster than before.

County health departments began to communicate with their state health departments by computer, further improving the process. By 2001, it was clear that if all large cities and counties had computer linkages to the system, reporting could finally move beyond the weekly reporting standard, which had been in place since 1912. Daily reporting would become possible, even reasonable to expect, and for terrorist events, instant reporting could occur. More epidemiologists will be needed to collect, enter, and send data; software and hardware will need to be developed and used; and more trained people will be needed to respond to the problems that are reported. In addition, reports from private-sector patient and laboratory data systems must be integrated into the system. CDC has begun working with states, territories, and large cities to establish standards for surveillance and reporting, and is funding demonstration projects that will create electronic linkages between medical-care data systems and public health departments. The groundwork has been laid for a truly modern, timely, and complete reporting system.

One of the goals of epidemiology is to contain an outbreak within one incubation period, thereby preventing unnecessary disease and disability. For example, to control measles, the outbreak must be reported, confirmed by the laboratory, and control measures completed within 7 to 10 days, before the second wave of cases strikes. This is difficult but not impossible to achieve. Hepatitis A, with an incubation period of approximately 30 days, allows more time to complete control measures. With current reporting procedures, gonorrhea or influenza, with much shorter incubation periods, cannot be controlled in the first wave of cases.

Airborne distribution of anthrax spores presents a new challenge to the surveillance system. The current standard of *weekly* reports does not provide data in a time frame that allows for prevention or intervention. Computer-based reporting offers a solution to the issue of timeliness. If *daily* reports can be established as the standard reporting interval, with *instant* reports from medical care providers when suspected cases are seen, unnecessary morbidity and mortality can be prevented. For this to become reality, the tools must be in place, with enough well-trained people to report and analyze data and immediately investigate suspicious occurrences. Funding and political will must be in place if this system is to work.

In the aftermath of the 2001 terrorist attacks, national political leaders began to recognize the role of public health in the recognition and control of terrorist events in the United States. Public health had been neglected for too long, and political leaders had lost sight of the meaning of public health. Public health is not medical care for the individual, or medical care for the indigent. Both are vital to the well-being of our country, but neither one is public health. Public health, in part, consists of the actions necessary to control problems with air, water, and food when the community—not the individual—is sick. This action occurs community-wide, and timely surveillance is vital if prevention efforts are to be successful. The goals of the CDC and the entire U.S. public health system now and for the past 50 years have been to provide teams of epidemiologists, high-quality public health laboratories, timely surveillance, and systems that encourage access to and sharing of relevant data with those who need to know. These goals are within reach, but the system must stretch to address current and future needs.

IMPROVING THE PUBLIC HEALTH LABORATORY

The terrorist attacks of 2001 demonstrated dangerous shortcomings of PHLs in the United States, both in capacity (the volume of samples that can be processed in time to provide data for intervention and prevention) and in capability (the ability to perform the specific testing needed by decision-makers). These shortcomings can be corrected with substantial investment, in both the short and the long term.

New and renovated buildings and equipment can be financed with one-time funding. Even training can be funded over a short period. Competent personnel are the greatest asset. Attracting and keeping them is the most difficult challenge. To hire and retain good laboratory scientists, PHLs will need sustained funding. At the time of this writing in early 2002, the economy is flat and many states are facing budget cuts—and especially deep cuts in public health programs and services—due to reduced revenue. While the terrorist events of 2001 have increased awareness of PHLs, funding for improved infrastructure and staffing will not be readily available through state budgets. The national political leadership has allocated funds to rebuild the infrastructure, and improve the capability and capacity of the nation's public health system to respond to terrorism. Often federal funds have been provided to states for a limited time, with the expectation that the state will assume the cost of maintaining the program when federal funding ends. It is extremely difficult, if not impossible, to hire high-quality staff members on "soft money" (limited-duration funding). Without a constant funding source, states will not be able to attract qualified people to work in these vital programs, or to keep them once hired.

Shortages of laboratory scientists, while difficult to quantify, occur at both the entry level and the doctoral level (Figure 14–3). Entry-level positions,

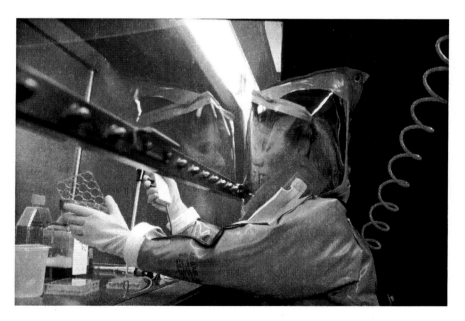

FIGURE 14–3. Strengthening the competencies of laboratory scientists and modernizing the equipment of state public health laboratories is necessary for developing better preparedness against bioterrorist threats and emerging infectious disease problems (Public Health Image Library, Centers for Disease Control and Prevention).

when advertised by state laboratories, often fail to attract qualified candidates. New graduates in the basic sciences or medical technology programs could fill these positions. Unfortunately, the number of graduates in these disciplines falls far short of the demand, salaries offered by states are often not competitive, and graduates do not consider public service when seeking a career. Even those who begin their careers in the public sector often leave state service. State laboratories provide excellent training, and their scientists are in demand by commercial entities. Retaining those trained scientists will require funding for improvements in salary. Estimates of the number of entry-level candidates needed range from 500 up to several thousand per year; the anticipated federal funding for terrorism preparedness will push the number toward the high end of this estimate.

Doctoral-level scientists with experience are also in short supply, both to lead individuals performing highly complex assays and applied research and to provide the next generation of PHL directors. Doctoral-level scientists will also benefit from federal funding to states and the LRN goal to move all state laboratories to a molecular testing platform. With the advent of genotypic assays, these scientists will be in demand to lead the implementation efforts. Additionally, expertise will be needed in states to provide validation of new tests and development of new assays.

PHL directors are also in demand. Qualification as a "high-complexity laboratory director" under the requirements of the federal Clinical Laboratory Improvement Act of 1988 (CLIA) is the baseline for most states. Experience in a diverse laboratory environment and with government practices, rules, and regulations is essential for a director's success. Currently, there are no programs to prepare PHL directors. A doctoral-level scientist needs at least five years of experience with increasing management responsibilities to qualify for these positions.

In order to successfully combat terrorism, the laboratory must have safe and secure facilities to work in, proper equipment, and well-trained and dedicated staff. Each state must have at least one laboratory with Biosafety Level Three (BSL3) capabilities, and staff trained to work with BSL3 procedures within that contained laboratory. As of February 2002, there were 23 states that had reported having a BSL3 facility in their PHLs. Programs to train people to work in contained laboratories are not readily available in the United States. The demand for personnel to work in these facilities will increase as state laboratories build new, or renovate old, facilities in order to meet safety guidelines.

More is necessary, however, for a functional system. Disaster plans and contingency plans must be developed and tested frequently. Proficiency testing, an essential for assessing the accuracy and reliability of analyses, must also be more readily available for the assays used to detect possible terrorist events. Also needed are laboratory supplies and reagents, computers, high-speed Internet access, and ongoing training. The laboratory must also be tied into a secure and reliable communications system with the state public health community and with local, state, and federal partners. In addition, it must have a laboratory information system with links to a secure public health network for both reporting and emergency communications.

CONCLUSION

Terrorism presents many new challenges to the nation's public health infrastructure. We have been complacent for the past 30 years and have let our basic structures of epidemiology, public health laboratory services, and disease control decline, while the challenges have become more sophisticated and elaborate. It is urgent that we now change and reinvest in our public health system to establish and maintain a strong disease-defense system—nationwide, competent, and modern. We must now train many more epidemiologists, laboratory scientists, and local health department staff members. Secure communications systems must be established to link surveillance data from public health offices in the smallest counties and towns to each other, to state health departments, to the CDC, and the nation as a whole in order to assure that accurate and timely information is available for making intelligent decisions for rapid disease control. Public health laboratories and epidemiologists are the cornerstones of this defense, and the nation's political leaders must recognize this to ensure that vital public health services are never again neglected and allowed to decay.

REFERENCES

1. Teutsch SM, Elliott CR. *Principles and Practice of Public Health Surveillance.* Oxford University Press: Oxford, 2000.
2. Council of State and Territorial Epidemiologists, 2872 Woodcock Boulevard, Suite 303, Atlanta, GA 30341-4015.
3. Centers for Disease Control Website: www.cdc.gov/od/hissb/docs.htm.
4. Gunn RA, et al. State epidemiology programs and state epidemiologists: results of a national survey. *Public Health Rep* 1989; 104:170–177.
5. Rosenfield R, Morse SS, Yanda K. September 11: The response and role of public health. *Am J Public Health* 2002; 92:10–11.
6. *The Epidemiology Monitor,* 2560 Whisper Wind Court, Roswell, GA 30076 or epimon@aol.com.

15

Improving vaccines, antimicrobials, and antitoxins through research

DOROTHY MARGOLSKEE

Vaccines, antimicrobials, and antitoxins play important roles in protecting the public from bioterrorism. Timely administration of these agents to affected or at-risk populations can prevent diseases caused by bioterrorist agents or minimize their adverse health effects.

This chapter covers vaccines, antimicrobials, and antitoxins, with a particular focus on potential research opportunities to improve the availability, efficacy, and safety of these medical interventions. Biological agents that could be used in terrorist attacks are covered in Chapter 10. They include the Category A high-priority agents identified by the Centers for Disease Control and Prevention (CDC), which are considered to have the greatest potential adverse impact on public health and require a broad-based level of preparedness to counteract them. Category A pathogens include three bacterial infections (anthrax, plague, and tularemia), one bacterial toxin (botulinum toxin), one specific virus (smallpox), and one disease syndrome (hemorrhagic fever) caused by a collection of viruses.[1] Each poses somewhat different scientific opportunities and challenges for those managing the impact of an intentional exposure (see Table 10–1).

Potential interventions for these and other diseases that may be spread through bioterrorism include specific drug therapies; immunological interventions (vaccines and passive immunizations with antibody preparations); and, for some diseases, antitoxins. Not all interventions are available for each pathogen. The existence of vaccines, antimicrobials, and/or antitoxins for the Category A high-priority agents and the diseases that they cause are noted in Table 15–1.

A systematic evaluation of society's ability to respond to potential bioterrorist agents can help identify and prioritize research and development needs. Critical elements of this ability to respond include: (a) early recognition of an intentional exposure; (b) rapid diagnosis with confirmation of the causative agent; (c) optimal treatment of the index case(s) and subsequent cases; (d) rapid institution of post-exposure prophylaxis for asymptomatic people who may have been exposed; and (e) when feasible and appropriate, pre-exposure prophylaxis for others.

Among the considerations in assessing research and development efforts are:

- *Incubation period duration.* The duration of the incubation period is important in evaluating the feasibility of successful post-exposure prophylaxis. Post-exposure prophylaxis will not be effective for a pathogen if the time taken to recognize a potential exposure and to start a specific prophylactic regimen exceeds the length of the incubation period.

TABLE 15–1. Current Existence of Vaccines, Antimicrobials, and Antitoxins for CDC Category A Agents and Diseases.

AGENTS/DISEASES	VACCINE	ANTIMICROBIAL	ANTITOXIN
Bacillus anthracis Anthrax	Yes[1,2]	Yes[3]	No
Smallpox virus Smallpox	Yes[1,2]	No	No
Clostridium botulinum toxin Botulism	No	No	Yes[1–4]
Yersinia pestis Plague	No	Yes[3]	No
Francisella tularensis Tularemia	Yes	Yes[3]	No
Viral hemorrhagic fevers Filoviruses	No	No	No

[1]Limited availability.

[2]Tolerability not optimal.

[3]Efficacy very time-dependent.

[4]Antitoxins not available for all toxin subtypes.

- *Pathogen virulence factors.* Unique characteristics of the virulence of pathogens may provide potential molecular targets for new antibiotics, antivirals, or vaccines.
- *Efficacy and tolerability.* The existence, efficacy, tolerability, and safety of therapeutic and prophylactic regimens are also important when prioritizing research efforts.

Table 15–2 highlights points to consider when devising a response for each pathogen.

There are a number of opportunities for research to enhance society's ability to respond to potential biological weapons (see Table 15–3). This chapter focuses on several research areas, including: (a) the need for rapid diagnosis and institution of appropriate antibiotic treatment for the bacterial pathogens that cause anthrax (*Bacillus anthracis*), pneumonic plague (*Yersinia pestis*), and tularemia *(Francisella tularensis)*; (b) the potential use of antitoxins to mitigate the effects of *B. anthracis* and *Clostridium botulinum* toxins; (c) considerations surrounding the availability and use of vaccines to prevent smallpox; and (d) the continued need for fundamental research on the viruses causing hemorrhagic fever.

THE NEED FOR RAPID DIAGNOSTIC TESTS FOR THE PATHOGENS THAT CAUSE ANTHRAX, PNEUMONIC PLAGUE, AND TULAREMIA

The anthrax outbreak in the United States in 2001 (see Chapter 6) dramatically highlighted general diagnostic and treatment challenges for the three Category A bacterial pathogens that can cause rapidly progressive, life-threatening infections if left untreated. The bacteria that cause pneumonic plague and tularemia could have had more serious and widespread consequences

TABLE 15–2. Transmission and Incubation Period Information for CDC Category A Agents

PATHOGEN	INFECTIVITY	PERSON-TO-PERSON TRANSMISSION	INCUBATION PERIOD	REFERENCES
B. anthracis	Low to moderate	No	4 to 60 days	2,64,65
F. tularensis	Very high	No	3 to 5 days	4,46,66
Y. pestis	High	Yes	2 to 4 days	3,67
C. botulinum	Not applicable	No	12 to 72 hours	18,68,69
Smallpox virus	Very high	Yes	12 to 14 days	35,39,41
Ebola virus	Low to moderate	Yes	Unknown	55,70

TABLE 15–3. Needed Research on Potential Bioterrorist Agents.

AREA OF RESEARCH	BACTERIAL PATHOGENS (B. ANTHRACIS, Y. PESTIS, AND F. TULARENSIS)	BOTULISM	SMALLPOX	HEMORRHAGIC VIRUSES (FILOVIRUSES)
Rapid detection assays needed	+++	+++	++	+++
Specific therapies (new antibiotics or antivirals) urgently needed	+*	–	++++	++++
Toxins identified and antitoxins needed or could be improved	+ to +++ (B. anthracis)	++	–	–
Potential to develop a vaccine with high impact to contain an outbreak	+ (B. anthracis)	–	++++	?+++

*To cover risk of resistant strains being engineered.

than those for anthrax: *Y. pestis* is spread person-to-person, whereas *B. anthracis* is not, while *F. tularensis* is more efficient than *B. anthracis* in causing infection.[2–4] For all three, the incubation periods—and opportunity for effective intervention—can be very short, especially for both *F. tularensis* and *Y. pestis* (Table 15–2). (See also Chapter 10.)

A review of the first ten cases of inhalational anthrax that occurred in 2001 illustrates the diagnostic challenges associated with this pathogen.[5] Patients sought medical care for nonspecific flu-like symptoms a few days after exposure. Initial chest x-rays were abnormal in all ten patients, but only seven patients had "classic" findings (mediastinal abnormalities, see Figure 6–5 in Chapter 6) and two had chest x-rays that were initially read as normal. Six of these ten patients were treated with multiple antibiotics active against *B. anthracis* and survived, while the four who had progressed to severe symptoms at the start of antibiotic treatment all died, reflecting the need for rapid diagnosis and early appropriate therapy for this potentially fatal disease.

A high level of clinical suspicion is needed to diagnose anthrax, pneumonic plague, or tularemia in patients who present with nonspecific symptoms (fever, cough, weakness, and malaise), and few physical signs. Routine evaluations may fail to identify the first patients affected by these diseases, since nonspecific symptoms in a community setting are much more likely to be associated with viral respiratory illnesses, such as influenza, rather than anthrax, pneumonic plague, or tularemia. Chest x-rays may show subtle changes. Blood cultures may take 12 to 18 hours (for *B. anthracis*)[2] or up to 48 hours (for *Y. pestis*)[3] to grow organisms. In addition, a positive blood culture for anthrax (Gram-positive *Bacillus* species) might be discarded as a presumed contaminant without further typing, unless the clinical laboratory is alerted. Finally, patients may be seen at different medical centers, making the recognition of a disease cluster more difficult.

The diagnostic hurdles posed by *B. anthracis*, *Y. pestis*, and *F. tularensis* extend to other unexpected infectious agents that have a high mortality potential. For example, surveillance studies conducted in the United States have estimated the incidence of unexplained critical illnesses and deaths potentially due to infection to be 0.5 to 8.9 cases per 100,000 per year in previously healthy people from 1 to 49 years of age[6,7]—probably an underestimate since misdiagnoses would not have been included. While progress has been made in strengthening the interactions across the network of clinical laboratories in the United States,[8,9] the limited access to specialized tests, including the polymerase chain reaction (PCR) test and immunohistochemical and serological assays available at the CDC and certain reference laboratories, causes an unavoidable time delay in diagnosis and risks the possibility that special tests will not be performed for index patients affected by serious, rare infectious diseases. In addition to putting these initial patients at high risk, delay in post-exposure prophylactic therapy can substantially increase the size of a potential outbreak, especially if the organism is highly infectious and transmitted person to person.[10]

Rapid-detection assays are critically needed for pathogens of highest concern. Optimally, these assays will be easy to use, reliable, sensitive (correctly determining the presence of a specific pathogen), specific (correctly determining the absence of a specific pathogen), and reasonably priced. Significant research effort is necessary to develop new technology for rapid detection assays.[11]

In addition, since there is a distinct potential for bioterrorists to genetically engineer drug resistance for the bacteria that cause anthrax, plague, and tularemia,[2–4] availability of new tests for rapid detection of drug-resistance markers would also be helpful in guiding initial treatment of cases. As new classes of broad-spectrum antibiotics become available from traditional industrial drug discovery and development programs, each should be tested for its activity against the pathogens that cause these three diseases, with promising candidate antibiotics then evaluated pre-clinically in animal models.

THE POTENTIAL ROLE OF ANTITOXINS

Anthrax Toxins

Distinct toxins released by *B. anthracis* and *C. botulinum* contribute to the very different clinical manifestations of anthrax and botulism. Concerning *B. anthracis*, three separate proteins (protective factor, lethal factor, and edema factor) work in concert with each other.[12,13] During the early phases of infection with *B. anthracis*, these toxins kill cells, especially macrophages, depressing the host's immune response to the infection and allowing rapid bacterial growth. Later, these toxins may have direct effects, causing edema and the release of cytokines, such as tumor necrosis factor and interleukin 1, and contributing to shock and ultimately death. There are currently no antitoxins available for *B. anthracis* toxins.

Recently, the crystal structures of the lethal and edema factors have been described.[14,15] In the current model, protective antigen forms a heptameric (seven-copy) ring that facilitates the entry of lethal and edema factors into cells. The importance of these toxins in disease is supported by the efficacy of the anthrax vaccine, which has previously been linked to the development of antibody against protective antigen.[16] The availability of crystal structures and an improved understanding of toxin protein–protein interactions should facilitate efforts to discover an antibody, peptide, or small-molecule inhibitor ("antitoxin") for anthrax.[17]

Botulinum Toxins

There are seven botulinum toxins (Types A through G),[18] any one of which could be used in a bioterrorist attack. All of these toxins have similar mechanisms of action, but they differ in their antigenic profiles and in their release from genetically diverse bacteria (primarily of the *C. botulinum* species). Lethal in very small quantities,[19] botulinum toxins have been included in bioweapon arsenals in Iraq and the former Soviet Union[18] and probably elsewhere.[20] Between 1990 and 1995, the Japanese cult Aum Shinrikyo dispersed toxin aerosols at various locations in Japan, but was unsuccessful in producing illness, perhaps for technical reasons (see Chapter 11).[21] Botulinum toxins are relatively easy to produce and can be disseminated as aerosols or (less likely) as contaminants in food.

All seven botulinum toxins work by preventing the delivery of acetylcholine from motor neurons to the corresponding muscle cells, causing paralysis.[22–24] These toxins are zinc-based proteases that initially bind and translocate into neuronal cells. They then cleave specific neuronal proteins responsible for fusing acetylcholine-containing vesicles released from the neurons with the plasma membranes of muscle cells. Once the toxin enters a neuron, it is no longer vulnerable to antibody neutralization. Three-dimensional protein structures have been determined for Type A and Type B toxins.[25–27] While both are zinc-containing proteases, each clips a different host protein involved in the fusion of the neuronal vesicles with muscle cells. There are corresponding differences in their three-dimensional structures that may help explain their different protein targets.

In general, antitoxin, in this case polyclonal antibody, minimizes the progression of paralysis caused by the matching botulinum toxin, although it does not change the course of resolution for affected neurons. Antitoxins against Types A, B, and E, which are obtained from horses immunized with type-specific botulium toxoid, are available from the CDC. Antitoxin supplies are limited, with only one supplier for the United States (Connaught) and variable availability in other parts of the world.[28] An additional investigational hexavalent antitoxin covering Types A through G has been used previously in a large Egyptian outbreak of Type E foodborne botulism.[29] Because of the foreign (equine) nature of the antibodies, hypersensitivity responses (urticaria, serum sickness, and anaphylaxis) are possible.

There are research needs in both diagnosis and therapy: (a) Currently, antitoxin is administered on the basis of clinical diagnosis because mouse bioassay confirmation may take days.[18] Rapid assays for laboratory confirmation and toxin typing are needed to assure the administration of the appropriately matched antitoxin, especially in the case of an intentional release. (b) In order to improve therapeutic options, the development of small-molecule protease inhibitors to cover all seven toxin types is unlikely, given the inherent difficulties of traditional drug development. On the other hand, it is feasible to develop a set of recombinant human monoclonal antibodies that, combined, neutralize the effects of all seven types of botulinum toxin.[30–32] The proof of therapeutic potential has been established with the effectiveness of the equine antitoxin; a recombinant source of human antibody would avoid the allergic reactions to foreign (equine) material and potentially provide sufficient volume to allow wider distribution to reference hospitals, in addition to the CDC and the U.S. Army.

THE POTENTIAL POST-EXPOSURE UTILITY OF VACCINES

Smallpox as an Example

While the smallpox virus is considered eradicated as a natural pathogen,[33] viral stockpiles exist in Russia and the United States and possibly elsewhere, making feasible the use of smallpox virus as a bioterrorist weapon.[34] An intentional exposure would most likely be by aerosol. Index cases would develop nonspecific symptoms and fever, followed by a very characteristic pustular rash.[35] Smallpox virus is highly infectious—person-to-person transmission would occur. (See also Chapter 10.)

There is no confirmed therapy for a patient with clinical smallpox. Cidofovir, an antiviral agent that inhibits viral DNA polymerase, is active *in vitro*.[36] While there is no animal model of smallpox to extend this observation, cidofovir is active against cowpox or vaccinia infections in mice.[37,38] There clearly is a need for more antiviral drugs to treat the viral infection, even if these drugs can only reduce the potential for, or period of, contagion.

Vaccine Safety and Efficacy

A protective vaccine was originally described by Edward Jenner in 1796.[39] This vaccine contains vaccinia (not smallpox) virus and was effective in protecting individuals from death if given within 3 to 4 days of exposure. From the 1950s through the 1970s, the smallpox vaccine was used in a concerted, worldwide campaign to eradicate smallpox, which featured detection of index cases and immunization of their potential contacts. With this combined approach, smallpox was declared eradicated worldwide as a natural infection in 1980.[33] The field experience during the smallpox eradication campaign established the effectiveness of the smallpox vaccine in post-exposure prophylaxis and outbreak containment.

Smallpox vaccine is administered by scarification of the skin with a bi-furcated needle.[39] A successful primary immunological response is assumed to have occurred if a vaccine recipient develops a typical skin response at the site of vaccination —development of a papule that evolves into a pustule (Figure 15–1), then a dried, crusted lesion, and ultimately a local scar. This primary reaction is often referred to as a "take." People vaccinated in the distant past may no longer be immune to smallpox infection;[40] therefore, in the event of an intentional exposure, prompt vaccination of all contacts would be potentially lifesaving.

Adverse health effects after vaccine administration can be significant. The most frequent adverse health effects include accidental auto-infection of other sites (eyes and mucosal membranes); eczema vaccinatum, in which vaccinia infection spreads to areas of pre-existing or prior eczema (Figure 15–2); and generalized vaccinia. Uncommon, but serious, complications include post-vaccinial encephalitis and, in immunosuppressed patients, progressive vaccinia, which is frequently fatal.[39,40] Vaccinia immune globulin (VIG) is recommended in the treatment of progressive vaccinia, severe generalized

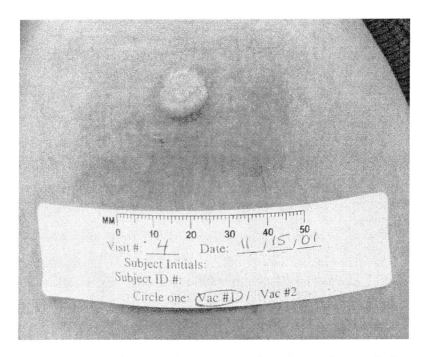

Figure 15–1. Typical primary reaction with pustule formation, erythema, and edema on day 7 after vaccination with vaccinia virus. (Frey SE, Couch RB, Tacket CO, et al. Clinical responses to undiluted and diluted smallpox vaccine. *New Engl J Med* 2002; 346:1270. Copyright © 2002 Massachusetts Medical Society.)

vaccinia, eczema vaccinia, and periocular auto-infection. VIG is recommended as prophylaxis if a patient with eczema or or an immunosuppressed patient requires vaccinia vaccination.[40] Based upon surveys in the 1960s of side-effects of the original smallpox vaccine, it has been estimated that one out of every one million people receiving primary vaccination would die of serious adverse effects of the vaccination.[41]

Current Recommendations for Vaccine Administration

CDC recommendations have been published, including non-emergency use of vaccine for laboratory workers occupationally exposed to vaccinia virus[40] and an interim updated bioterrorist response plan.[42] (These can be accessed at www.bt.cdc.gov.) A covert release of smallpox would probably go undetected until the first cases presented with the typical rash about 1 to 2 weeks after exposure. In order to limit secondary transmission, the CDC has recommended isolating these index cases and vaccinating and closely following known contacts (a "ring-vaccination" approach), since vaccination within the first few days of exposure could prevent severe disease. In addition, health care workers and essential disaster response personnel should also be vaccinated, assuming no medical contraindications. Because of the potential for severe adverse health effects of vaccination, especially in immunosuppressed patients such as those who are HIV-positive and those with a history of eczema, mass immunization has not been recommended, although there is considerable ongoing debate and discussion on this issue.[43,44]

A recent analysis modeled the impact of an intentional release of smallpox virus to a susceptible human population.[45] The results suggest that the timing of interventions in relation to exposure, the quarantine of symptomatic patients, and the availability of vaccine to administer to contacts would all have a significant impact on containing the spread of infection. In order to adequately cover vaccination needs, it has been estimated that 40 million doses should be stockpiled.[35] This estimate, however, may be too low a number. While approximately 10,000 people received post-exposure treatment during the recent anthrax outbreak,[46] anthrax is not transmitted person-to-person, so household contacts did not necessarily require prophylaxis. In addition, the effectiveness of a "ring vaccination" approach has been questioned in the setting of an unexpected attack on a susceptible population that could include simultaneous bioterrorist attacks in multiple cities.[43,44] (See Chapter 10.)

Opportunities and Challenges Related to Vaccine Development

Smallpox vaccine and VIG supplies are currently limited. Routine smallpox vaccination was gradually halted and then discontinued throughout the world

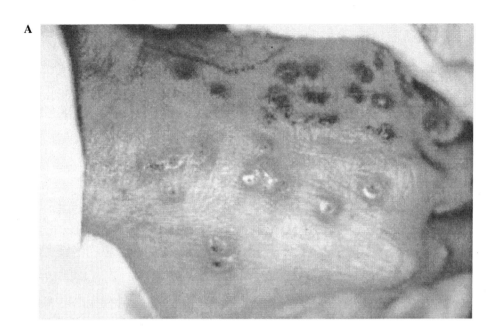

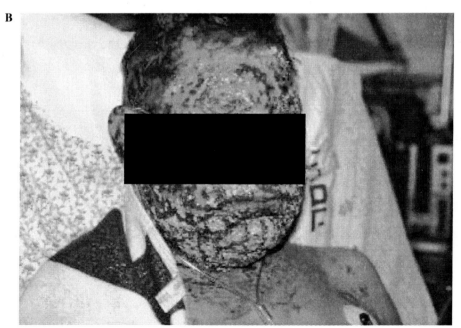

FIGURE 15–2.

after 1980, with subsequent discontinuation of the manufacture of vaccinia vaccine. A limited supply (about 15.4 million doses) of vaccine (Dryvax), produced by Wyeth Laboratories in the 1970s, is stored at the CDC.[47] An additional 85 million doses of 40-year old vaccine was donated in early 2002 to the United States by the vaccine manufacturer Aventis Pasteur.[48]

An effective vaccine against smallpox is an important component in the coordinated efforts required to contain a smallpox outbreak. There are two current avenues being pursued to expand the supply of smallpox vaccine.

First, recently completed clinical studies reported that 1:5 and 1:10 dilutions of the original vaccine resulted in successful immunization, as assessed by the development of an appropriate skin response, in 97 to 99 percent of volunteers.[49,50] Thus, if the U.S. Food and Drug Administration (FDA) concurs, current vaccine supplies could be expanded to cover initial containment needs and potentially an initial mass vaccination, if deemed necessary.

Second, there is an ongoing effort to manufacture new vaccinia vaccine. There are several challenges associated with this effort since the original process of vaccine manufacture is no longer acceptable for new vaccine release. Historically, vaccinia vaccine was produced by inoculation into the hides of calves, with subsequent harvest of lesion fluids. These fluids ("lymph") were then minimally purified and freeze-dried.[39] Current manufacturing strategies for live virus vaccines have employed cell culture systems, including diploid lines, such as MRC-5 or WI-38, or primary chick embryo fibroblast cultures. Vaccinia virus replicates well in several cell lines and a manufacturing process has been developed.[51]

Delivering new vaccine doses for stockpiling will be only part of the effort. Demonstrating the safety and efficacy of the newly manufactured vaccine will also be important, since the characteristics of live viruses can change

---

FIGURE 15–2. Ten days after being vaccinated against smallpox, a 27-year-old man, with a history of atopic dermatitis, was hospitalized with a high fever, facial edema, and an umbilicated, vesicular, crusting rash on his face, neck, upper chest, and hands (Panel A). He was diagnosed with eczema vaccinatum. As the vesicular rash became disseminated, supraglottic edema with shortness of breath developed. The patient was transferred to the intensive care unit and received vaccinia immune globulin and supportive care. Over the next 2 weeks extensive crusting of the facial lesions occurred (Panel B). Cultures of vesicular fluid grew vaccinia virus, and skin biopsy showed necrotic epidermal cells with intranuclear inclusions compatible with the diagnosis of eczema vaccinatum. Three weeks after admission, the patient was discharged, with deep facial and chest scars. Eczema vaccinatum is a rare complication of smallpox vaccination. It develops in patients with a history of eczema who are given the vaccine or who are in close contact with vaccinated persons. (Moses AE, Cohen-Poradoosu R. Eczema vaccinatum—a timely reminder [Images in clinical medicine]. *New Engl J Med* 2002; 346:1287 Copyright © 2002 Massachusetts Medical Society.)

with the type of cell culture and number of passages. The FDA will expect a full clinical program to evaluate the vaccine.[51] A successful Phase 1–2 clinical evaluation will require demonstration of acceptable safety and tolerability, as well as immunological responses—that is, an acceptably high percentage of subjects with local cutaneous "takes" and the development of serum-neutralizing antibody. Phase 3 will be primarily for obtaining additional clinical safety and tolerability data. Subsequent clinical studies to further evaluate any tolerability issues may be required, especially if reinstitution of routine immunization comes under consideration. Traditional efficacy studies are not possible, given the lack of naturally circulating disease and the inherent danger associated with a smallpox challenge study.

Finally, there are currently limited supplies of VIG available, owned mainly by the U.S. Department of Defense, with small quantities available from the CDC. In the event of an intentional smallpox release, significant quantities of VIG would be required. In the short term, a possible source would be by hyperimmunizing volunteers with Dryvax and harvesting their sera. Long term, the generation of monoclonal antibodies could be considered, although it may be difficult to demonstrate that a monoclonal antibody is as efficacious as a polyclonal set of antibodies from immunized individuals, given the lack of animal models to verify that the selected monoclonal antibodies are protective. In any event, adequate supplies of VIG would be urgently needed if the need for vaccinations were anticipated.

Considerations for Use of Vaccine for Prophylaxis for the General Population

Discussions of re-initiating smallpox vaccinations for the general public have intensified as vaccine supplies have improved; this debate should be considered in the context of general vaccine use. Most of the vaccines currently approved by the FDA are used as routine prophylaxis to prevent symptomatic infection. Currently recommended childhood immunizations, which cover 13 different pathogens, comprise 20 injections for each infant in the first two years of life.[52] Vaccines recommended for adults include those to protect against hepatitis A virus, hepatitis B virus, and influenza infection. Travelers' vaccines, tetanus boosters, and vaccines for special circumstances, such as rabies exposure, are also available.

When a vaccine is approved by the FDA for general use, very careful consideration is given to the potential benefit offered by the vaccine's efficacy in comparison to its potential for adverse effects.[52] Also considered are the method and consistency of manufacture, and the quality and safety of the final product. Modern vaccines approved for general use are highly effective and very well tolerated. Typical adverse reactions are generally transient and mild, such as fever and tenderness at the site of administration. Serious re-actions, such as anaphylaxis, are very infrequent, occurring in less than one in 100,000 immunizations. In some instances, however, rates even lower than one in one million immunizations are of concern; for example, an incidence rate of one case of oral vaccine-associated paralytic poliomyelitis in 2.4 mil-lion doses prompted changes in U.S. immunization practices[53] and an even-tual switch to inactivated polio vaccine.[54]

The effectiveness of the original vaccinia vaccine was demonstrated through the worldwide eradication of circulating smallpox in the 1970s. Ev-idence of cutaneous "take"—once demonstrated—will probably indicate similar protection by the newly manufactured vaccine, although this pro-tection will not be proven in the absence of a smallpox outbreak. On the other hand, there are frequent, known adverse effects associated with small-pox vaccination in healthy individuals; identified high-risk groups, includ-ing people with undiagnosed immunosuppression, such as those with un-diagnosed HIV infection; and a relatively high incidence of severe and life-threatening adverse effects when compared to current "routine" im-munizations. As the debate continues, the likelihood of a bioterrorist ac-tion will need to be weighed carefully by informed parties against the cer-tainty of dealing with adverse health effects of smallpox vaccination. If mass vaccination is undertaken, the public will need to be carefully edu-cated about what to expect.

THE NEED FOR FUNDAMENTAL RESEARCH ON THE VIRUSES THAT CAUSE HEMORRHAGIC FEVER

Of the viruses causing hemorrhagic fever, filoviruses have received consid-erable public attention. Two groups of these single-stranded RNA viruses have been identified: the Marburg and Ebola strains. The Marburg virus was first identified in 1967 in Marburg, Germany, from laboratory staff working with African green monkeys. Four subtypes of Ebola virus have been identified by the site of initial isolation: Zaire, Cote d'Ivoire, Sudan, and Reston (Virginia). Mortality is highest with Ebola-Zaire, ranging from 50 to 80 percent.[55]

The natural reservoir(s) for Ebola virus is not known. With the exception of occupationally related infections in laboratory workers (Marburg and Re-ston),[56,57] there have been sporadic, limited epidemics in Central Africa over a period of at least 25 years, occurring in Zaire, Sudan, Cote d'Ivoire, Gabon, and the Republic of the Congo (DRC).[55] Non-human primates, including chimpanzees and gorillas, are likely intermediate hosts but not reservoirs, given the extent of disease and high mortality rate when infected. Multiple species—arthropods, bats, even plants—have been suggested as potential chronic hosts, but there is no concrete evidence as yet.[58]

Little is known about the pathophysiology of hemorrhagic fever. The clinical course is typically severe and rapid. When it occurs, death is within 2 weeks of the start of symptoms, with the development of diffuse bleeding from mucosal surfaces, multi-organ failure, and shock.[55] There is no treatment or vaccine; the use of hyperimmune serum has not been proven to be effective. Effective barrier precautions and quarantine of infected patients have been successful in stopping outbreaks.[59]

There is considerable research interest on the Ebola virus, although the need for high-level containment (Biosafety Level 4) has limited the number of participating laboratories. The viral genes and proteins have been identified,[60] although the reason for the extreme pathogenicity (especially associated with Ebola-Zaire) is not known. Factors contributing to the clinical syndrome may include cell toxicity associated with the envelope glycoprotein (GP); infection and replication in white blood cells (monocytes and macrophages), with subsequent cytokine release; and, in fatal cases, destruction of the immune system, including lymphocytes.[60–63]

Emerging Infectious Diseases and the Potential to Cause Harm

Unlike smallpox, transmission of Ebola virus appears to require direct contact with infected body fluids for effective person-to-person transmission, limiting the extent of an intentional outbreak. Yet intentional introduction of such a severe and potentially lethal disease would have a significant psychological impact on the general public. In many ways, the circumscribed extent of an outbreak would favor the choice of Ebola virus over smallpox virus as an agent, although gaining access to the virus would be a challenge.

Even without potential bioterrorist use, emerging infectious diseases are a clear threat to a mobile society and therefore require focused attention. In addition to new entities, re-emergence or spread of known diseases, such as yellow fever and dengue, and the development of antibiotic or antiviral resistance in existing pathogens are serious concerns. In the case of filoviruses, remaining important research initiatives include continued efforts to elucidate their molecular biology, pathogenesis and virulence, epidemiology, and natural reservoirs, and to develop specific treatments and vaccines against them.

CONCLUSION

Consideration of the Category A pathogens highlights the general criteria for an effective response to bioterrorism:

- Early recognition of an intentional exposure is critical to allow effective medical intervention for index cases and their contacts. Rapid diagnosis of the infectious agents associated with significant, persistent, but initially non-specific, symptoms will require continued development, frequent updating, and widespread use of rapid diagnostic tests for rare and emerging pathogens.
- Even with accurate diagnosis, many infections—especially viral ones—cannot currently be treated. The development of antiviral agents is an important research goal. In addition, the ability to bioengineer common bacterial and viral pathogens for antimicrobial resistance requires the continued development of new classes of anti-infective drugs.
- Vaccine research is also a high priority. Given the challenges of vaccine development, careful choice of infectious disease targets is mandatory. In addition, for each vaccine, considerations for use—general immunization versus post-exposure prophylaxis—will demand that we carefully weigh the potential benefits of preventing infection versus the risks of causing vaccine-associated adverse effects.
- Most important, the bioterrorist events in the United States in 2001 have highlighted the public's general vulnerability to exposure to new and emerging infectious agents. A renewed emphasis on public health surveillance, diligent case follow-up, and early diagnosis is critical, since these activities comprise the first line of a broadly effective defense.

REFERENCES

1. Rotz LD, Khan AS, Lillibridge SR, et al. Public health assessment of potential biological terrorism agents. *Emerg Infect Dis* 2002; 8:225–230.
2. Inglesby TV, Henderson DA, Bartlett JG, et al. for the Working Group on Civilian Biodefense. Anthrax as a biological weapon. *JAMA* 1999; 281:1735–1745.
3. Inglesby TV, Dennis DT, Henderson DA, et al. for the Working Group on Civilian Biodefense. Plague as a biological weapon. *JAMA* 2000; 283:2281–2290.
4. Dennis DT, Inglesby TV, Henderson DA, et al. for the Working Group on Civilian Biodefense. Tularemia as a biological weapon. *JAMA* 2001; 285:2763–2773.
5. Jernigan JA, Stephens DS, Ashford DA, et al. and members of the Anthrax Bioterrorism Investigation Team. Bioterrorism-related inhalational anthrax: the first 10 cases reported in the United States. *Emerg Infect Dis* 2001; 7:933–944.
6. Perkins BA, Flood JM, Danila R, et al. Unexplained deaths due to possibly infectious causes in the United States: defining the problem and designing surveillance and laboratory approaches. The Unexplained Deaths Working Group. *Emerg Infect Dis* 1996; 2:47–53.
7. Haijeh RA, Relman D, Ciesiak PR, et al. Surveillance for unexplained deaths and critical illnesses due to possibly infectious causes, United States, 1995–1998. *Emerg Infect Dis* 2002; 8:145–153.

8. Klietmann W, Ruoff KL. Bioterrorism: implications for the clinical microbiologist. *Clin Micro Rev* 2001; 14:364–381.

9. Robinson-Dunn B. The microbiology laboratory's role in response to bioterrorism. *Arch Pathol Lab Med* 2002; 126:291–294.

10. Kaufmann AF, Meltzer MI, Schmid GP. The economic impact of a bioterrorist attack: are prevention and postattack intervention programs justifiable? *Emerg Infect Dis* 1997; 3:83–94.

11. Niiler E. Bioterrorism—biotechnology to the rescue? *Nature Biotech* 2002; 20:21–25.

12. Friedlander AM. Tackling anthrax. *Nature* 2001; 414:160–161.

13. Liddington RC. Anthrax: a molecular full nelson. *Nature* 2002; 415:373–374.

14. Pannifer AD, Wong TY, Schwarzenbacher R, et al. Crystal structure of the anthrax lethal factor. Nature 2001; 414:229–233.

15. Drum CL, Yan S-Z, Bard J, et al. Structural basis for the activation of anthrax adenylyl cyclase exotoxin by calmodulin. *Nature* 2002; 415:396–402.

16. Stepanov AV, Marinin LI, Pomerantsev AP, Staritsin NA. Development of novel vaccines against anthrax in man. *J Biotechnol* 1996; 44:155–160.

17. Mourez M, Kane RS, Mogridge J, et al. Designing a polyvalent inhibitor of anthrax toxin. *Nature Biotech* 2001; 19:958–961.

18. Arnon SS, Schechter R, Inglesby TV, et al. Botulinum toxin as a biological weapon. *JAMA* 2001; 285:1059–1070.

19. Gill MD. Bacterial toxins: a table of lethal amounts. *Microbiol Rev* 1982; 46:86–94.

20. Cole LA. The specter of biological weapons. *Sci Am* December 1996; 275:60–65.

21. WuDunn S, Miller J, Broad WJ. How Japan germ terror alerted world. *New York Times.* May 26, 1998:A1, A10.

22. Halpern JL, Neale EA. Neurospecific binding, internalization, and retrograde axonal transport. In: Montecucco C, ed. *Clostridial Neurotoxins. Current Topics in Microbiology and Immunology,* vol. 195. New York: Springer; 1995. 221.

23. Singh BR. Intimate details of the most poisonous poison. *Nature Struct Biol* 2000; 7:617–619.

24. Shapiro RL, Hatheway C, Swerdlow DL. Botulism in the United States: a clinical and epidemiologic review. *Ann Intern Med* 1998; 129:221–228.

25. Lacy DB, Tepp W, Cohen AC, et al. Crystal structure of botulinum neurotoxin type A and implications for toxicity. *Nature Struct Biol* 1998; 10:898–902.

26. Swaminathan S, Ewaramoorthy S. Structural analysis of the catalytic and binding sites of Clostridium botulinum neurotoxin B. *Nature Struct Biol* 2000; 7:693–699.

27. Hanson MA, Stevens RC. Cocrystal structure of synaptobrevin-II bound to botulinum neurotoxin type B at 2.0 A resolution. *Nature Struct Biol* 2000; 7:687–692.

28. Shapiro RL, Hatheway C, Becher J, Swerdlow DL. Botulism surveillance and emergency response. *JAMA* 1997: 278:433–435.

29. Hibbs RG, Weber JT, Corwin A, et al. Experience with the use of an investigational F(ab')$_2$ heptavalent botulism immune globulin of equine origin during an outbreak of type E botulism in Egypt. *Clin Infect Dis* 1996; 23:337–340.

30. Amersdorfer P, Marks JD. Phage libraries for generation of anti-botulinum scFv antibodies. *Methods Mol Biol.* 2000; 145:219–240.

31. Green LL, Hardy MC, Maynard-Currie CE, et al. Antigen-specific human monoclonal antibodies from mice engineered with human Ig heavy and light chain YACs. *Nat Genet* 1994; 7:13–21

32. Bavari S, Pless DD, Torres ER, et al. Identifying the principal protective antigenic determinants of type A botulinum neurotoxin. *Vaccine* 1998; 16:1850–1856.

33. Fenner F, Henderson DA, Arita I, et al. *Smallpox and Its Eradication.* Geneva: World Health Organization, 1988.
34. Henderson DA. Countering the posteradication threat of smallpox and polio. *Clin Inf Dis* 2002; 34:79–83.
35. Henderson DA, Inglesby TV, Bartlett JG, et al. for the Working Group on Civilian Biodefense. Smallpox as a biological weapon. *JAMA* 1999; 281:2127–2137.
36. De Clercq E. Vaccinia virus inhibitors as a paradigm for the chemotherapy of poxvirus infections. *Clin Micro Rev* 2001; 14:382–397.
37. Bray M, Martinez M, Smee DF, et al. Cidofovir protects mice against lethal aerosol or intranasal cowpox virus challenge. *J Infect Dis* 2000; 181:10–19.
38. Smee DF, Bailey KW, Sidwell RW. Treatment of lethal vaccinia virus respiratory infections in mice with cidofovir. *Antivir Chem Chemother* 2001; 12:71–6.
39. Henderson DA, Moss B. Smallpox and vaccinia. In: Plotkin SA and Orenstein WA, eds. *Vaccines.* Philadelphia: WB Saunders, 1999:74–97.
40. Centers for Disease Control and Prevention. Vaccinia (Smallpox) Vaccine. Recommendations of the Advisory Committee on Immunization Practices (ACIP), 2001. *MMWR* 2001; 50:1–25.
41. Breman JG, Henderson DA. Diagnosis and management of smallpox. *N Engl J Med* 2002; 346:1300–1308.
42. Interim smallpox response plan and guidelines. Atlanta: Centers for Disease Control and Prevention, 2001. (Accessed April 1, 2002, at http://www.bt.cdc.gov/DocumentsApp/Smallpox/RPG/index.asp).
43. Fauci, A. Smallpox vaccination policy—the need for dialogue. *N Engl J Med* 2002; 346:1319–1320.
44. Bicknell, WJ. The case for voluntary smallpox vaccination. *N Engl J Med* 2002; 346: 1323–1325.
45. Meltzer MI, Damon I, LeDuc JW, Millar JD. Modeling potential responses to smallpox as a bioterrorist weapon. *Emerg Infect Dis* 2001; 7:959–969.
46. Centers for Disease Control and Prevention. Evaluation of postexposure antibiotic prophylaxis to prevent anthrax. *MMWR* 2002; 51:59.
47. LeDuc JW, Becher J. Current status of smallpox vaccine. *Emerg Infect Dis* 1999; 5:593–4.
48. Connelly C. French firm giving stores of smallpox vaccine to U.S.; 85 million doses a huge boost for bio-defense. *San Francisco Chronicle*, March 30, 2002; A-3.
49. Frey SE, Couch RB, Tacket CO, et al. for the NIAID Smallpox Vaccine Study Group. Clinical responses to undiluted and diluted smallpox vaccine. *N Engl J Med* 2002; 346:1265–1274.
50. Frey SE, Newman FK, Cruz J, et al. Dose-related effects of smallpox vaccine. *N Engl J Med* 2002; 346:1275–1280.
51. Rosenthal SR, Merchlinsky M, Kleppinger C, Goldenthal KL. Developing new smallpox vaccines. *Emerging Inf Dis* 2001; 7:920–926.
52. Parkman PD, Hardegree MC. Regulation and testing of vaccines. In: Plotkin SA and Orenstein WA, eds. *Vaccines.* Philadelphia: WB Saunders, 1999:1131–1143.
53. Poliomyelitis prevention in the United States: introduction of a sequential vaccination schedule of inactivated poliovirus vaccine followed by oral poliovirus vaccine: Recommendations of the Advisory Committee on Immunization Practices (ACIP). *MMWR* 1997; 46:1–25.
54. Poliomyelitis prevention in the United States: updated recommendations of the Advisory Committee on Immunization Practices (ACIP). *MMWR* 2000; 49:1–22.

55. WHO-recommended guidelines for epidemic preparedness and response: Ebola Haemorrhagic Fever. WHO, Emerging and Other Communicable Diseases, Surveillance and Control, 1997 (WHO/EMC/DIS/97.7). Accessed April 1, 2002 at http://www.who.int/emc-documents/haem_fevers/whoemcdis977c.html.

56. Smith CE, Simpson DI, Bowen ET, Zlotnik I. Fatal human disease from vervet monkeys. *Lancet* 1967; 2:1119–1121.

57. Centers for Disease Control and Prevention. Update: filovirus infection among persons with occupational exposure to nonhuman primates. *MMWR* 1990; 39:266–7.

58. Monath TP. Ecology of Marburg and Ebola viruses: speculations and directions for future research. *J Inf Dis* 1999; 179 (suppl 1):S127–38.

59. Peters CJ, LeDuc JW. An introduction to Ebola: the virus and the disease. *J Inf Dis* 1999; 179 (Suppl 1):ix–xvi.

60. Wilson JA, Bosio CM, Hart MK. Ebola virus: the search for vaccines and treatments. *Cell Mol Life Sci* 2001; 58:1826–1841.

61. Feldmann H, Volchkov VE, Volchkova VA, et al. Biosynthesis and role of filoviral glycoproteins. *J Gen Vir* 2001; 82:2839–2848.

62. Takada A, Kawaoka Y. The pathogenesis of Ebola hemorrhagic fever. *Trends Microbiol* 2001; 9:506–511.

63. Gibb TR, Bray M, Geisbert TW, et al. Pathogenesis of experimental Ebola Zaire virus infection in BALB/c mice. *J Comp Path* 2001; 125:233–242.

64. Pile JC, Malone JD, Eitzen EM, Friedlander AM. Anthrax as a potential biological warfare agent. Arch Intern Med 1998; 158:429–434.

65. Centers for Disease Control and Prevention. Update: Investigation of bioterrorism-related anthrax and interim guidelines for exposure management and antimicrobial therapy, 2001. *MMWR* 2001; 50:909–919.

66. Perez-Castrillon JL, Bachiller-Luque P, Martin-Luquero M, et al. Tularemia epidemic in northwestern Spain: Clinical description and therapeutic response. *Clin Inf Dis* 2001; 33:573–576.

67. Feldman KA, Enscore RE, Lathrop SL, et al. An outbreak of primary pneumonic tularemia on Martha's Vineyard. *N Engl J Med* 2001; 345:1601–6.

68. Hughes JM, Blumenthal JR, Merson MH, et al. Clinical features of types A and B food-borne botulism. *Ann Intern Med* 1981; 95:442–445.

69. St. Louis ME, Peck SH, Bowering D, et al. Botulism from chopped garlic: delayed recognition of a major outbreak. *Ann Intern Med* 1988; 108:363–368.

70. Disease outbreaks reported: Ebola haemorrhagic fever in Gabon/The Republic of the Congo. Update 21. WHO, Emerging and other Communicable Diseases, Surveillance and Control. (Accessed April 1, 2002 at http://www.who.int/disease-outbreak-news/n2002/march/22march2002.html).

16

Protecting food, water, and ambient air

CRAIG W. HEDBERG, JEFFREY B. BENDER,
AND DONALD VESLEY

Protecting food, water, and the ambient air are primary functions of the public health system. These functions are important in preventing terrorist acts and in minimizing the health consequences of terrorist acts that do occur. This chapter focuses on many aspects of this broad subject.

PROGRESS DURING THE 20TH CENTURY

During the first half of the 20th century, environmental health measures in the United States substantially reduced the spread of infectious agents through food and water, contributing to greatly reduced rates of death and markedly increased life expectancy—from approximately 47 years in 1900 to approximately 76 years in 2000.[1] Measures such as the provision of sanitary sewage disposal, chlorination and filtration of drinking water, pasteurization of milk, and refrigeration of perishable food helped control typhoid fever, tuberculosis, botulism, scarlet fever, and many other infectious diseases.[2]

So successful were these measures that during the second half of the 20th century the safety of food and water in the United States was largely taken for granted by the general public and policy-makers. New infectious disease threats emerged during this period, however. For example, in 1976, Legionnaire's disease emerged as a public health threat in the air and ventilation systems of buildings.[3] During the next 20 years, *Escherichia coli* O157:H7, *Listeria, Campylobacter*, and *Cryptosporidium* emerged as important foodborne and waterborne pathogens.[4,5] These emerging infectious diseases highlighted weaknesses in public health surveillance systems and led public health and regulatory agencies to undertake actions that focused on environmental sources of contamination of food, water, and air. These actions provide a framework for protecting food, water, and air from bioterrorism.

CHALLENGES

Food production and distribution systems extend from farms to retail grocery stores and restaurants. There are many potential targets for bioterrorism throughout these systems, depending on the goals of the terrorist. The one confirmed event of bioterrorism targeted at food in the United States involved the intentional contamination of restaurant salad bars with *Salmonella* in an attempt to disrupt a local election[6] (see Box 10–2 in Chapter 10). Although this contamination did not achieve the perpetrators' objectives, it caused 751 cases of salmonellosis. Numerous other outbreaks of plant, animal, and human diseases from unintentional contamination highlight the vulnerabilities of these food production and distribution systems, and the potential impact of bioterrorism on these systems. Some examples of these are highlighted in Table 16–1.

Much of the discussion about bioterrorism before October 2001 focused on potential mass-casualty situations resulting from aerosolization of the agents that cause anthrax, smallpox, and plague. But the mailing of a few letters containing or contaminated with anthrax spores demonstrated that a relatively low-tech and inefficient delivery device could elicit widespread fear and disrupt routine activities, even without causing many cases of illness or death (see Chapter 6).[7] Similarly, disruption of food distribution systems could be achieved by use of hoaxes, terrorist spread of non-lethal foodborne disease agents, or terrorist spread of highly contagious animal or plant pathogens.

Potential agents and bioterrorism targets can be identified throughout the food-production and food-distribution systems, from farm to table. A hazard analysis for food, water, and air can identify many points of interaction among these systems. For example, water is used in irrigating crops and processing fresh fruits and vegetables. In food-processing plants, ventilation systems are potential sources for contamination.

TABLE 16-1. Outbreaks that Demonstrate the Potential Impact of Bioterrorism Events on Food, Water, and Air.

SYSTEM	AGENT	CRITICAL CONTROL POINT FAILURE	OUTCOME OF OUTBREAK
Ambient air	*Legionella pneumophila*	Aerosol-generated from unchlorinated whirlpool spa	188 confirmed and probable cases of Legionnaire's disease at a flower show in the Netherlands.[42]
Animal agriculture	Foot-and-mouth disease virus	Apparently contaminated refuse used as feed ingredients on pig farm	10,135 farms affected and more than 4 million animals destroyed in the United Kingdom.[41]
Food processing and distribution	*Salmonella enteritidis*	Pasteurized ice cream pre-mix contaminated by raw egg in tanker trailer	Estimated 224,000 cases in 41 states in the United States.[18]
Water	*Cryptosporidium parvum*	Apparent failure or partial by-pass of filtration at water treatment plant	Estimated 403,000 cases in Milwaukee, WI.[5]

THREATS TO CROPS AND LIVESTOCK

There have been numerous incidents in which biological agents have been directed against animals and crops.[8,9] During World War II, the United Kingdom had stockpiled five million anthrax cakes to be delivered by parachute to grazing cattle in Germany. During the Cold War, the United States had weaponized the viruses that cause hog cholera and Newcastle disease (a respiratory disease of poultry) to be delivered by virus-coated feathers from balloons. In the same period, the Soviet Union developed biological weapons directed against livestock, poultry, and crops that contained the agents that cause foot-and-mouth disease, rinderpest, classic swine fever, African swine fever, wheat rust, karnal bunt, and fusarium.

The intentional introduction of an agent or chemical directed at animals or crops in order to disrupt local economies is called agroterrorism. Bioterrorists would probably choose infectious agents that are easy to acquire or reproduce, are disseminated easily, persist in the environment, elicit disease, spread easily from person to person, and do not cause disease in perpetrators. Table 16–2 lists some biological and chemical agents that can be directed against animal or agricultural targets. The intentional introduction of these agents may cause disease outbreaks that cannot be differentiated from natural disease events (see Chapters 10 and 11).

The introduction of exotic, highly infectious disease agents could have dire consequences for U.S. agriculture and commerce. Agriculture, including food exports, is an important component of the economy in many countries. Agriculture employs over 24 million people in the United States, accounting for

TABLE 16–2. Illustrative Agents that Could Be Directed Against Animal or Agricultural Targets.*

ANIMAL AGENTS	PLANT PATHOGENS	CHEMICALS
African swine fever virus	Wheat rust	Pesticides
Avian influenza virus	Rice blast	Nitriles
Blue tongue virus	Karnal bunt	Cyanide
Foot-and-mouth disease virus	Fusarium	Heavy metals
Classic swine fever virus		Dioxin
Newcastle disease virus		
Pseudorabies virus		
Rift Valley fever virus		
Rinderpest virus		
Sheep and goat pox viruses		
Venezuelan equine encephalitis		

*Agents/chemicals identified are based on economic trade impact and ease of transmission. This is not an all-inclusive list.

one of the largest sectors (13 percent) of the U.S. economy.[8,9] In 1998, the United States exported $54 billion of agricultural products.[10]

Recent natural outbreaks have had significant economic impact on affected countries. Examples include the foot-and-mouth disease (FMD) outbreaks in Taiwan and the United Kingdom.[11,41] These diseases curtailed animal and human movements, disrupted the local and national economies, dramatically reduced tourism, and adversely affected mental health, which was demonstrated, in part, by increases in suicides and depression. This does not take into account the direct impact on animals or farms lost. The disease does not kill the animals, but due to economic factors—to maintain access to world markets—animals were sacrificed. In the 1997 FMD outbreak in Taiwan, the disease spread throughout the island within 4 months. Four million pigs (38 percent of Taiwan's pig population) were destroyed. The total economic impact of the outbreak was estimated at $1.6 billion.[12] The FMD outbreak in the United Kingdom in 2001, which required the slaughter and disposal of over four million animals from 10,135 premises, resulted in an estimated economic impact of £3 billion.[41] Other recent animal and plant diseases have also had direct human impacts. During the 1998–1999 outbreak of the Nipah virus associated with swine in Malaysia, 265 human cases of encephalitis were reported.[12] Such pathogens could be engineered by terrorists for mass dissemination, and they have been identified as Category C biological agents by the CDC's Strategic Planning Work Group in Preparedness and Response to Biological and Chemical Terrorism.[13]

To protect livestock or agriculture products, there are many challenges, including limited farm or commodity security, large production units, and the inability to control the movement of people, products, or animals across borders.[9,10] A key area for disease dissemination is the rapid movement of animals through auctions or sale barns, as was demonstrated in the recent FMD disease outbreaks in the United Kingdom and Taiwan.[11] Large production units allow for rapid dissemination of disease through a concentrated number of animals in limited geographical areas. In addition, imports of infected animal products may introduce exotic diseases, highlighting the need for improved biosecurity protocols for animal and agricultural products and human movement.

Another area of concern is the vulnerability of animal feed.[14,15] It is estimated that 110 million tons of feed are manufactured annually in the United States. There are numerous access points for potential perpetrators to feed elevators, transport containers, or bulk finished products. These feeds are widely distributed locally, nationally, and internationally. Contamination of feed products requires some working knowledge of both feed manufacturing processes and the survivability of the agent or the persistence of the chemical during processing.[15] The occurrence of multinational outbreaks of human salmonellosis associated with internationally distributed alfalfa seeds highlights the potential for pathogen survival on cereal grains.[16] For crops, the lack of genetic diversity of certain plant species may make them highly susceptible to the introduction of a biological threat[17]—especially a problem with short-incubation-period diseases that can spread rapidly during a growing season.

THREATS TO FOOD PROCESSING AND DISTRIBUTION

Many of the major foodborne disease outbreaks that occurred in the United States during the 1990s highlighted vulnerable points in food processing and distribution that could possibly be exploited by bioterrorists. In 1994, an outbreak of *Salmonella enteritidis* infections affected an estimated 224,000 people in 41 states; pasteurized ice-cream mix was contaminated from unpasteurized eggs during transportation.[18] An estimated 16,000 cases of *Salmonella agona* infections occurred after contamination of toasted oat cereals; environmental contamination was documented within the plant in a pattern that followed the movement of the cereal dust.[19] Airborne spread of contamination within a processing plant most likely accounted for a multistate outbreak of listeriosis associated with hot dogs; cooked hot dogs were apparently contaminated with *Listeria* that was aerosolized as a result of remodeling and construction within the plant.[20] In 1998, a multi-state outbreak of shigellosis was associated with parsley imported from a single farm in Mexico.[21] Eight separate outbreaks in restaurants were linked to this source as a result of molecular subtyping and epidemiological analysis. Water used in harvesting and packing the parsley was taken from a municipal system that was susceptible to contamination and was not adequately treated. The import from other countries of more than half of the fresh produce consumed in the United States presents great challenges, as illustrated, in part, by this outbreak.

The scale of contemporary food production and distribution means that contamination events that occur at the point of production can result in large, geographically dispersed outbreaks that may be difficult to detect, whether the contamination was intentional or not. The potential impact of single contamination events in these settings makes them important bioterrorist targets.

Most ready-to-eat foods are packaged in ways that limit their potential vulnerability to intentional contamination. Most fresh fruits and vegetables, however, are transported and displayed as bulk commodities that are susceptible to contamination up to the point of sale.

The intentional contamination of salad-bar items has already occurred. Although salad bars are widely available and vulnerable to intentional contamination, the limited impact of such events, in terms of number of persons potentially exposed, makes them likelier targets for disgruntled employees, local pranksters, copy-cats, and hoaxes.

THREATS TO WATER

Water is used for agricultural and recreational purposes as well as for drinking. Drinking-water supplies provide the most visible targets, and water treatment and distribution systems may be targets. Agricultural water and recreational water may provide easier access for contamination by potential bioterrorists, and be more difficult to protect against.

Potential threats to the water supply include some of the chemicals and biological agents listed in Tables 10–1 and 11–1 that are at least potentially capable of being transmitted through water.[22] The latter include the agents that cause anthrax, botulism, Q fever, tularemia, brucellosis, melioidosis, and glanders. Stability in water and chlorine tolerance characteristics of these agents varies, however. For example, anthrax spores are stable in water and resistant to chlorine, while the vegetative form of the organism is not likely to survive in water or to survive chlorination. Although botulinum toxin is extremely potent, it will probably break down rapidly with conventional chlorination treatment or become attached to particulates removed by the filtration process.[23] Specific information about chlorine resistance of the less-common pathogens is often unknown, speculative, or based on limited and often obsolete data.

One other prominent toxin is ricin, a constituent of the castor bean, which can be readily extracted in high concentrations and is also heat-stable and relatively resistant to chlorine. Its ease of extraction probably accounts for its inclusion on "most likely" lists, such as the CDC's Category B list (Tables 10–1 and 10–3 in Chapter 10). Its toxicity varies considerably among species with horses most susceptible. However, it is relatively poorly absorbed from the intestinal tract with an LD_{50} (median lethal dose) of 20 mg/kg.[23] Thus, dilution factors would likely be protective against ricin unless huge quantities could be introduced into the water supply.

Fungal toxins, such as the trichothecene mycotoxin T-2, are still another potential threat to the water supply. They are extremely heat-resistant but are apparently susceptible to standard alkalinized household bleach (5.25 percent hypochlorite).[23] As with ricin, however, the LD_{50} is high, and dilution effects mitigate against a sufficient injection into a public water supply to cause significant human disease.

Other toxins that are of concern include abrin, aflatoxins, *Clostridium perfringens* epsilon toxin, conotoxin, diacetoxyscirpenol, saxitoxin, shigatoxin, and tetrodotoxin. Most of these toxins are relatively heat-stable and have varying susceptibility to chlorination as practiced in municipal water treatment plants. Thus, for the most part, we must rely on tight security arrangements to deny access to water treatment facilities and downstream mains, while high dilution factors are protective against attempts to contaminate watersheds and reservoirs.

Water is generally not conducive to microbial growth and multiplication. Thus, large quantities of any agent would have to be introduced into the system to bypass the safeguards and cause a significant adverse health impact. The same principles would apply to other potential chemical agents, such as heavy metals, organophosphate pesticides, and cyanide. Yet successful penetration of the system could affect many individuals if the protective mechanisms failed. In addition, the sheer number of public water systems in the United States implies a formidable security challenge. There are approximately 60,000 municipal systems and another 140,000 small-scale systems, serving such places as trailer parks and resorts, that meet the "public water supply" definition of more than 15 connections. Potential targets within the water system are listed in Table 16–3.

THREATS TO AMBIENT AIR

Widespread dissemination of airborne agents is limited by dilution and dispersion of agents. The outbreak of inhalation anthrax in 1979 in Sverdlovsk in the former Soviet Union that followed an accidental release is widely used

TABLE 16–3. Potential Bioterrorism Targets in the Water System.

POINT OF VULNERABILITY	COMMENTS
1. Irrigation water	Could potentially contaminate food supply. Usually independent of drinking water supply.
2. Food-processing water	Could potentially contaminate food supply. Frequently connected to drinking water supply.
3. Recreational water	Could potentially expose large numbers of people under heavy-use conditions.
4. Drinking water	
a. Semi-private supply	Multiple systems, minimal treatment, more difficult to secure.
b. Municipal surface reservoirs	Large dilution factor is protective
c. Community water towers	Easier to secure than reservoirs.
d. Municipal wells	Require security and monitoring. Often receive minimum treatment.
e. Major supply lines	Could disrupt major municipal supply.
f. Municipal treatment plants	Security and monitoring essential.

to model the intentional release by a bioterrorist.[24] The epidemiological model of this event predicted mass casualties that would potentially overwhelm the capacity of local medical and public health professionals to respond. The intentional release of anthrax through letters presented a very different scenario, however: the outbreak may not have been recognized without the heightened awareness that followed the events of September 11 (see Chapter 6).

Airborne dissemination of anthrax spores from sealed envelopes had not been anticipated. But four postal workers at a mail-processing and distribution center developed inhalation anthrax, and two died, 7 to 9 days after one contaminated letter went through an automated sorter at the facility.[25] Environmental samples collected 12 days after the contamination event revealed widespread contamination with *Bacillus anthracis* spores throughout the facility, with the greatest concentrations along the path followed by the contaminated letter. No spores were collected in air samples, and only eight (7 percent) of 114 surface swabs were positive for *B. anthracis*. *B. anthracis*, however, was isolated from 27 (69 percent) of 39 vacuum dust samples, at concentrations ranging from 3 CFU/g to 9.7 million CFU/g.[25]

The widespread dissemination of anthrax in this mail-processing facility and the occurrence of Legionnaire's disease outbreaks attributed to aerosolization of water from whirlpool spas suggests that many indoor environments could be vulnerable to a bioterrorist attack. A primary lesson to be taken from these events is that our previous experience in dealing with the natural transmission of potential bioterrorism agents may not predict the outcome of their intentional release. Although inhalational anthrax is a recognized occupational disease of persons who have worked with natural animal hides or hair, several investigators have documented tannery workers who have had substantial exposure to *B. anthracis* spores without any apparent ill effects,[26] suggesting that acquired immunity probably modified the risk of exposure among workers in these settings. In contrast, isolated cases have been reported in persons with apparently minimal exposure to some of the same contaminated environments.[26] The relative immunity of tannery workers could have led public health officials to underestimate the infectivity of anthrax during its dissemination after September 11, and to discount the exposure potential at the contaminated mail-handling facility. Knowledge of history may not always be a reliable guide to dealing with future events.

RECOMMENDATIONS AND RESOURCES

Responding to the threat of bioterrorism against air, food, and water requires: (a) a strong public health surveillance system with the capacity to rapidly detect and investigate disease outbreaks (Chapter 14); (b) a rapid communication system to potentially affected communities and industries (Chapter 7); and (c) an industry-based risk management system that identifies intentional contamination as a potential hazard. Key recommendations are summarized in Table 16–4.

Public Health Surveillance

Improved public health surveillance is a necessary step in any strategy to deal with threats of bioterrorism. Information from past surveillance can provide a baseline of the "expected" frequency of events, with which "observed" events possibly due to bioterrorism may be compared. The CDC has operated a national surveillance system for foodborne disease outbreaks since 1966, and one for waterborne disease outbreaks since 1971.[27,28] It has periodically published summaries on outbreaks attributed to food, drinking water, and recreational water.

Although these outbreak summaries provide important compilations of public health investigations, their publication is usually not timely. For example, at the time of this writing in early 2002, the most recently published CDC summary of foodborne disease outbreaks includes outbreaks reported to the CDC from 1993 to 1997, and of waterborne disease outbreaks reported to the CDC from 1997 to 1998. In response to concerns over the emergence of foodborne disease agents such as *E. coli* O157:H7, the Clinton administration started a food safety initiative that included several efforts to improve the sensitivity, specificity, and timeliness of foodborne disease surveillance.

TABLE 16–4. Key Recommendations for Protecting Food, Water and Air.

GENERAL	SPECIFIC
Improve capacity of public health surveillance to detect potential bioterrorism events.	1. Increase routine submission of isolates to PulseNet laboratories, and link laboratory and epidemiological data on real-time basis. 2. Initiate industry-based surveillance of workers' health through occupational health programs.
Incorporate concepts of Critical Infrastructure Protection (CIP) on permanent basis.	1. Consider intentional contamination as a potential hazard to be controlled under Hazard Analysis and Critical Control Point (HACCP) plans. 2. Develop a "farm-to-table" food industry Information Sharing and Analysis Center (ISAC) to increase security awareness and share information on security threats.

The most important of these efforts has been PulseNet, the national molecular subtyping network for foodborne disease. PulseNet includes a molecular subtyping protocol that can be used at all public health laboratories, and an electronic communications network so that information about subtype patterns and potential outbreaks can be shared rapidly by all participants.[29] Virtually all public health laboratories in the United States participate in PulseNet. Not all routinely receive isolates to subtype, or link laboratory and epidemiological data on a real-time basis, though. Improvements in these areas are needed before PulseNet can serve as the basis for national foodborne disease surveillance and a defense against bioterrorism.

In addition, surveillance of workers through an occupational health program may be an important indicator of contamination events. For example, workers in feed manufacturing can serve as sentinels for unusual contamination events, especially for intentionally introduced zoonotic agents or chemicals that impact human health. In many foodborne disease outbreaks, foodhandlers are also exposed to contaminated food, get ill along with the patrons, and serve as secondary sources for propagating the outbreak. Thus, surveillance for workers' health is important throughout food production and distribution systems.

A second major preventive action is to incorporate the concepts of Critical Infrastructure Protection (CIP) as a permanent response. This concept is based on a presidential directive issued by President Bill Clinton in May 1998 and reaffirmed by an executive order issued by President George W. Bush in October 2001. CIP is a comprehensive program "to identify physical and cyber infrastructures critical to the health, security and economic welfare of the nation, to assess their vulnerability to being degraded or denied and to initiate actions to mitigate those risks." The presidential directive encourages the owners and operators of the critical services to establish private-sector Information Sharing and Analysis Centers (ISACs) to increase security awareness, share information on security practices, and contribute anonymous or attributed incident information to the system concerning security threats.

An ISAC has been organized among the nation's public water-supply systems. Members are provided with early trend data on threats, vulnerabilities, and incidents affecting public water supplies. An ISAC that would provide comprehensive coverage of food production and distribution systems from farm to table is being developed.

Animals and Agriculture

Prevention requires a "common-sense" systematic approach for assessing threats and vulnerabilities and for designing risk-management strategies. The agricultural industry is familiar with the Hazard Analysis and Critical Control Point (HACCP) system, which can be used not only to identify weak links in food production, but also to identify areas of concern for security on farms, and at feed manufacturers or processors. This system includes the identification of critical areas or hazards, measures to reduce the risk, and procedures to verify that the implemented security programs are working. These prevention steps may include securing and locking feed or ingredient storage areas, restricting access of non-employees, devising a mechanism to report suspicious activity, and developing a response plan, if and when evidence of tampering occurs.

Other activities on a local or national level include improving surveillance activities, education of key personnel, and resources to monitor for potential terrorist activities. Disease-surveillance activities include educating extension-service personnel about prompt reporting of crop-related diseases, educating veterinarians to recognize and report foreign or unusual animal diseases, developing rapid diagnostic tests for key diseases of concern, and improving the infrastructure of regional veterinary diagnostic laboratories.[30–32]

Other measures include better communication between federal, state and local agencies, tools for rapid outbreak analysis, and personnel dedicated to security-related issues and disease surveillance. Clear lines of communication are needed among animal and plant producers, veterinarians, and public health officials.[33] Some agricultural risk analyses are currently underway. As part of these educational efforts, livestock, poultry, and crop producers need to evaluate their on-farm security policies, including those on the physical security of buildings, visitors, commodity suppliers, feed biosecurity, and pre-hire screening of employees. Various organizations and agencies have devised guidelines to improve biosecurity at the farm level.[34–37] Often the first recommendation for improving security is recognizing vulnerabilities.

Food Processing and Distribution

The primary approach to protecting food production and distribution systems is embodied in the application of HACCP system, as described above, with specific consideration given to intentional contamination as a potential hazard. In response to concerns about bioterrorists targeting food, the U.S. Food and Drug Administration (FDA) has issued specific guidance documents for food producers, processors, transporters, and retailers.[37] Specific prevention measures have been recommended for all aspects of food establishment operations:

1. Actively manage food security procedures; assign responsibility for security to qualified individuals; provide an appropriate level of supervision for all employees; and develop response strategies to terrorist events.

2. Screen employees before hiring; establish a positive identification system; limit employee access to only those areas necessary for job function; and restrict employee access to computer control systems.
3. Restrict and monitor access of visitors to the physical facility; secure doors, windows, and other access points with locks and perimeters with fencing; secure storage areas for hazardous chemicals; secure access to water sources, storage, and handling facilities; and secure access to air intake points.
4. Use only known and approved sources for all ingredients; coordinate food security measures, such as using locked and sealed vehicles, with suppliers and transporters; and inspect incoming ingredients to reconcile receipts with orders.
5. Secure finished products; and investigate missing or surplus stock.

The FDA also developed and is promoting a process called operational risk management (ORM) to help food processors prioritize the preventive measures that are most likely to have the greatest impact on reducing the risk of terrorist actions.[38] ORM involves six steps: (a) identify hazards, (b) assess risk, (c) analyze risk-control measures, (d) make control decisions, (e) implement risk controls, and (f) supervise and review. The principles of ORM resemble the principles of the HACCP system. Each of these systems requires a commitment from management to maintain ongoing monitoring activities and to reassess operations as conditions change.

Water Protection

Community systems serve about 90 percent of the U.S. population, about equally divided between surface water and ground water sources. Vulnerability of public water supplies to bioterrorism is limited by a number of factors. First, any agent injected into the system will be diluted by the volume of water flowing through the system. Second, existing treatment regimens will be effective against many potential agents—assuming that they are added upstream of the treatment facility. Third, it is possible to provide a high level of security for centralized treatment plants. Thus, while large-scale terrorist acts face formidable hurdles, concrete steps must be taken to prevent deliberate contamination of drinking water. Tight security at treatment facilities, including thorough background checks of all employees to prevent insider complicity, is necessary and will have to be continued into the indefinite future. While deliberate contamination of the supply with chemical or biological agents is a major concern, sabotage of a principal feeder-main is also a viable scenario that can be prevented only by diligent security efforts.

Primary reliance on chlorination to destroy bacterial and viral pathogens continues to be effective, but has been supplemented in many systems by the additional use of ozone. Upgraded and well-maintained pressure-sand filtration can prevent or remove contamination with parasitic agents such as *Cryptosporidium*. A comprehensive investigation of the susceptibility of potential bioterrorist agents to chlorination or other forms of disinfection should be conducted. Currently available treatment systems and the significant dilution factors that occur in water distribution mitigate against successful terrorist acts. Heightened security and vigilant surveillance should be carried out—not only to thwart terrorists, but also to assist in preventing traditional waterborne disease and infectious agents that emerge in the future.

Because botulinum toxin is relatively stable in water and is among the most virulent toxins known, it must be considered a potential threat.[39] Monitoring for this toxin may be desirable to evaluate a potential threat or hoax situation. PCR technology can detect the toxin within 2.5 hours.[23] A 5-hour ELISA test is also available. Should botulinum toxin be detected in a community supply, boiling for a few minutes will inactivate it and effectively protect the public until the system can be cleared.

Ambient Air

In the fall of 2001, the CDC issued interim recommendations for protecting workers from exposure to *B. anthracis* in worksites where mail is handled and processed.[41] These recommendations included a combination of engineering, administrative, and housekeeping controls, as well as personal protective equipment for workers. They were developed in response to a specific threat, but many are applicable to the prevention of exposure to a variety of biologic aerosols in occupational settings. Engineering controls include industrial vacuums with high-efficiency particulate air (HEPA) filters, local exhaust systems, and laminar air flow to direct potential contaminants away from workers. Housekeeping controls include limiting the use of dry sweeping and dusting, which may spread contamination rather than remove it. Workers are advised to wear appropriate protective clothing, to avoid touching their mucous membranes and their eyes, and to wash their hands thoroughly with soap and water after removing gloves and before eating.[40]

CONCLUSION

Traditional public health measures designed to detect and control outbreaks of emerging infectious diseases provide a framework for protecting food, water, and ambient air from bioterrorism. Specific modifications to these measures are needed to anticipate terrorist threats and attacks and to respond effectively.

REFERENCES

1. Centers for Disease Prevention and Control. Achievements in Public Health, 1900–1999: Control of Infectious Diseases. *MMWR* 1999; 48:621–629.
2. Centers for Disease Prevention and Control. Achievements in Public Health, 1900–1999: Safer and Healthier Foods. *MMWR* 1999; 48:905–913.
3. Fraser DW, Tsai TR, Orenstein W, et al. Legionnaires' disease: description of an epidemic of pneumonia. *N Engl J Med* 1977; 297:1189–1197.
4. Tauxe RV. Emerging foodborne diseases: an evolving public health challenge. *Emerg Infect Dis* 1997; 3:425–434.
5. MacKenzie WR, Hoxie NJ, Proctor ME, et al. A massive outbreak in Milwaukee of cryptosporidium infection transmitted through the public water supply. *N Engl J Med* 1994; 331:161–167.
6. Török TJ, Tauxe RV, Wise RP, et al. A large community outbreak of salmonellosis caused by intentional contamination of restaurant salad bars. *JAMA* 1997; 278:389–95.
7. Centers for Disease Control and Prevention. Update: Investigation of bioterrorism-related anthrax and interim guidelines for clinical evaluation of persons with possible anthrax. *MMWR* 2001; 50:941–948.
8. Brown C, Bolin CA. *Emerging diseases of animals.* Washington, DC: ASM Press, 2000.
9. Horn FP, Breeze RG. Agriculture and food security. *Ann N Y Acad Sci* 1999; 894:9–17.
10. Dunn MV. The threat of bioterrorism to U.S. agriculture. *Ann N Y Acad Sci* 1999; 894:184–188.
11. Yang PC, Chu RM, Chung WB, Sung HT. Epidemiological characteristics and financial costs of the 1997 foot-and-mouth disease epidemic in Taiwan. *Vet Rec* 1999; 145:731–734.
12. Parashar UD, Sunn LM, Ong F, et al. Case-control study of risk factors for human infection with a new zoonotic paramyxovirus, Nipah virus, during a 1998–1999 outbreak of severe encephalitis in Malaysia. *J Infect Dis* 2000; 181:1755–1759.
13. Centers for Disease Prevention and Control. Biological and chemical terrorism: strategic plan for preparedness and response. Recommendations of the CDC Strategic Planning Workgroup. *MMWR Recomm Rep* 2000; 49(RR-4):1–14.
14. Neher NJ. The need for a coordinated response to food terrorism. The Wisconsin experience. *Ann N Y Acad Sci* 1999; 894:181–183.
15. von Bredow J, Myers M, Wagner D, et al. Agroterrorism. Agricultural infrastructure vulnerability. *Ann N Y Acad Sci* 1999; 894:168–80.
16. Mahon BE, Ponka A, Hall WN, et al. An international outbreak of Salmonella infections caused by alfalfa sprouts grown from contaminated seeds. *J Infect Dis* 1997; 175:786–882.
17. Rodgers PWS, Dando M. Biological warfare against crops. *Scient Amer* 1999; 280:70–75.
18. Hennessy TW, Hedberg CW, Slutsker L, et al. A national outbreak of *Salmonella enteritidis* infections from ice cream. *N Engl J Med* 1996; 334:1281–1286.
19. Centers for Disease Control and Prevention. Multistate outbreak of *Salmonella*

serotype Agona infections linked to toasted oats cereal–United States, April–May, 1998. *MMWR* 1998; 47:462–464.

20. Centers for Disease Control and Prevention. Multistate outbreak of listeriosis-United States, 1998. *MMWR* 1998; 47:1085–1086.

21. Centers for Disease Control and Prevention. Outbreaks of *Shigella sonnei* infections associated with eating fresh parsley-United States and Canada, July–August, 1998. *MMWR* 1999; 48:285–289.

22. Khan AS, Swerdlow DL, Juranek DD. Precautions against biological and chemical terrorism directed at food and water supplies. *Public Health Reports* 2001; 16:3–14.

23. Madsen JM. Toxins as weapons of mass destruction: A comparison and contrast with biological-warfare and chemical-warfare agents. *Clinics in Laboratory Medicine* 2001; 21:593–605.

24. Inglesby TV, Henderson DA, Bartlett JG, et al. Anthrax as a biological weapon. Medical and public health management. *JAMA* 1999; 281:1735–1745.

25. Centers for Disease Prevention and Control. Evaluation of *Bacillus anthracis* contamination inside the Brentwood Mail Processing and Distribution Center—District of Columbia, October 2001. *MMWR* 2001; 50:1129–1133.

26. Watson A, Keir D. Information on which to base assessments of risk from environments contaminated with anthrax spores. *Epidemiol Infect* 1994; 113:479–490.

27. Olsen SJ, MacKinnon LC, Goulding JS, et al. Surveillance for foodborne disease outbreaks—United States, 1993–1997. *MMWR* 2000; 49:SS-1.

28. Centers for Disease Control and Prevention. Surveillance for waterborne disease outbreaks—United States, 1997–1998. *MMWR* 2000; 49:SS-4.

29. Swaminathan B, Barrett TJ, Hunter SB, et al. PulseNet: the molecular subtyping network for foodborne bacterial disease surveillance, United States *Emerg Infect Dis* 2001; 7:382–389.

30. Franz DR. Foreign animal disease agents as weapons in biological warfare. *Ann N Y Acad Sci* 1999; 894:100–104.

31. Frazier TW. Natural and bioterrorist/biocriminal threats to food and agriculture. *Ann N Y Acad Sci* 1999; 894:1–8.

32. Williams JL, Sheesley D. Response to bio-terrorism directed against animals. *Ann N Y Acad Sci* 2000; 916, 117–120.

33. Fitzpatrick AM, Bender JB. Survey of chief livestock officials regarding bioterrorism preparedness in the United States. *J Am Vet Med Assoc* 2000; 21:1315–1317.

34. American Feed Industry Association. Guide to biosecurity awareness, American Feed Industry Association. Available at: http://www.afia.org, 2002.

35. College of Veterinary Medicine. Farm security for visitors, University of Minnesota, available at: http://www.cvm.umn.edu/anhlth_foodsafety/farmvisitors.html, 2002.

36. Biosecurity of dairy farm feedstuffs. Bovine Alliance on Management and Nutrition. Available at: http://aphis.usda.gov/vs/ceah/cahm/Dairy_Cattle/dairy.htm, 2002.

37. Food and Drug Administration. Guidance for Industry. Food Producers, Processors, Transporters, and Retailers: Food Security Preventive Measures Guidance. Food and Drug Administration, Washington, D.C., available at: http://www.cfsan.fda.gov/~dms/secguid.html, 2002.

38. Food and Drug Administration. Food Safety and Security: Operational Risk Management Systems Approach, November 26, 2001. Available at: http://www.cfsan.fda.gov.

39. Arnon SS, Schechter R, Inglesby TV, et al. Botulinum toxin as a biological weapon. Medical and public health management. *JAMA* 2001; 285:1059–1070.

40. Centers for Disease Control and Prevention. CDC interim recommendations for protecting workers from exposure to *Bacillus anthracis* in work sites where mail is handled and processed, October 31, 2001, available at: http://www.bt.cdc.gov.
41. Department for Environment, Food and Rural Affairs. Tackling the impact of foot-and-mouth disease on the rural economy. October, 2001.
42. Den Boer JW, Yzerman EP, Schellekens J, et al. A large outbreak of Legionnaires' disease at a flower show, the Netherlands, 1999. *Emerg Infect Dis* 2002; 8:37–43.

17

Protecting civil liberties

H. JACK GEIGER

Throughout American history, the civil liberties embedded in the Constitution and the Bill of Rights—properly regarded as bedrock structures of the nation's political system, and defined and expanded by decades of subsequent federal and state legislation, as well as volumes of judicial interpretation—have been periodically limited and eroded by perceived threats to national security. These threats have included wars against other nations (both declared and undeclared), "police actions," and wars fought by international coalitions in which the United States has been the prime military participant (such as in the Korean War, the Vietnam War, and the Persian Gulf War). These perceived threats also include situations of intense international ideological conflict with only limited or covert direct military engagement, except through surrogate nations (such as in the 50-year Cold War with the Soviet Union). In each of these situations, there have been domestic consequences that have threatened civil liberties.

Historical examples abound. The Alien and Sedition Acts of 1796, aimed at President John Adams' domestic opponents, (a) targeted immigrants; (b) gave the President power to imprison or deport aliens suspected of activities posing a threat to national security; and, most strikingly, (c) broadly banned spoken or written criticism of the government, the Congress, or the President—virtually nullifying freedom of speech and freedom of the press. During the Civil War, President Abraham Lincoln suspended the right of *habeas corpus* and imprisoned newspaper editors critical of the Union cause. In the early 1900s, the Congress and state legislatures passed laws against "anarchy," so vaguely defined as to permit arrest and imprisonment of people with a wide range of unpopular political views. Restrictions on speech were common during World War I and, in 1920, were followed by the Palmer Raids (named for then–Attorney General A. Mitchell Palmer), which utilized 500 Federal Bureau of Investigation (FBI) agents to target immigrants, union members, and war protestors for arbitrary searches and seizures, arrests without warrants, and deportations.

During World War II, President Franklin D. Roosevelt established an alternative, judicially unreviewable justice system—with military tribunals conducting secret trials—to convict and execute a small group of Nazi saboteurs. He also ordered the internment into camps of thousands of Japanese-American citizens and non-citizens. Both actions were declared constitutional in wartime by the U.S. Supreme Court. During the Cold War and the McCarthy era (in the 1950s), violations of civil liberties were commonplace, including (a) the criminalization of political dissent (in the name of anti-Communism); and (b) unauthorized surveillance, and illegal wiretaps and break-ins by the FBI, culminating in COINTELPRO, a secret and illegal FBI program of political sabotage and disinformation.[1]

Abuses were not limited to the executive branch. Congress passed the Smith Act, making membership in the Communist Party a crime and facilitating alien deportations. The House Un-American Activities Committee held a long series of widely publicized hearings—in effect, show trials—in which witnesses felt compelled to seek Fifth Amendment protections against self-incrimination. These hearings, in turn, set the stage for a massive private-sector campaign of blacklisting, job firings, and other economic sanctions.

There is a discernable pattern in these responses. All of them were characterized by unilateral, and often sweeping, expansions of presidential and executive-branch powers, ignoring or limiting congressional participation and oversight, and limiting or obliterating judicial review—fundamentally altering the checks and balances provided by the Constitution.[2] In all of these responses, it was alleged that national security and national emergency required expansions of government secrecy and limitation of governmental accountability to the public. Most of the responses were accompanied by nongovernmental action, in which private-sector organizations, including some news-media organizations, not only supported civil liberties violations, but also participated in them. Frequent targets were immigrants, other non-citizens, faculty members and their academic institutions, and members of disfavored political, religious, racial, and ethnic minority groups. Fueled by repetitive government assertions of threats to national security (sometimes real and specific, sometimes vague and ephemeral), both public anxiety and patriotic fervor were enlisted to create and maintain substantial support for these changes. Dissent and debate were often labelled as being unpatriotic (at best) or conspiratorial, or giving aid and comfort to an enemy (at worst). There has often been a long lag before corrective action restored support of constitutional protections; for example, almost five decades passed before the Japanese-American internment camps were retroactively ruled unconstitutional. In sum, national security often trumps civil liberties.

THE BILL OF RIGHTS

In order to understand the constitutional problems posed by the response to terrorism, it is useful to review briefly the core civil-liberties protections provided by key sections of the Bill of Rights, the first 10 Amendments to the Constitution.[3]

The First Amendment sweepingly guarantees (a) freedom of religion; (b) freedom of speech and freedom of the press; and (c) the rights of peaceful assembly and "to petition the government for redress of grievances"—in effect, the right of unfettered political association and political action.

The Fourth Amendment (a) asserts the right of the people to be secure in their persons, houses, papers, and effects; (b) prohibits unreasonable searches and seizures; and (c) requires a showing of probable cause for, and mandates specificity of, such (judicial) warrants for search and seizure.

The core of the Fifth Amendment (a) bars deprivation "of life, liberty, or property" without due process of law; (b) requires a showing of evidence to, and indictment by, a grand jury as a prerequisite for criminal charges in "a capital, or otherwise heinous crime"; and (c) bars both double jeopardy and compulsory self-incrimination—except for the military "in time of war or public danger."

The Sixth Amendment mandates (a) the right, in all criminal prosecutions, to a speedy and public trial by an impartial jury; and (b) the rights of the accused (1) to be informed of the charges and evidence, (2) to be confronted by the witnesses against him or her, (3) to obtain defense witnesses, and (4) to have the assistance of legal counsel.

The Seventh Amendment (a) asserts the right of trial by jury in civil cases, and (b) establishes a process for appeals. The Eighth Amendment (a) prohibits cruel and unusual punishment, and (b) bars excessive bail and fines.

Collectively, these amendments to the Constitution are the fundamental statements of American personal, political, and religious freedoms. In the contemporary response to terrorism, the rights defined by each of these amendments are once again in jeopardy.

UNIQUE ASPECTS OF THE "WAR ON TERRORISM"

American wars and military and ideological conflicts in the 20th century pitted the United States against existing or aspiring nation-states: Spain during the early 1900s; Germany and its allies in World War I; Germany, Italy, and Japan in World War II; the Soviet Union and its allies during the Cold War; and, later, North Korea, China, North Vietnam, and Iraq. During most of these wars and conflicts, enemies could be clearly specified, victory or defeat could be defined, and an endpoint could be established.

The current "war on terrorism" is different. With the possible transient exception of Afghanistan and a variable list of nations accused of harboring terrorists or sponsoring terrorism, the enemy is defined as an international— and largely still unidentified—network of non-state forces, armed and trained, but not organized as conventional, uniformed military units, and committed not to conventional battle, but to assaults on civilian populations and institutions. The very definition of *terrorism* is variable and changeable over time (see Chapter 1). And there is no clear-cut endpoint or definition of victory in a war that is announced as requiring decades to complete. These shadowy uncertainties have shaped both legislative-branch and executive-branch responses to terrorism, as have (a) the acute and unprecedented national sense of ongoing domestic vulnerability produced by the September 11 attacks, (b) the anthrax dissemination and fears of further bioterrorism, and (c) the repeated government announcements of ongoing, but unspecified, terrorist threats. All of these developments have had an adverse impact on civil rights.

TERRORISM LEGISLATION AND CIVIL LIBERTIES

New anti-terrorist legislative efforts *preceded* the events of September 11. They actually began in response to domestic terrorism—the bombing of the Oklahoma City Federal Office Building in 1995. In 1996, three new federal laws accelerated a process of "court-stripping"—that is, limiting or removing meaningful judicial review of the exercise of executive authority. The Anti-Terrorism and Effective Death Penalty Act granted the federal government new powers while protecting its enforcement actions—especially death sentences—from effective judicial review. The Illegal Immigration Reform and Immigrant Responsibility Act and the Prison Litigation Reform Act either (a) flatly denied courts the authority to even hear certain types of cases, such as death-penalty cases and cases involving deportation of long-time legal residents; or (b) permitted federal judges to hear the claims of such disfavored litigants, but deprived them of any effective intervention. Either way, according to the American Civil Liberties Union

(ACLU), the result was "no process for some, superficial process for others and due process for none."[4]

These provisions pale, however, in comparison with those of the USA Patriot Act, which was passed hastily in October 2001 after a single congressional hearing shortly after the September 11 attacks. The Act gave the federal government new powers that can be used "against those whose First Amendment activities are deemed to be threats to national security by the Attorney General." It expands the definition of terrorism to include raising money for a "terrorist group," whether or not the donor knows that the group is engaged in terrorism. *Terrorist activity* is broadened to include any foreigner who uses "dangerous devices." The Act allows the federal government to detain indefinitely any foreigner whom the Attorney General certifies as endangering national security on the basis of "reasonable grounds to believe" that he or she might be a threat.

Although the Bill of Rights makes no distinction between citizens and non-citizens, the USA Patriot Act and its regulations effectively deny to 20 million resident non-citizens the protections of the Fifth and Sixth Amendments against prolonged detention and for the right to a speedy trial.[5] (To expand these provisions, the Justice Department has also asked a federal court for a broad ruling to authorize the use of secret evidence in efforts to detain or deport immigrants it contends are in the United States illegally.) Other provisions permit "delayed notification" of initially secret physical searches and allow the seizure of personal or organizational assets—ostensibly to prevent money-laundering by terrorist groups—on the basis of evidence that would ordinarily be inadmissible in U.S. courts.[6] Any such evidence, furthermore, can be kept secret if the federal government alleges that its disclosure would compromise national security or ongoing investigations.

These provisions justified the rapid round-up and arrest, soon after September 11, of more than 1,200 people (in what future historians will surely call "the Ashcroft Raids"), all but a rumored handful of whom proved to have no connection to terrorist activity—although more than 700 lingered in detention for months on charges of immigration law violations. The numbers, like the charges, are uncertain because the Justice Department persistently (a) failed to release exact figures, (b) refused to release the names of detainees (claiming that to do so would either endanger national security or constitute an invasion of privacy, despite existing laws mandating the rapid public identification of all those held in prison), and (c) hampered detainees' access to human-rights lawyers.

These actions were paralleled by the "voluntary" questioning of approximately 5,000 immigrants who had entered the United States legally after January 2000. Despite numerous state and local laws prohibiting racial and ethnic profiling, almost all those singled out for such interviews were persons of Middle Eastern descent and/or Muslim faith. In a classic euphemism, Attorney General John Ashcroft chose to describe them as persons who fit "a generic set of parameters."[7]

TERRORISM, EXECUTIVE POWER, AND CIVIL LIBERTIES

In addition to legislation, there are at least two other routes to the expansion of government power in the name of national security against terrorist conspiracy and attack in ways that limit or threaten constitutional safeguards.

The first of these routes is to issue an executive order, most controversially manifested by President George W. Bush's October 2001 edict establishing secret military tribunals, involving procedures that would be unconstitutional in civilian courts, for the trial of anyone he alone defines as a terrorist—without the right of appeal to any court.

The second route is to write federal regulations, requiring only the publication of a decree in the Federal Register, and sometimes ignoring a legally mandated period of public comment before it takes effect. The most controversial example is a new federal regulation giving the government power—without any requirement for judicial review and authorization—to monitor or eavesdrop on conversations between prison inmates and their attorneys, based solely on the Attorney General's determination that there exists reasonable suspicion that an attorney-detainee conversation may be used to further acts of terrorism. No further definition of any of these terms is provided. This regulation applies not only to convicted prisoners, but to all persons in federal custody (presumably including those unconvicted and thus presumed innocent), material witnesses, and immigration detainees not accused of any crime. Civil-liberties organizations have observed that this "renders attorney-client privilege worthless and essentially guts the right to counsel guaranteed by the Constitution."[8]

Other intrusive powers have received less public attention. The Justice Department now has the right to conduct what might be called "literary profiling"; as the American Booksellers Foundation for Free Expression has warned its members, the Justice Department now has the authority to secretly search for the titles of books purchased by individual customers.[9] An existing federal software program called "Carnivore" can, with only perfunctory judicial approval, seize voicemail messages, monitor e-mail correspondence, and track Web sites visited by any Internet user.[10]

Still other expansions of executive-branch powers are pending. In December 2001, the Attorney General was reported to be considering a plan to ease existing restrictions or guidelines that prohibit the FBI from spying on domestic religious and political groups or investigating organizations that meet in places like churches or mosques, unless investigators first find probable cause that laws have been broken.[11] In addition, the Model State Emergency Health Powers Act has been proposed for state legislatures to consider. The Act would facilitate the detection, management, and containment of public health emergencies, including those resulting from terrorist attacks (see Box 13–2). The proposed Act, in the view of many, however, would further erode civil liberties and constitutional protections (see Box 17–1).

The other side of the coin of government intrusiveness is government secrecy. The primary mechanism for public accountability of government is the Freedom of Information Act (FOIA), passed by Congress in 1974 in response to the secrecy and cover-ups of the Watergate scandals. The FOIA gives ordinary citizens, journalists, watchdog groups, and historians access to all public records, except for those that have been classified. In an October 2001 memo, the Attorney General urged all federal agencies to resist most FOIA requests, and promised that the Justice Department will defend decisions to withhold records, in whole or in part. We are thus presented with the extraordinary spectacle of the federal government's chief law enforcement officer urging federal government agencies to "resist" a federal law.[12] This attempt to increase government secrecy is, however, only one part of a larger pattern. Maryland, Virginia, and nearly a dozen other states, as of this writing in February 2002, are actively considering legislative or gubernatorial decrees to drastically limit their own freedom-of-information statutes,[13] and President Bush has issued an executive order allowing him to seal all presidential records since 1980, thereby limiting access to documents from the Reagan, Clinton, and both Bush administrations.

DISSENT AND ACADEMIC FREEDOM

The horrifying loss of life and property on September 11 and the administration's subsequent summons to the nation to unite in a war on terrorism have understandably produced and sustained a climate of patriotic fervor akin to the national response to the Japanese attack on Pearl Harbor in 1941. This patriotic fervor has been intensified by (a) the recognition that in this assault, unlike previous assaults on American embassies overseas, the homeland itself—an American city, civilian lives—was assaulted; and (b) the perception that the fabric of everyday life—airline flights, mail delivery, football games—was vulnerable to terrorist assault, in addition to strategic targets, such as nuclear-power plants, reservoirs, bridges and tunnels. The World Trade Center site was almost immediately termed "Ground Zero"—a term borrowed, without apparent irony, from the bombing of Hiroshima that killed more than 100,000 civilians—and accorded the status of a national war shrine.

Box 17–1. Public Health and Civil Liberties: A Critique of the Model State
Emergency Health Powers Act.

In response to the health threat of chemical and biological weapons attacks, state and
federal health agencies themselves are now enmeshed in the conflict between the Bush
administration's draft proposal for a medical and public health response and the
prospect of further erosions of civil liberties and constitutional protections.

The proposal—the Model State Emergency Health Powers Act (MSEHPA)—is briefly
described and defended, on both operational and legal grounds, by one of its authors elsewhere in this book (see Box 13–4). But some of its most controversial features are set
forth in blunter language in a journalist's report in the *Detroit Free Press*: "In the event
of a deadly bio-terrorist attack using a deadly and contagious disease such as smallpox,
public heath officials want to be able to close roads and airports, herd people into stadi-
ums, and, if necessary, quarantine whole cities." Other provisions would, in the event of
a public heath emergency, provide the legal authority to compel the testing, examination,
and treatment of individuals; close or seize hospitals; and ration medical supplies.

Not all authorities agree, however. In a letter to Secretary of Health and Human Services Tommy Thompson, the New England Coalition for Law and Public Health, a
group of distinguished public health physicians and lawyers, argued that there is no
lack of present legal authority for public health departments to respond effectively.
The real problem, they contend, is a longstanding lack of money, facilities, and staffing-
neglect that has profoundly weakened the public health infrastructure. Furthermore,
the Coalition pointed out that: (a) the MSEHPA's definition of "emergency" is so broad
that "an emergency declaration authorizing the use of coercive powers could be made
every flu season," and that there is neither provision for review nor the suggestion of
less drastic measures; (b) there is neither a standard nor adequate due-process provisions for imposing a quarantine, and the arbitrary use of such extreme powers can effectively imprison ill people who have committed no crime; and (c) most of all, the
Model Act views public health "as an arm of law enforcement rather than as an independent health protection profession," and treats the American public, not biological
or chemical weapons, as the source of the problem, in ways that will destroy public
confidence in the system and afford little protection.

Others have expressed concern about the possibility that quarantines and other restrictions will be imposed selectively on the poor, immigrants, and people of color—
as has happened in the past—and are worried about the fate of the estimated 900,000
Americans who have HIV/AIDS and some 200,000 others, who are immunosuppressed
as a result of organ transplantation, cancer treatment, and other conditions, people who
are particularly vulnerable to infection, but for whom vaccination may be lethal.

Such fears are not relieved by the statement of one of the proposed Act's authors,
who intimated that the use of lethal force—that is, shooting to kill—could be justified
for anyone attempting to evade a quarantine. (As of late July 2002, more states had
rejected or stalled MSEHPA than had adopted it.)

—H. Jack Geiger

National emergencies and wartime states of mind have always had a profound impact on the ordinary democratic process of political debate and public discussion. Criticism of government policies, opposition to specific administrative measures and actions, and expression of alternative views of the origins of conflict and the appropriateness of response all become susceptible to attack—not on their merits, but as, at best, "harmful to a war effort," and, at worst, "unpatriotic and disloyal." Dissent is a consistent casualty of war. In the aftermath of September 11, when members of Congress and civil-rights activists criticized on constitutional grounds provisions of the USA Patriot Act, military tribunals, immigrant detentions, and other executive-branch actions, Attorney General Ashcroft repeatedly attacked such criticisms as aiding terrorism and giving aid and comfort to the enemy.[14] When Senator Patrick Leahy demanded Senate Judiciary Committee hearings and congressional oversight of Department of Justice actions, one conservative journal called him "Osama's enabler in Congress."[14]

As in the past, the news media have often been vulnerable. Many major newspapers have published vigorous editorial criticisms. The *New York Times*, for example, called executive-branch actions "an end run around the Constitution" and the President's establishment of military tribunals "a crude and unaccountable system that any dictator would admire."[15] However, some reporters, columnists, editorial writers, and cartoonists of smaller newspapers have been fired for expressing critical views. And major television-network news programs were accused by federal government officials of "lack of patriotism" for reporting on civilian deaths in Afghanistan.[16]

Colleges and universities have traditionally provided forums for free speech and unfettered debate, teach-ins and other demonstrations, and other opportunities for the expression of dissent and unpopular views. They have therefore been particularly vulnerable to what one historian has called "self-appointed guardians who are engaging in private blacklisting . . . , trying to intimidate individuals who hold different points of view."[9] Less than two months after the September 11 attack, the American Council of Trustees and Alumni, a private organization, published a report entitled "Defending Civilization: How Our Universities Are Failing America, and What Can Be Done about It." Most of the report described 114 examples of faculty or student statements during campus discussions, student chants at demonstrations, and other criticisms of the war on terrorism. The report characterized them as revealing a "dominant campus ideology" and "expressions of pervasive moral relativism," and claimed that "the message of much of academe was clear: Blame America first."[17] While acknowledging that "professors should be passionately defended in their right to academic freedom," the report made little mention of attempts by trustees, presidents, or other officials at the City University of New York, the Massachusetts Institute of Technology, the University of Texas, the University of South Florida, and other institutions to denounce or even dismiss faculty members who publicly criticized the U.S. government's domestic or foreign policies.[18] While insisting that "if both sides are heard, students and all of us will benefit," the report failed to cite any incidents such as one at the California State University-Sacramento campus, in which a commencement speaker who criticized Bush administration policies involving civil liberties and racial profiling was booed off the stage.

CIVIL RIGHTS UNDER SIEGE: POLLS AND THE PUBLIC

Public support for the Bill of Rights has always been strong in the abstract, but weaker, even in peacetime, when respondents have been asked to judge specific protections or when these protections have been considered in relation to disfavored groups, such as immigrants or prisoners. Recent national surveys document the power of national security concerns and personal fears to erode support for civil rights. For example, in a *New York Times*/CBS poll reported just two months after the World Trade Center attack, 77 percent of respondents approved of *indefinite* detention of non-citizens "if the government thinks the person is a threat to national security." The same percentage approved of government eavesdropping on conversations between "suspected terrorists in jail" and their lawyers. Most ominously, 64 percent of respondents said that the President should "have the authority to make changes in the rights usually guaranteed by the Constitution." Only about one-third of those polled, however, felt that such changes would affect their own rights.[19]

Similarly, an elaborately detailed survey by National Public Radio (NPR) News, the Kaiser Family Foundation, and Harvard University's Kennedy School of Government found that Americans hold strong beliefs "in principle" about civil liberties—but substantial majorities of Americans support giving law enforcement broader authority to wiretap telephones (68 percent); intercept mail (57 percent); intercept e-mail (72 percent); and examine people's Internet activity (82 percent), telephone records (82 percent), bank records (89 percent), and credit card records (75 percent). Approximately two-thirds of Americans, however, according to this survey, want law enforcement to obtain court orders before utilizing any of these powers, suggesting, the survey report states, that "Americans want the courts to provide a check on the executive branch." But nearly 60 percent of survey respondents stated that they trust the government to do what is right most of the time; in contrast, only 29 percent felt that way in a survey in June 2001—3 months before the September 11 attacks. Although there were differences among survey respondents in their intensity of support of these statements, these majorities came from the entire spectrum of political affiliation and belief.[20]

TERRORISM AND THE FUTURE OF CIVIL LIBERTIES

Now is not the first time in our national history in which civil liberties have been under siege, nor is it likely to be the last. In previous wars, hot and cold, civil liberties have similarly been subjected to what the ACLU currently describes as "a frontal assault." Our history suggests that when the war is over, or the perceived threat no longer exists, Americans gradually see that national security and civil rights seem less in conflict with each other, and view as dangerously excessive responses that once had their overwhelming support. Even in the worst of times, over the past 50 or more years, the work of many civil-rights and human-rights organizations, and of the independent news media, has kept alive concern for constitutional safeguards.

That history, however, is a less than perfect guide to the present. As noted earlier in this chapter, the present war on terrorism is unique in several key respects. For the first time in almost 200 years, the homeland itself has been attacked, and the driving force behind public support for restrictions of liberty is a public demand that the government be enabled to protect us. Any further terrorist attacks, therefore, are almost certain to produce public support for ever more draconian measures. Furthermore, the shadowy nature of *terrorists* and *terrorism* facilitates expanded definitions of these terms, for partisan political or other reasons, to disfavored groups and organizations and their activities. This evolution makes patriotism the first, rather than the last, refuge of political scoundrels, and taps into sadly familiar racial, religious, or ethnic biases. Finally, during a war on terrorism that has already been proclaimed to last for decades, civil liberties restrictions are more likely to become entrenched, and constitutional balances may be distorted for far longer periods of time than during past conflicts.

More intensely than in the past, then, the containment of these threats will test, under stress, the durability of the American public's concept of fairness. The durability of this concept of fairness, as in the past, will require unyielding support of domestic civil-rights organizations and international human rights organizations, the latter a new resource for the invocation of international human-rights law as a check on domestic violations. The durability of this concept of fairness will require legislative independence, always difficult in times of patriotic conformity. Most of all, it will require a campaign for the restoration of effective judicial oversight, affirming the rule of law and restoring the checks and balances of our constitutional system. The Bill of Rights has weathered many such storms over time—a cause for guarded optimism; but its only real defense, however transiently unpopular, is unremitting vigilance.

This vigilance is a task for public health professionals and students: first, in their roles as citizens who, like all other citizens and non-citizen residents, have a profound stake in the protection of their own civil rights. For public health professionals and students, this vigilance will also require resistance to militarization and inappropriate involvement with, or subservience to, non-civilian authority in the ordinary conduct of their work. It will also require thoughtful opposition to any sweeping government proposals to censor scientific publication and restrict the free flow of scientific information. Finally, it will require public health teachers and students to re-emphasize, with other members of academe, the obligation to preserve academic freedom and unfettered debate, including both support and criticism of government policies.

Public health professionals and students need to join with others, particularly those focused on civil rights and human rights, to inform the public, to seek redress in the courts when necessary, and to take vigorous political action. Such activities may come at a price; it is predictable that dissent and criticism will be labeled by some people as unpatriotic. Members of the public health community who undertake this work, however, will be acting in the tradition of 19th-century German pathologist Rudolf Virchow, recognizing the principle that the public health is, ultimately, the product of the social, political, and economic order.

(*Editor's note:* In July 2002, the U.S. Department of Justice announced its Terrorism Information and Prevention System (TIPS). As an editorial in the *New York Times* summarized TIPS: "The Bush administration plans to enlist millions of Americans to spy on their fellow Americans, and to feed that information into a centralized database." The editorial warned: "This ill-considered domestic spying program should be stopped before it starts."[21])

REFERENCES

1. Schrecker E. *Many Are the Crimes: McCarthyism in America.* Princeton, NJ: Princeton University Press, 1999.
2. *Upsetting Checks and Balances: Congressional Hostility Toward the Courts in Times of Crisis.* New York: ACLU, 2001.
3. Accessed at *http://memory.loc.gov/const/bor.html.*
4. *New Anti-Terrorism Law Further Strips Federal Judiciary of Authority.* ACLU Online, Newsletter of the American Civil Liberties Union. November 8, 2001, p. 2. (Accessed at *www.ACLUOnline@aclu.org*).
5. Bush's new rule to fight terror transforms the legal landscape. *New York Times*, November 25, 2001, p. A1.

6. Higgs R. Letter to the editor. *Wall Street Journal*, January 21, 2002, p. A19.

7. Rich F. Wait until dark (op-ed column). *New York Times*, November 24, 2000, p. A27.

8. Broad coalition calls on Attorney General to rescind "unprecedented assault" on attorney-client confidentiality. Accessed at *http://www.acky.irg/action/attorney 197.html.*

9. Rothschild M. The new McCarthyism. *Progressive*, January 2002. Accessed at *http://www.progressive.org/0901/roth 0102.html.*

10. Justice tells prosecutors how to make use of new anti-terror laws. Associated Press. October 31, 2001.

11. Ashcroft seeking to free FBI to spy on groups. *New York Times*, December 1, 2001, p. A1.

12. The day Ashcroft censored freedom of information. Editorial, *San Francisco Chronicle*, January 6, 2002.

13. Maryland, Virginia consider limits on public records. *Washington Post*, January 23, 2002, p. B04.

14. ACLU appalled by Ashcroft statement on dissent. Washington: ACLU. December 10, 2001.

15. A travesty of justice (editorial). *New York Times*, November 16, 2001, p. A27.

16. Network coverage a target of fire from conservatives. *New York Times*, November 16, 2001, p. B2.

17. Martin JL, Neal AD. *Defending Civilization: How Our Universities Are Failing America and What Can Be Done About It.* Washington, D.C.: American Council of Trustees and Alumni. November 2001.

18. Academic Freedom Statement, Center for Economic Research and Social CHange, Chicago, Ill. Accessed at *academicfreedomnow@hotmail.com*

19. Mixed views on civil liberties. *New York Times*/CBS News Poll. *New York Times*, December 12, 2001, p. B9.

20. NPR/Kaiser/Kennedy School Poll on Security Trumps Civil Liberties. Kaiser Family Foundation, Menlo Park, Calif. November 2001.

21. A nation of spies? (editorial). *New York Times,* July 25, 2002.

18

Exploring the roots of terrorism

CHERYL E. EASLEY AND CAROL EASLEY ALLEN

Since any discussion of the roots of terrorism runs the significant risk of being misunderstood as a justification for terrorist acts, we feel that we must begin with a disclaimer and a caveat. As a disclaimer, we assert that there is no justification for terrorism in any form or by any person or group—reasons for terrorist acts do not provide moral bases or excuses for them. As a caveat, we assert that the context in which terrorism is conceived and perpetrated cannot be ignored—to do so could lead to an endless cycle of terrorism, which some people and groups view as the only available response to intolerable conditions in the face of overwhelming power.

For us, as U.S. citizens, to understand the roots of terrorism, we must be willing to examine critically our often-idealized perception of our country's policies and actions. The events of September 11 did not occur in a contextual vacuum. In trying to understand these events, we may view them as either the aberrant, random, and unexplainable acts of an extremist minority, or as acts reflecting, to some extent, shared anger and frustration of many other people in their countries or cultures.

People become terrorists for various reasons: many become terrorists because of strongly held philosophical, ideological, or religious beliefs. Some become terrorists because of perceived oppression or economic deprivation. Other terrorists are simply criminals or mercenaries for hire. U.S. foreign policy specialists and public health workers must address why people become terrorists.[1]

HISTORICAL AND POLITICAL ROOTS OF TERRORISM

Terrorism as Historical Warfare Against Civilians

Caleb Carr, author of *The Lessons of Terror*, suggests an interesting perspective on terrorism, viewing it not as a crime or a uniquely modern phenomenon, but as a form of warfare with ancient roots.[2] He defines terrorism as "simply the contemporary name given to, and the modern permutation of, warfare deliberately waged against civilians with the purpose of destroying their will to support either leaders or policies that the agents of such violence find objectionable." Using this definition, Carr classifies a number of historical and contemporary figures as terrorists, such as the Roman emperor Augustus, King Louis XIV of France, Otto von Bismarck of Germany, and former U.S. President Richard Nixon and former Secretary of State Henry Kissinger. Carr's first conclusion is that terrorism in the long run has always failed to achieve its ends and will always fail, whatever its motivation: hatred, revenge, greed, or political or psychological insecurity.

Carr's second conclusion is that attacks against civilians are only appropriately met by military action. Here, instead of a destructive, retaliatory war against civilians, he advocates a preemptive military response that is progressive and limited. His maxim is: "Terror must never be answered with terror; but war can only be answered with war."[2] Answering terror with terror only leads to a cycle of terrorism that can last for generations. The tactics of terror must never be viewed as expedient or controllable; they are self-sustaining.

As the only remaining superpower and as the widely viewed propagator of a particularly Western economic system and popular culture, the United States has become the target for those who would perpetrate terrorist acts against the West. In defense of their traditional cultures, modern terrorists often resort to weapons of mass destruction, which they feel will best attract the attention of the U.S. public and counter U.S. military might. The international response to the attacks of September 11 demonstrates, however, that terrorism is self-defeating.

Carr questions whether the United States possesses the political will to wage a war against terrorism that is strategically limited and decisive. It remains to be seen whether the United States will control the impulse to answer terror with terror; if it does not, there could be an escalation of destructive engagement. Carr's analysis is clear and well-reasoned, but deeply troubling for those who hold a moral position against all war or against any but the most limited "defensive defense," as do many people in the public health community.

United States Foreign Policy and the Perception of the United States Abroad

In the wake of September 11, 2001, many U.S. citizens wondered why the United States is not universally loved, despite the widely held perception that it is the most consistent defender of human rights and the most generous international benefactor. The words used repeatedly by many in the "Two-Thirds World" to characterize the United States have been arrogance, indifference, hypocrisy, insensitivity, and decadence. (We do not use the pejorative term *Third World* to refer to the so-called developing countries. Instead, we prefer the term *Two-Thirds World*, which accurately describes the proportion of the planet's land mass occupied primarily by peoples of color in the Southern Hemisphere.)

From the end of the Cold War in 1989 to the terrorist attacks in 2001, people in the United States had generally become more internally focused and more indifferent to events in other parts of the world that were perceived as not substantially affecting U.S. security.[3] In the absence of a countervailing superpower, the United States saw little need for full-partner allies and forged ahead unilaterally with policies based on its own perceived self-interest.

In its interactions with foreign countries, the United States has often exerted preemptive rights to act with little attention to the impact on others. Examples of what many see as U.S. arrogance are found in the facility with which it chooses and discards allies. Our recent history with Iraq and Al Qaeda are cases in point.[4] In these cases, U.S. support for Saddam Hussein in Iraq's conflict with Iran and for Osama bin Laden in the conflict with Russia in Afghanistan was followed by disaffection and conflict. The U.S. history of lending financial, logistical, and political support to various repressive regimes around the world, when it suited U.S. interests, has been recognized by other nations,[5] as has the U.S. record of delayed payments to the United Nations, and its very low amount of development assistance as a percent of Gross National Product. Other unilateral actions by the United States, such as its withdrawal of support for strengthening the Biological Weapons Convention and unilateral abrogation of the Anti-Ballistic Missile Treaty, have raised suspicions about its actions.

Political Roots of Terrorism

Terrorism may be viewed as a pragmatic political strategy of the weak who lack political or military power. Time may be a factor in their choosing terrorism: would-be terrorists may be impatient to achieve political aims or they may perceive a window of opportunity when a state or regime appears vulnerable. Terrorists also may be encouraged to act by the acquisition of resources or a strategic innovation that makes action possible or more likely to be successful.[4] Unfortunately, the means of violence and destruction may be readily available and relatively inexpensive. The disintegration of the Soviet Union has meant that former Soviet scientists may be motivated by financial need to work for terrorist groups seeking weapons of mass destruction[7] (see Chapters 9 through 12).

Political factors have influenced the development of terrorism in many parts of the world. The remainder of this section focuses on the Middle East. Similar and analogous political factors have contributed to the development of terrorism elsewhere.

In the post-colonial period, Arab states have tried to cobble together national identities from disparate ethnic and cultural groups. The powerless masses found common cause in opposition to Zionism and its embodiment in the modern state of Israel. The establishment and persistence of Israel have been seen by some Arab states as the current manifestation of a centuries-long enmity of the West against Muslims. Indeed, public expression of anti-Zionist sentiment may have served some Arab state governments as a safety valve for the pent-up frustration of their populations due to political and social repression, economic hardships, and loss of hope for the future.[8,9]

For nearly three decades, Arab wealth has been firmly based on the oil resources of the region, but the continued stability of many Arab nations is undermined by the needs of rapidly expanding populations and the failure of their economies to diversify. None of the Islamic countries has succeeded in providing its people with realistic hope for the future. Middle Eastern youth, especially young men, seem to suffer from a pervasive sense of humiliation and failure of identity. This results from the political and economic weakness of their nations, as seen in high birth rates, unequal distribution of wealth, high unemployment, government inefficiency and corruption, and widespread serious health problems.[10]

Failure of the Arab states to succeed politically can be attributed, in part, to the Islamic unified model of church and state that has proved incompatible with ideas of statehood. Traditional Muslim ideas of governance involve the concept of *umma*, or community, which transcends all national boundaries, and the rule of *shari'a*, law that is based on a literal reading of the Koran. The mere existence of nation-states is, strictly speaking, illegitimate and evidence of non-Islamic practice. Along with unsuccessful attempts to establish a pan-Arabic state, the above factors have inhibited the full participation of the Arab states in the international community of nations.[8]

Muslim solidarity against the West was fueled by the 1979 Iranian Revolution, which established the paradigm of martyrdom rooted in the tradition of Shi'a Islam. The radicalization of Islam in the 1980s inspired a generation of young Muslims, including Osama bin Laden and some of his lieutenants. Violent events, including the siege of Mecca in 1979 and the assassination of Anwar Sadat in 1981, reflect a history of Muslim extremism.[10]

Resources

Although terrorism is a relatively inexpensive form of violence, resources are necessary for its conduct.[6] In addition to funding, terrorist organizations need state support; space and facilities; weaponry; means of communication; leadership and training; military, financial, and technical expertise; and transportation. A number of countries, sometimes termed "rogue states" by the U.S. government, are willing to provide support and/or sanctuary to terrorist groups because these groups will indirectly further national aims, or because these countries hope, in this way, to protect themselves from terrorist attacks.[7]

While much is made of the use of Osama bin Laden's personal fortune, his most substantial contribution to terrorism has been through the development of a global financial network whose first beneficiaries were the mujahideen in Afghanistan. Bin Laden profited from legal businesses and investments; grand and petty crimes, including the drug trade; solicitation of rich Arabs; and fund-raising for charitable organizations and other nongovernmental organizations (NGOs). He was able to recruit individuals from within some charitable organizations and NGOs to divert contributions to terrorism. Al Qaeda has transferred its funds by money smuggling and the use of banking havens and the underground Arab banking networks (*hawalas*), where, through cash transfers based on trust, money does not cross national borders and paper trails are not created. The diversity of bin Laden's financial operations made them very difficult to detect and shut down.[11]

ECONOMIC AND SOCIAL ROOTS OF TERRORISM

Poverty and Waste

Ubiquitous news media continually reveal Western affluence and waste to people in the Two-Thirds World, many of whom live in poverty and despair. Despite increased economic development, technological advancement, and wealth generation, the rich are growing richer and the poor, poorer. Poverty has been described as "a colossal powder-keg that can explode without most of the industrialized countries and the rest of the world realizing its debilitating and negative consequences."[12]

There are gross economic disparities in the world. The richest one-fifth of the world's population own about 85 percent of the world's wealth; the poorest one-fifth, about 1 percent (Figure 18–1). The 400 richest Americans have $1 trillion in wealth—more than the gross domestic product of China.[13] One-third of the extremely poor people in the world subsist on less than $1 per day.[14] Ninety percent of global health resources are concentrated on 10 percent of the world's health problems.[15]

The health of many people is compromised or at risk because of reduced access to resources and of inadequate environmental conditions. Daily, more than one billion people drink unsafe water. Infectious diseases remain the leading cause of death in the world, killing nearly 50,000 per day, mostly

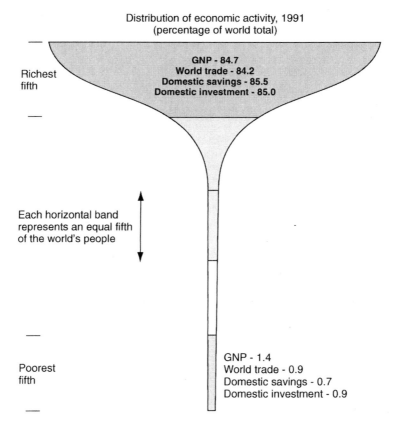

Distribution of economic activity, 1991
(percentage of world total)

Richest
fifth

GNP - 84.7
World trade - 84.2
Domestic savings - 85.5
Domestic investment - 85.0

Each horizontal band
represents an equal fifth
of the world's people

GNP - 1.4
World trade - 0.9
Domestic savings - 0.7
Domestic investment - 0.9

Poorest
fifth

FIGURE 18–1. Global economic disparities. (United Nations Development Program, *Human Development Report 1994*. New York: Oxford University Press, 1994, p. 63.)

children. Three million die from diarrheal disease each year and one million from malaria. One billion people are without adequate shelter. Three billion people lack adequate sanitation. The caloric and protein intake of the people of many countries is declining, despite economic improvement. While 840 million people, including 200 million children, suffer hunger, 27 percent of the food in the United States is wasted: about one pound per person each day. Five percent of the food wasted in the United States could feed, if transported to places in need of it, 4 million people.[16]

International poverty may be increasing, based on an analysis of wealth per capita that incorporates the depreciation of capital assets, including the deterioration of natural resources.[17] While sub-Saharan Africa has been in a declining economic state, with an average 0.2 percent decline in per-capita gross national product (GNP) between 1965 and 1996, the GNP for the Indian subcontinent has demonstrated growth. If wealth per capita is calculated, however, the average change between 1970 and 1993 for the Indian subcontinent is also negative (Table 18–1). While the GNP of a country may be increasing, quality of life may actually be declining.

The misleading picture created by the widespread use of the GNP (and Gross Domestic Product) may influence the World Bank, national governments, and development organizations to reduce the amount of development aid to specific countries. Under pressure from international financial institutions to adopt structural economic reforms, countries may exacerbate the erosion of natural assets through the adoption of policies and programs that increase the GNP in the short run while decreasing wealth-per-capita, including destroying natural resources for the future. For example, some countries, under pressure from these financial institutions, have increased timber export to meet export quotas—and debt payments—without consideration of the long-term consequences of deforestation.[17]

TABLE 18–1. Average Annual Change in Per-Capita Gross National Product (GNP) and Wealth per Capita, in Selected Asian Countries and Sub-Saharan Africa.

COUNTRY OR REGION	GNP 1965–1996	WEALTH PER CAPITA 1970–1993
Bangladesh	+1.0%	−2.6%
India	+2.3%	−0.1%
Nepal	+1.0%	−3.0%
Pakistan	+2.7%	−1.9%
Sub-Saharan Africa	−0.2%	−3.4%
China	+6.7%	+0.8%

("World Sinks Into Deeper Poverty." Friday, June 8, 2001. Accessed at http://news.bbc.co.uk/hi/ english/ business/newsid_1375307.stm.)

Role of the World Bank and the International Monetary Fund

The perception of the International Monetary Fund (IMF) and the World Bank is generally negative among many people in the Two-Thirds World, who have firsthand experiences with these institutions. To the extent that people perceive the IMF and the World Bank to be controlled by the West in general, and the United States in particular, the attitudes towards and grievances against them are associated with the overall perception of the United States.

While attempting to resolve the issues between the IMF and the World Bank and their detractors is beyond the scope of this chapter, there is strong criticism of these institutions[18-20] that is at variance with their self-perception and self-presentation.[21-24] A major target of World Bank and IMF criticism is their structural adjustment program (SAP), the standard IMF/World Bank policy package borrower countries must agree to in order to receive loans. Requirements imposed by SAPs include decreasing government spending, privatizing national enterprises, and opening countries to foreign investment. Critics maintain that such policies have led to deepening poverty throughout the world and increases in income inequality and wealth inequality within and among nations.

Environmental Justice Issues

The IMF and the World Bank have profound influence over developing countries in the Two-Thirds World and Central and Eastern Europe, with the potential to alter the lives of individuals as well as local and global ecosystems. Critics charge that IMF and World Bank policies and practices have for too long usurped local priorities, and have demonstrated "short-term vision, obliviousness to local conditions, failure to consider longer-term implications for biodiversity, the natural resource base and society itself."[25] Much of the annual $22 billion World Bank budget supports programs in the environmentally sensitive areas of energy, agriculture, and transportation. The record of World Bank lending and its accompanying advice and guidance are characterized, in our opinion, by needless environmental destruction and missed opportunities for environmentally friendly alternatives.

Even more problematic are many World Bank loans to projects that require forced resettlement, which leads to a lower quality of living for those affected. World Bank policies and programs have often undermined sustainable development, one of its stated goals.[25,26]

PHILOSOPHICAL, IDEOLOGICAL, AND
RELIGIOUS ROOTS OF TERRORISM

Religious Roots of Terrorism

Religious totalitarianism influences terrorism in a number of societies, including that of the United States. During the 1990s, several terrorist acts against the United States were apparently influenced by religious extremism: the attacks on the U.S. embassies in Kenya and Tanzania; the bomb blast at the Atlanta Olympics; the destruction of a U.S. military barracks in Dhahran, Saudi Arabia; the bombing of the Federal Building in Oklahoma City; and the first attack on the World Trade Center.

A characteristically U.S. form of religiously justified terrorism has been the bombing of abortion clinics and murderous attacks on their professional staff members. To rationalize their actions, these terrorists cite the concept of "just war" and the example of Dietrich Bonhoeffer, a German Lutheran pastor, who opposed Nazi policies and was hanged during World War II for his involvement in a plot to kill Hitler. Other extremists espouse the theology of a United States–based extremist group called the Christian Reconstruction and believe that Christians are obliged to take over society and usher in the millennium that will precede the second coming of Christ. Timothy McVeigh was, in part, influenced by the Christian Identity, an extremist group founded on ideas of racial supremacy and biblical law whose members seek a revolution that will result in the establishment of a religious state in America.[27]

Violence against civilians has historically been perpetrated by both sides of the Arab-Israeli conflict. Even before the establishment of Israel as a national state, Jewish settlers in Palestine were protected by two armed groups. Known as the Irgun and the Stern Gang, these organizations introduced paramilitary violence to the region and enabled thousands of Jews to enter Palestine illegally. The method to achieve the goal of establishing the state of Israel was illustrated by the logo of a raised fist holding a rifle over the words "Only thus."[27]

Al Qaeda arises, in part, from an Islamic movement called *Salafiyya* or "the venerable forefathers," referring to the generation of the Prophet Mohammad. Salafis regard most of the Islam currently practiced around the world to be polluted and in need of reform. Emphasis is placed on the idea of *jihad* (holy war) and the emulation of the Prophet Mohammad in his mortal struggle against idolatry. Some devoted members of Al Qaeda are willing to make martyrs of themselves, since they feel that they, like Mohammad, are engaged in struggle against unbelief that has implications for the future of religion and the world. Representatives of Salafiyya can be found in every Sunni Muslim country, where they work to force the state to apply the shari'a (Islamic law). Extremist Salafis regard Western civilization as a source of evil that spreads idolatry throughout the world in the form of secularism.[28]

Hamas, the Palestinian extremist organization, springs from the same roots of Salafiyya, but its nationalistic aims raise difficult problems. According to Salafiyya, with its emphasis on the universal Muslim community, nationalism constitutes polytheism and idolatry. Hamas has attempted to justify this conflict by emphasizing the importance of Jerusalem as an Islamic holy place and focusing on Zionism and the United States as the common enemies of Islam.[28]

Concepts of Honor and Shame

The value system of a culture provides insight into why individuals and groups commit themselves to particular courses of action. Honor and shame are significant keys to understanding several cultures worldwide, including those in Japan and other Asian countries, and in members of modern Mediterranean societies, such as Cypriot villagers, Egyptians, Bedouins, and Lebanese peasants.[1,29–33]

In a society based on honor and shame, the primary goal is accruing honor and avoiding shame. Honor as a cultural value is the positive evaluation of a person—both in his or her own eyes and those of society. Honor is increased by causing shame to others through ridicule and other rhetorical strategies.

In Mediterranean cultures, male honor is associated with authority over the household, strength in public dealings, daring and boldness, and sexual competence. Important aspects of male honor include integrity, nobility of spirit, problem-solving ability, economic capacity, and ability to protect the "sexual purity" of females in the family. Refusal to submit to any humiliation is an important element of maintaining honor.[32,34,35] In some Middle Eastern countries, national narratives that emphasize manhood and masculinity in addition to feminization of the land contribute to increasing secular nationalism.[36]

Occidentalism

Some modern-day terrorists are motivated by Occidentalism—a rejection of, and hostility towards, the values of the West. Occidentalism, which played a significant role in the events of September 11, takes the form of "a cluster of images and ideas of the West in the eyes of its haters."[37] Four targets of Occidentalism are: the city, reason, the bourgeoisie, and feminism.

To some people, the city symbolizes all the facets of modern urban civilization: commerce, diverse populations, artistic freedom, sexual license, scientific pursuits, leisure, personal safety, wealth, and power. A negative reaction to the city can hold religious meaning: urban sinfulness, as contrasted with the purity, self-denial, and obedience of idealized rural simplicity. The wealth of the city can incite their rage and envy. Images of an urban skyline, most notably that of Manhattan, evoke for these people the greed and selfishness of the marketplace.

Reason, as exemplified by science and higher education, contrasted with natural spirit, warmth, feeling, community, and relationship. Reason is seen as cold, fragmented, essentially corrupt, and lacking idealism. Many who reject reason as a governing principle wish to link religion more closely with public life.

Fundamentalists who aspire to heroism reject the settled bourgeoisie. Everyday workers are characterized as cold, decadent, mediocre, lifeless, and rarely heroic, in contrast to the holy warrior who submerges himself or herself in a mass movement that leads to greatness. Honor gained from self-sacrifice in the war against the West is the antithesis of bourgeois fear.

The fourth and final target of Occidentalism is feminism. Occidentalism, which exalts manhood, opposes the freedom of women. Female sexuality is a provocation to holy men and to those who seek exaltation through death for a higher cause. Revealing images of Western women in movies and advertisements, which represent an unreachable and sinful world, are enraging.

THE PSYCHOLOGY OF TERRORISTS

While comparative research on the psychology of terrorists fails to demonstrate a major psychopathology or a particular personality profile, a review of informal and anecdotal information and rare interviews suggests that men and women with certain psychological traits tend to be drawn to terrorism. Terrorists are described as action-oriented, aggressive, and stimulus-hungry, with tendencies to use the psychological mechanisms of "externalization" and "splitting." They are likely to have experienced psychological damage during childhood that has led to a self-concept in which the perceived good and bad aspects of their personalities are not integrated: good aspects are idealized, while bad aspects are projected onto others. The rhetoric of terrorism is highly attractive to such persons.[38]

Often characterized as springing from fragmented families, these people may find in terrorist groups their first experiences of belonging and identity. They are, therefore, particularly susceptible to pressures for conformity to group norms and for group cohesiveness that are increased by the perception of external threats. The absolutist ideology of terrorist groups becomes the intellectual justification for their morality—doubters are not tolerated.[38]

In contrast to others who attribute terrorist violence to the drive to achieve instrumental political goals, Jerrold Post argues that terrorist violence is not the means, but the end in itself; "the cause is not the cause"; and "individuals become terrorists in order to join terrorist groups and commit acts of terrorism."[38] The very existence of terrorist groups is justified by acts of terrorism. Success in achieving their ostensible aims would undermine group survival.

Albert Bandura describes the psychological mechanisms of moral disengagement that provide self-exoneration for inhumane conduct. Euphemistic language may be employed to disguise repugnant acts or to attribute them to nameless forces. Comparisons with contemporary or historical events may be made to justify terrorist acts. The media may be used to gain sympathy and support by portraying terrorists as self-sacrificing heroes who champion the causes of the helpless. Group decision-making, collective action, and efforts to decrease the perceived human impact or scope of terrorism may serve to diffuse a terrorist's sense of personal culpability for violent behavior.[39]

Suicidal Terrorist Attacks

The suicidal attacks of September 11 in the United States and suicidal bombings in Israel have drawn attention to this type of terrorist attack, but suicide as a method of terror dates back at least to the 11th-century Assassins who used it in their struggle to advance Islam in India. Muslims in India, Sumatra, and the Philippines in the 18th century also resorted to suicidal assaults in the face of colonialist repression. Such attacks present several advantages over conventional terrorism: They are simple and inexpensive, deliver maximum destructive power, leave no captives to reveal secret information, and have tremendous impact on the public, which feels helpless to defend itself.[40]

Prohibitions against suicide are found in Catholicism, Islam, and Judaism, although the promise of life after death may encourage suicide if it is committed for a righteous cause. Catholicism and Judaism teach that people who commit suicide are bound for Hell. The Islamic promise of paradise for those killed in jihad is generally considered to be reserved for those who are killed in battle, not for those who kill themselves.[41]

Indoctrination by parents, teachers, or charismatic religious or political leaders may play a role in terrorist suicide, as may the presence of the mass media and a desired audience. The formation of the "Black Tigers," a suicide unit within the Liberation Tigers of Tamil Eelam in Sri Lanka, was based on a personality cult of a brutal leader, who was inspired by the actions of Hezbollah in Lebanon.[15] Study of the personality characteristics of persons who have killed themselves during terrorist acts is difficult. The only frequently described factor in their life histories seems to be a broken family background.[41]

Since 1990, Hamas has developed a complex organization divided into a policy wing and a military wing that contains secret cells where young men are trained for suicide operations.[27] The wave of suicide bombings against Israel in the winter and spring of 2002, however, were largely carried out by young men and women attached to secular terrorist organizations who emulated the tactics of Hamas. These attacks sprang from desperation and the lack of effective government in Palestine.[42]

PREVENTING TERRORIST ATTACKS

With some understanding of the roots of terrorism, public health workers may be able to identify approaches for preventing future terrorist attacks.

Prevention of terrorism may involve general and specific measures to thwart planned terrorist attacks or to deny terrorists access to resources such as sanctuary, funding, and weapons. More fundamental is the need to address social and economic conditions underlying terrorism. Reduction of international poverty and of economic and other disparities would deprive terrorist movements of a pool of susceptible recruits. Even more important may be giving people realistic hope for political solutions to problems and genuine participation in the decisions that affect their lives. Initial steps toward allowing poor nations to begin to build more prosperous and hopeful societies include debt relief and substantial foreign aid from richer nations. Provision of education and employment opportunities for young men and women in the Two-Thirds World would help improve their quality of life and help dispel feelings of humiliation and despair that provide terrorist movements with public support.

Concerned people in the United States must seek to understand, at a much deeper level, the ideas, values, and aspirations of other people, especially those in the Two-Thirds World. While it is heartening that bookstores in the United States are selling more materials on Islam, it is unfortunate that it took a terrorist attack to interest many Americans in the beliefs of Muslim Americans even though Islam has the fastest-growing number of adherents of all the religions in the United States.

Extremists and fanatics who rationalize terrorism on a narrow interpretation of religious texts spring from various belief systems. Leaders and adherents of all faith communities must be strong public voices to emphasize tenets that lead to respect and caring for others, whatever their belief or practice. Schools that foster extremist views and hatred, sometimes even among young children, should be discouraged, within the bounds of First-Amendment protections.

As informed citizens, all of us must demand policies from our leaders that emphasize long-term international peace and progress, rather than immediate military or political gains. Concomitant with the hegemonic power that the United States now seems to exercise is the responsibility for wise rhetoric and actions that look beyond only what seems to be in our immediate national interest. A unilateral approach to world politics is a liability in the face of threats that transcend national borders. The United States should aim for consistent, principled decision-making in its interaction with other nations.

Once terrorist acts have occurred, prompt and effective protective response should be accompanied by measures to abort a deadly cycle of retaliation, as has been tragically demonstrated in the Israeli-Palestinian and Northern Ireland conflicts. Responses to terrorist acts should not themselves constitute terrorism that alienates and embitters those affected. Excessive and misdirected military action can doom all involved to an endless cycle of violence, which can marginalize potential allies and nullify any claims for the justice of a cause.

Reactions to the threat of terrorism should not lead to the adoption of laws or other policies that abrogate civil rights or human rights (Chapters 17 and 19). These rights include the rights to due process of law, freedom of speech and assembly, and privacy.

Active attention should also be given to developing public attitudes free of racism and religious bigotry. Vulnerable immigrant and ethnic minority populations in the United States should be protected from discrimination or violence resulting from misdirected attempts at revenge. (See Box 3–2 in Chapter 3.)

Successful confrontation of the post–September 11 world requires new ways of thinking and new capabilities from everyone. Primarily, people in the United States need to understand ourselves and the world more clearly and comprehensively. Then we must demonstrate the creativity and wisdom to respond to the challenges we now face in ways that help build a freer, more secure future for all people throughout the world.

REFERENCES

1. National Commission on Terrorism. Countering the changing threat of international terrorism. *Report of the National Commission on Terrorism*, Pursuant to Public Law 277. 105th Congress, June 2000.
2. Carr C. *The lessons of terror: a history of warfare against civilians*. New York: Random House, 2002.

3. Nye JS, Jr. *The paradox of American power: why the world's only superpower can't go it alone.* New York: Oxford University Press, 2002.
4. Judt T. America and the war. *The New York Times Review of Books.* November 15, 2001. Accessed at http://www.nybooks.com/articles/14760.
5. Jones CF. Terrorism: its cause and cure. *American Diplomacy.* Fall 1997. Accessed at http://www.unc.edu/depts/diplomat/articles/jones_terrorism/jones_terrorism.html.
6. Crenshaw M. The logic of terrorism: terrorist behavior as a product of strategic choice. In: Reich W (ed.). *Origins of terrorism: psychologies, ideologies, theologies, states of mind.* Washington, D.C.: Woodrow Wilson Center Press, 1998.
7. Loy JH, Ross RG. Meeting the homeland security challenge: a principled strategy for a balanced and practical response. ANSER Institute of Homeland Security. September 2001. Accessed at *www.homelandsecurity.org.*
8. Amanat A. "Empowered through violence: the reinventing of Islamic extremism." In Talbott S, Chanda N (eds.). *The age of terror: America and the world after September 11.* New York: Basic Books, 2001.
9. Hill C. "A Herculean task: the myth and reality of Arab terrorism." In Talbott S, Chanda N (eds.). *The age of terror.*
10. Talbott S, Chanda N (eds.). *The age of terror.*
11. Wechsler WF. "Strangling the hydra: targeting Al Qaeda's finances." In Hoge JF, Rose G (eds.). *How did this happen? terrorism and the new war.* New York: Public Affairs, 2001.
12. United Nations. "Poverty Is Colossal Powder Keg Which Can Explode Without Most of World Realizing Its Negative Consequences, Assembly President Says." Press Release GA/SM/168, 1 June 2000.
13. ABC News, September 24, 1999.
14. United Nations Development Programme. *1999 Human Development Report.* Geneva: United Nations, 1999.
15. Bunyavanich S, Walkup RB. US public health leaders shift toward a new paradigm of global health. *Am J Public Health* 2001; 91:1556–1558.
16. US Department of Agriculture. More than one-fourth of U.S. food wasted, USDA study finds. Release No. 0212.97. Accessed at http://www.usda.gov/news/releases/1997/06/0212.
17. BBC News. "World Sinks into Deeper Poverty." Friday, June 8, 2001. Accessed at http://news.bbc.co.uk/hi/english/business/newsid_1375307.stm.
18. Debt. Fact Sheet. *50 Years Is Enough.* Accessed at www.50years.org.
19. MacCuish D. World Bank should stop acting like a loan shark. *Montreal Gazette,* July 24, 2001.
20. Dawson TC. Poor countries don't want more debt relief (letter to the editor). *Montreal Gazette,* July 28, 2001.
21. International Monetary Fund. The IMF at a glance: a factsheet. August 17, 2001. Accessed at www.imf.org.
22. International Monetary Fund. Social dimensions of the IMF's policy dialogue: a factsheet. March 2001. Accessed at www.imf.org.
23. World Bank. 10 things you never knew about the World Bank. Accessed at www.worldbank.org.
24. World Bank. About us. Accessed at www.worldbank.org.
25. The environment. *50 Years Is Enough.* Accessed at www.50years.org.
26. Institute for Policy Studies. New database calculates lifetime greenhouse gas emissions from nine years of World Bank fossil fuel projects: first-of-its-kind resource

catalogues $20 billion in dirty energy projects since 1992. October 29, 2001. Accessed at http://www.seen.org.

27. Juergensmeyer M. *Terror in the mind of God: the global rise of religious violence.* Berkeley, Calif: University of California Press, 2000.

28. Doran MS. Somebody else's civil war: ideology, rage, and the assault on America. In Hoge JF, Rose G (eds.), *How did this happen? Terrorism and the new war.* New York: Public Affairs, 2001.

29. Gilmore DD. *The people of the plain: class and community in lower Andalusia.* New York: Columbia University Press, 1982.

30. MacMullen R. *Roman social relations: 50 B.C. to A.D. 284.* New Haven: Yale University Press, 1974.

31. Persitany JG (ed.). *Honour and shame: the values of Mediterranean society.* Worcester, UK: Trinity, 1965.

32. Rabichev R. *The Mediterranean concepts of honour and shame as seen in the depiction of biblical women.* South Africa: Unisa Press, 2000.

33. Schneider J. Of vigilance and virgins: honour, shame and access to resources in Mediterranean societies. *Ethnology* 1971; 9:1–24.

34. Malina BJ, Neyrey JH. Honour and shame in Luke-Acts: pivotal values in the Mediterranean world. In Neyrey JH (ed.). *The social world of Luke-Acts, models for interpretation.* Peabody, Mass.: Hendrickson, 1991.

35. Pitt-Rivers J. *The fate of Shechem of the politics of sex: essays in the anthropology of the Mediterranean.* Cambridge: Cambridge University Press, 1977.

36. Katz SH. Adam and Adama, 'Ird and Ard: engendering political conflict and identity in early Jewish and Palestinian nationalisms. In Kandyoti D. *Gendering the Middle East.* Syracuse: Syracuse University Press, 1996.

37. Margalit A, Buruma I. Occidentalism. *New York Review of Books,* January 17, 2002.

38. Post JM. Terrorist psycho-logic. In Reich W (ed.). *Origins of terrorism: psychologies, ideologies, theologies, states of mind.* Washington, D.C.: Woodrow Wilson Center Press, 1998.

39. Bandura A. Mechanisms of moral disengagement. In Reich W (ed.). *Origins of terrorism.*

40. Sprinzak E. Rational fanatics. *Foreign Policy.* September/October 2000. Accessed at http://www.foreignpolicy.com/issue_SeptOct_2001/sprinzak.html.

41. Merari A. The readiness to kill and die: suicidal terrorism in the Middle East. In Reich W (ed.), *Origins of terrorism: psychologies, ideologies, theologies, states of mind.* Washington, D.C.: Woodrow Wilson Center Press, 1998.

42. Telhami S. Why suicide terror takes root. *New York Times.* April 4, 2002. Accessed at www.NYTimes.com.

19

Promoting international law

PETER WEISS

"Terror—it's all in the eyes of the beholder." Thus reads the headline of a news feature in the mainstream Israeli newspaper Haaretz.[1] And by way of exposition, it asks in the subhead, "Why is the attack on the Twin Towers called terrorism, while the bombing of a hospital in Kabul is not?"

The question, in infinite guises, has plagued international lawyers for over a century. It poses not only the dilemma of state terrorism versus terrorism by non-state actors, but also the question of whether a distinction should be drawn between violence in pursuit of a just cause and an unjust one. One person's terrorist is another person's freedom fighter, in the words of the hoary cliché (see Chapter 1).

As a result, there is currently no generally agreed-upon definition of *terrorism* in international law. There are a number of conventions that deal with terrorist acts such as hijacking and hostage-taking, without, however, defining terrorism. Diplomats have had to make do with formulations like that of Sir Jeremy Greenstock, the British ambassador to the United Nations, in his post–September 11 speech to the General Assembly: "What looks, smells and kills like terrorism is terrorism." Ironically, a proposal by the 119-member Non-Aligned Movement for a major United Nations conference to be held for the purpose of drafting a Comprehensive Convention on International Terrorism was sidetracked by the events of September 11, as well as by the opposition of the United States to discussing a comprehensive definition of terrorism.[2]

There are, however, perfectly serviceable definitions of terrorism in domestic law (see Chapter 1). The Criminal Code of the United States defines *international terrorism* as activities that:

(a) involve violent acts or acts dangerous to human life that are a violation of the criminal laws of the United States or any State;

(b) appear to be intended to intimidate or coerce a civilian population; to influence the policy of a government by intimidation or coercion; or to affect the conduct of a government by assassination or kidnapping; and

(c) occur primarily outside the territorial jurisdiction of the United States, or transcend national boundaries in terms of the means by which they are accomplished.[3]

The Federal Bureau of Investigation (FBI) definition says it all in fewer words: "Terrorism is the unlawful use of force or violence against persons or property to intimidate or coerce a government, the civilian population, or any segment thereof, in furtherance of political or social objectives."[4]

Both of these definitions, literally read, would apply to state terrorism as well as non-state terrorism, although one may doubt that this was the intention of their drafters. In a legal sense, the debate about "justifiable" terrorism, which raged in the second half of the 20th century in the context of anti-colonialism and wars of liberation, has been largely laid to rest. The Taliban leader Mulla Omar may have been the last person in a position of government authority to endorse violence against innocent civilians as a way of achieving political goals. Others in official capacities may continue to practice it, while disavowing any intention to do so, and the Osama bin Ladens of this world will both continue the practice and proclaim its justification.

In 1996, the United Nations General Assembly adopted without a vote—that is, without dissent—a resolution stating: "Criminal acts intended or calculated to provoke a state of terror in the general public, a group of persons or particular persons for political purposes are in any circumstances unjustifiable, whatever the considerations of a political, philosophical, ideological, racial, ethnic, religious or other nature that may be invoked to justify them."[5]

RESPONSES

Does a terrorist act justify full-scale war as a response? It is doubtful that, before the events of September 11, many international lawyers would have answered this question in the affirmative. But the enormity and brutality of those events have led facts to intrude on and muddy the clarity of abstract principles, as is frequently the case in the interplay between law and reality. Nevertheless, it is important not to lose sight of the principles involved, lest the force of law suffer a mortal wound from the law of force. As former ambassador to the United Nations Jeanne Kirkpatrick famously said, "International law is not a mutual suicide pact." To this, it is necessary to reply with the commonplace saying: "Hard cases make bad law."

Bad law was made by President George W. Bush when he characterized September 11 as an act of war. In a metaphorical sense, he was right; in a legal sense, he was treading on dangerous ground. He was certainly not within the parameters of the United States criminal code, which, in order to distinguish it from terrorism, defines an "act of war" as "Any act occurring in the course of: (a) a declared war; (b) armed conflict, whether or not war has been declared, between two or more nations; or (c) armed conflict between military forces of any origin."[6]

Bad law was again made by President Bush when he announced that any country that harbors terrorists would suffer the fate of terrorists. There can be no doubt that September 11 was a crime against humanity of enormous proportions whose perpetrators must be punished. In a properly functioning world order, whose outlines are clearly delineated though inadequately implemented, the perpetrators would be brought to justice before the nascent International Criminal Court or, pending its imminent establishment, before an ad hoc international tribunal, on the model of the Yugoslav and Rwandan tribunals or those being discussed for East Timor and Sierra Leone. In such a world order, punishment would also be meted out to nations that encourage or facilitate acts of terrorism.

But war, in a world rife with weapons of mass destruction, is serious business. The consequences of the U.S. anti-terrorist doctrine are already alarmingly evident in places such as the Middle East and South Asia, where, if terrorism is not halted, Israel threatens war against Palestine (which is not yet even a state) and India against Pakistan. A similar phenomenon is manifesting itself in the eagerness of many countries to follow the lead of the United States in enacting emergency measures that violate constitutional and international human rights norms.

Equally worrisome is the general acceptance of the just war theory by the public and the media. A *New York Times* editorial, "Terrorism's Other Battlefields," while advising caution in carrying the war against terrorism beyond the borders of Afghanistan, blandly stated that President Bush "rightly warned governments around the world that offering sanctuary to international terrorists could expose their countries to American military action."[7] A host of moral, political, and legal problems is contained in these few words, which represent the conventional wisdom of the moment, such as:

- By what right? Not the Charter of the United Nations, Article 51 of which limits the right to use armed force to situations of self-defense "if an armed attack occurs" and only "until the Security Council has taken measures necessary to maintain international peace and security." In customary international law, the right of self-defense is further limited to circumstances where "the necessity of that self-defense is instant, overwhelming, and leaving no choice of means, and no moment for deliberation."[8]
- What does "offering sanctuary," or "harboring," in the words of the President, mean? For several years, Emmanuel "Toto" Constant, a founder and Secretary General of FRAPH, a terrorist paramilitary group guilty of torture, rape, and other heinous human rights violations committed in Haiti, has been living in the United States. Extradition requests from the Haitian government have been ignored, as has a final deportation order from the Immigration and Naturalization Service. As of this writing (February 2002), Constant is still living in New York. If Haiti had the means, would it be justified in launching a military attack on the United States?[8a]
- What is an "international terrorist" in this context? Is it only a person planning a terrorist attack on the United States from another country, or also one of the tens—perhaps hundreds—of thousands of people engaged in cross-border attacks against civilians anywhere in the world?
- "American military action"? Even if not sanctioned by the United Nations or approved by our allies in the anti-terrorist coalition? What happened to "The United States cannot nor will not be the world's policeman?"

Hard cases make not only bad law, but also bad and dangerous policies.

SOLUTIONS

It is incumbent on critics of all-out war as the response to terrorism to propose alternative responses. Fortunately there is no dearth of such proposals, either at the national level or at the level of international law and cooperation, with which this chapter is particularly concerned.

In the wake of September 11, the U.N. Security Council adopted two resolutions, 1368 and 1373. The first condemned "in the strongest terms the horrifying terrorist attacks," recognized "the inherent right of individual and collective self-defense in accordance with the Charter," called on all states to "bring to justice the perpetrators, organizers and sponsors" of the attacks, and stressed that those responsible for "aiding, supporting or harbouring the perpetrators, organizers and sponsors of these acts will be held accountable." It is by no means clear that this constituted the authorization required by the Charter for the war on Afghanistan, much less the extension of the war to other terrorist-harboring states, although it has been so interpreted by the United States and its principal allies.

Resolution 1373 is a different matter. It sets out, in considerable detail—three single-spaced pages—a series of non-military steps designed to fight terrorism by cutting off the flow of funds and weapons to terrorists, increasing international cooperation in intelligence and law enforcement, and controlling the movement of suspected terrorists across national borders. While the implementation of these aims may lead to abuses, they are certainly commendable in principle and should serve as a guide to counter-terrorism without plunging the world into war without end.

The curious aspect of 1373 is that it is worded as a command issued to the world at large by the 15 ambassadors who compose the Security Council at any one time, including the five permanent members. The operative words are, "The Security Council decides that all states *shall* (emphasis added) prevent and suppress (a) the financing of terrorist acts. . . ." Then come 10 other specific measures that "all states shall" take, followed by seven more that all states are, in the more traditional language of the Security Council, *called upon* to take. Thus, one thing that has changed after September 11 is that we now have the Security Council as supreme lawgiver of the world, and this pursuant to a resolution drafted and sponsored by a United States administration not known, before or after September 11, for its enthusiasm for the United Nations.

In fact, much has already been done by many countries in carrying out the mandate of 1373; some good and some bad. The Resolution also created a special committee to monitor its implementation, chaired by Sir Jeremy Greenstock.[9,10] It remains to be seen how the Security Council proposes to deal with states that fail to do what the Council has decided they shall do.

"UNLAWFUL COMBATANTS" AND "MILITARY COMMISSIONS"

Thanks to enterprising journalism and bad public relations, the pictures of the hooded, manacled, and shackled prisoners arriving at the Guantanamo base in Cuba, and news about their drugged state during the long trip from Afghanistan, provoked a veritable firestorm of criticism from around the world, including most of the partners of the United States in the "coalition against terror." The first reaction from the United States was that the prisoners were "unlawful combatants," not entitled to the protection of the Geneva Conventions. In a statement characteristic of the cavalier attitude of the Bush administration toward international law, Secretary of Defense Donald Rumsfeld announced, "Unlawful combatants do not have any rights under the Geneva Convention. We have indicated that we do plan to, *for the most part*, treat them in a manner *reasonably consistent* with the Geneva Conventions, *to the extent they are appropriate*"[11] (emphases added).

The term *unlawful combatant* is not a part of the Geneva Conventions. It derives from the case of the eight Nazi saboteurs who landed in Florida and on Long Island in June 1942 and were quickly apprehended and then tried by a military commission appointed by President Franklin D. Roosevelt. The Supreme Court, in affirming the jurisdiction of the military commission in the *Quirin* case said that, as persons who had entered the country "for the commission of hostile acts involving destruction of life or property" and had discarded their military uniforms upon entry, they had "the status of unlawful combatants punishable as such by military commission."[12]

The prisoners taken by the United States and its allies during the short Afghan war, however, fall into at least two entirely different categories: soldiers of the Taliban armed forces and volunteers of Al Qaeda who were captured in Afghanistan. A third category, the only one fitting the description of the defendants in *Quirin*, would have been the 19 hijackers who went to their suicidal deaths on September 11. Their alleged co-conspirators found in the United States also fall into this category, but so far only one, Zacarias Moussaoui, has been charged, and he, curiously, is being tried in a regular federal court. Richard Reid, the "shoe bomber" charged with attempting to blow up a plane en route to the United States, also comes close to the *Quirin* facts, but he, as well, will be tried in federal court.

The notion that the Geneva Conventions do not apply to Taliban prisoners never made any sense. Secretary of State Colin Powell, remembering his days as Armed Forces Chief of Staff and looking forward to situations where such an illogical precedent might be used against American soldiers, urged President Bush to reconsider. His efforts were crowned with success: on February 7, the President announced that the Taliban prisoners, but not the Al Qaeda prisoners, would be entitled to all the protections of the Geneva Conventions. The reasoning behind this decision was still tortured, to say the least: the Conventions would be applied, said the President, because Afghanistan was a party to them. The Taliban prisoners, however, were not prisoners of war because the Taliban regime was never recognized by the United States.[13]

As for the Al Qaeda prisoners, their status is more ambiguous. What is not ambiguous is that, under Article 5 of the Third Geneva Convention, any person captured in the course of a belligerent action is entitled to the protection of the Convention until his status has been determined "by a competent tribunal" and that the President of the United States cannot appoint himself to fill that role. It is also unambiguous that, whether the Conventions apply or not, "everyone," and that means every last terrorist or suspected terrorist, is entitled not to be subjected to cruel, inhumane, or degrading treatment or punishment, under the International Covenant on Civil and Political Rights, to which both Afghanistan and the United States are parties. In this connection, it is noteworthy that, under the glare of public opinion, the conditions of the Guantanamo prisoners have become, if not humane, at least less inhumane (Figure 19–1). Observers for Physicians for Human Rights have charged that, of 3,500 prisoners held in Afghanistan, many have already died and many more are at risk of dying due to enormous overcrowding and "grossly inadequate food and medical care."[14]

It remains to be seen, in any case, whether membership in, or association with, Al Qaeda is equivalent *per se* to an intent to destroy American lives or property. It may emerge that many of the Arabs, Pakistanis, Uzbeks, Chechens, Chinese, and others who joined Al Qaeda did so for the main or sole purpose of defending the Taliban against its internal opponents and did not receive terrorist training in Osama bin Laden's camps. Presumably, the trial of John Walker Lindh will shed some light on this issue. (*Epilogue, July 2002:* That is precisely what has happened since this chapter was written; the terrorism charges against Lindh have been dropped.)

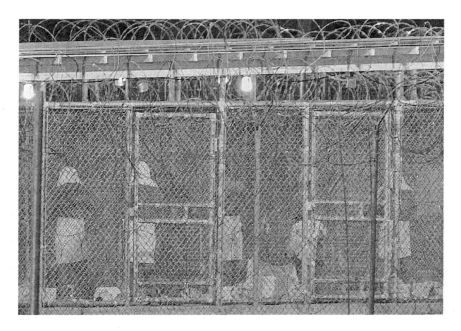

FIGURE 19–1. Detainees are seen in their cells facing towards Mecca during evening prayer at Camp X-Ray at the U.S. naval base on Guantanamo Bay, Cuba, on March 4, 2002 (AP/Wide World Photos).

The Bush Administration has also incurred severe criticism at home and abroad for the rules of procedure proposed by presidential order for the military commissions. As a member of the American armed forces at the end of World War II, I was assigned to a unit charged with separating "real Nazis" from mere collaborators among German prisoners of war in the United States, and I remember well the difficulties inherent in that task. Today, no one wants to see an O.J. Simpson trial for each of the thousands of Al Qaeda prisoners, but fundamental norms are just that; they are intransgressible prescriptions for countries that consider themselves civilized, whatever that much-abused term may mean.

In this respect also, President Bush has had to backtrack from his original announcement: the death penalty can no longer be imposed by a two-thirds vote; the right to counsel of the defendant's choice has been restored, at least in principle. But the President's authority to designate a person a terrorist subject to trial by military commission still stands, and the detailed guidelines for the operation of the commissions have not been announced as of this writing (February 2002). The American Bar Association (ABA), in a resolution overwhelmingly approved by its House of Delegates this month, has urged that the commissions be used only in limited circumstances and under established legal and constitutional rules. Among the ABA recommendations is that the commissions operate in accordance with Articles 14 and 15 of the International Covenant on Civil and Political Rights, which set out in some detail, for international observance, the contents of what in the Anglo-American system is called "due process of law."[15]

Even in emergency situations, even when dealing with individuals who would not hesitate to use the most brutal methods to kill their perceived enemies, including those who may sit in judgment on them, basic due process must be observed. In the words of Evan Davis, President of the New York City Bar Association, "We want to bring these terrorists to justice with justice." That is what America has preached to dictators invoking the same excuses for their derogation of fundamental norms in "states of siege." That is what America must practice today, lest it set a precedent by which past and future dictators will be excused for their transgressions against justice and human rights.[16,17]

Epilogue, July 2002: Details have begun to surface of the Bush administration's plans to attack Iraq to bring about a "regime change"—another instance of war as a response to terrorism. This term has apparently now been redefined to include "potential possession of weapons of mass destruction." As of now, war on Iraq would be a violation of both the United Nations Charter, which forbids aggression, and the U.S. Constitution, which forbids Presidential warmaking without Congressional authorization.

REFERENCES

1. Horowitz N. *Haaretz*, November 18, 2001.
2. Deen T. US shies away from un treaties on terrorism. International Press Service, September 11, 2001.
3. 18 USC 2331(1).
4. Website of the Terrorism Research Center, http://www.terrorism.com/index.html.
5. United Nations General Assembly. A/RES/51/210, 17 December 1996.
6. 18 USC 2331(4).
7. Terrorism's other battlefields (editorial). *New York Times*, January 9, 2002.
8. *The Caroline Incident.* 29 British and Foreign State Papers 1129, 1138. Cf. *The Corfu Channel Case*, 1949 I.C.J. Reports 4.
8a. Letter of December 11, 2000, to Attorney General Janet Reno and Secretary Madeleine Albright from a number of human rights organizations. Accessed at http://www.hrw.org/press/2000/12/constant1211.html.
9. The country reports submitted to the committee, including the United States report, are available at www.un.org/Docs/sc/committees/1373/.
10. Critiques of some of the actions taken by governments can be found at www.hrw.org.
11. *New York Times*, January 12, 2002.
12. *Ex parte Quirin*, 317 U.S. 1, 35.
13. Seelye KQ. In shift Bush says Geneva rules fit Taliban captives but not Qaeda members. *New York Times*, February 8, 2002.
14. Leaning J, Heffernan J. Forgotten prisoners of war (op-ed.). *New York Times*, February 2, 2002.
15. ABA Resolution and related articles available at www.law.com, keyword *military tribunals*.
16. Safire W. Seizing dictatorial power. *New York Times*, November 15, 2001.
17. Safire W. Kangaroo courts. *New York Times*, November 26, 2001.

Epilogue

BARRY S. LEVY AND VICTOR W. SIDEL

The chapters for the first printing of this book were written in 2002, within months of the 9/11 attacks on the World Trade Center (WTC) and the Pentagon and the dissemination of anthrax spores that followed soon after. These events and terrorist attacks in other countries, which led to widespread fear of future attacks, caused the U.S. government to initiate a "war on terror" and widespread efforts to prevent and prepare for possible terrorist attacks. This epilogue updates and adds to information in the first printing of *Terrorism and Public Health,* with references to material published since mid-2002.

U.S. law defines *terrorism* as "premeditated, politically motivated violence perpetrated against noncombatant targets by subnational groups or clandestine agents."[1] This definition of terrorism does not include acts committed by nation-states (see our broader definition of terrorism on page 4). Based on this definition, the National Counterterrorism Center reported that during 2005, there were approximately 11,000 terrorist attacks worldwide that resulted in more than 14,600 deaths and about 25,000 people wounded. Suicide bombings increased in some countries, with 360 suicide bombings accounting for about 20 percent of the deaths. About 30 percent of the terrorist attacks and 55 percent of the deaths occurred in Iraq. Almost 54 percent of attacks were against facilities and/or resulted in no casualties.[2]

Among major terrorist attacks since 2002 have been the detonation of bombs on a train in Madrid in March 2004 that killed 191 people and injured 1,700, and on local public transport in London in July 2005, that killed 56 people, including four perpetrators, and injured 700 people; the occupation of a theater in Moscow in October 2002 by Chechen guerillas in which 170 people were killed, including 41 of the guerillas—deaths that were mainly caused by fentanyl and halothane used in gaseous form by the police in a rescue attempt;[3] and the seizure of a public school in Beslan in southern Russia in September 2004 by a Chechen group that led to the death of 332 people, mostly students, teachers, and parents.

9/11 FOLLOW-UP STUDIES

Several studies have been, and are being, performed to assess adverse health effects on people exposed to airborne contaminants during and after 9/11 (Chapter 4). In the 2 to 3 years after 9/11, survivors of the WTC attack who had been caught in the dust and debris cloud of the collapsing towers experienced substantial physical and mental health problems, including significantly more injuries; respiratory symptoms; severe headaches; skin rash/irritation; hearing problems or loss; heartburn; diagnosed stroke; self-reported depression, anxiety, or other emotional problems; and, at the time of follow-up, serious psychological distress. The long-term significance of these findings is not known.[4]

In the 2 years after 9/11, firefighters in the New York Fire Department (FDNY) experienced a five-fold increased rate of sarcoidosis, which has declined since then; however, the New York Police Department did not find an increase in sarcoidosis among police working at the WTC site.[5]

Intense, short-term exposure to materials generated during the WTC collapse was associated with increased bronchial responsiveness and cough, with physiological severity related to intensity of exposure.[6-8] Workers in the dust cloud at the time of the WTC collapse had significantly higher risks of persistent lower respiratory symptoms (an almost 10-fold increased risk), mucous membrane symptoms, depressive symptoms, and symptoms of post-traumatic stress disorder (PTSD).[9]

During the 6 months after the attacks, 332 firefighters had WTC-related cough severe enough to require 4 or more consecutive weeks of medical leave. During the 11 months after 9/11, there were 1,277 stress-related incidents observed among FDNY rescue workers.[10]

Forty percent of rescue and recovery workers and volunteers at the WTC site had persistent lower respiratory symptoms and 50 percent, upper respiratory symptoms, which were related to work at the site. On spirometry testing, 33 percent had abnormal findings, most suggestive of restrictive disease.[11] Follow-up investigations found that approximately 70 percent of nearly 10,000 workers tested from 2002 to 2004 reported new or substantially worsened respiratory problems during the time they worked at Ground Zero (the WTC site) or afterward.[12]

Samples of total settled dust and smoke collected at locations east of the WTC 5 and 6 days after the attack identified: (a) inorganic materials, including metals, radionuclides, and asbestos; and (b) organic materials, including polycyclic aromatic hydrocarbons (PAHs), polychlorinated biphenyls (PCBs), polychlorinated dibenzodioxins and dibenzofurans (PCDD/F), pesticides, and other hydrocarbons.[13]

Residents near the WTC site had significantly higher (more than double) rates of new-onset upper respiratory symptoms after 9/11, most of which persisted 1 year after 9/11 in the affected area.[14] Among residents of central and southern Manhattan with a previous diagnosis of asthma, 27 percent reported worsening of asthma symptoms after 9/11.[15]

Eight percent of adults residing in central or southern Manhattan reported symptoms consistent with PTSD related to 9/11 and 10 percent, symptoms consistent with depression; 20 percent of those who lived near the WTC had PTSD symptoms.[16] Most PTSD symptoms resolved within 6 months after 9/11.[17] Forty percent of Pentagon employees had mental health symptoms in the 4 months after 9/11, including PTSD (8 percent of employees), depression (18 percent), panic attacks (23 percent), and generalized anxiety (27 percent).[18]

Term infants born to women who were pregnant on 9/11 and had been living within 2 miles of the WTC during the month after 9/11 had significant decrements in term birth weight and birth length, possibly due to pollutants and/or stress related to the disaster.[19] A follow-up of pregnant women who were either inside or near the WTC on 9/11 demonstrated a doubling in small-for-gestational-age (SGA) infants.[19]

In September 2006, the New York City Department of Health and Mental Hygiene began mailing to every physician in the city guidelines to diagnose and treat physical and mental health problems related to the 9/11 attacks.[20]

PUBLIC HEALTH PREPAREDNESS IN THE UNITED STATES

Since 9/11, billions of dollars have been spent by the federal government as well as state and local governments in the United States on emergency preparedness and response capabilities for potential terrorist attacks. While some of this huge allocation of money has helped to improve public health capabilities, these efforts to prepare for low-probability events have diverted attention and resources from many, widespread existent public health problems, such as smoking-related diseases, alcoholism and other forms of substance abuse, domestic and community violence, diabetes, and environmental health problems.[21,22] A recently published book, *Are We Ready? Public Health Since 9/11*, documents how public health workers responded effectively to the 9/11 attacks and the anthrax dissemination soon afterward, and also explores how needed reforms to the nation's public health system have been undermined since then.[23]

An overall assessment of terrorism preparedness in the United States performed in December 2005 indicated many gaps and inadequacies.[24] Recent cuts and ongoing disparities in anti-terror funding have led to the perception that the funding has been based on politics rather than on the level of threat.[25,26]

The Centers for Disease Control and Prevention (CDC) has extensive useful information on its Web site at: http://www.bt.cdc.gov. This includes information on bioterrorism, chemical emergencies, radiation emergencies, mass casualties, natural disasters and severe weather events, and recent outbreaks and incidents. This Web site also provides useful links to information on a variety of related subjects, including disaster mental health, the Laboratory Response Network, and the *Public Health Emergency Response Guide for State, Local, and Tribal Public Health Directors*. Many other Web sites have useful information on these and related issues, including the Health Resources and Services Administration (HSRA) Web site (http://www.hrsa. gov), which includes information on the National Bioterrorism Hospital Preparedness Program.

There are many examples of dysfunctional "preparedness" that have taken place. For example, a campaign of mass smallpox vaccination was announced by President George W. Bush in December 2002, despite there not having been any known cases of smallpox anywhere in the world since 1981. The campaign was to focus on vaccinating 500,000 military personnel, 500,000 health workers, and as many as 10 million emergency responders. Many public health workers expressed concerns about the risk of smallpox vaccination and diversion of public health resources to implement this program.[27] Smallpox vaccination, although implemented on a much smaller scale than planned, resulted in less than 40,000 health workers and emergency responders being vaccinated, with at least 145 serious adverse events and at least three deaths.[28] The diversion of resources for this campaign led to neglect of other urgent public health problems, such as tuberculosis, for which an increase in incidence occurred.[29,30]

The U.S. Department of Defense (DoD) had ordered, in 1997, that all U.S. service members be immunized against anthrax (Chapters 6 and 10). Reports of adverse reactions and doubts about the effectiveness of the current vaccine against inhalation anthrax led some service members to refuse vaccination, resulting in their demotion, dismissal from military service, or conviction at court-martial for "refusal to obey a lawful order." In response to a class-action lawsuit on behalf of the refusers, the U.S. District Court for the District of Columbia in 2004 issued an injunction against further administration of the vaccine. When the injunction was lifted in 2005, on the basis of an Emergency Use Authorization issued by the Food and Drug Administration (FDA), the Court ordered that the immunizations be voluntary rather than compulsory; the DoD resumed immunizations to service members, who were given an option to refuse. A total of 1.1 million service members have received the vaccine manufactured by the Bioport Corporation, the only licensed U.S. supplier of anthrax vaccine.

The most dysfunctional consequence of U.S. "preparedness" programs and their political use has been widespread fear.[31] The identification of levels of "terrorism risk," dramatized by use of five color codes and the frequent unnecessary mobilization of first-responders and military and national guard forces, led to a climate of fear that enabled the Bush administration to gain approval of the Congress for additional major funding for Project Bioshield 2003, a well-funded program that authorizes U.S government purchase and stockpiling of vaccines and drugs, and other counter-terrorism programs. Fear of people who "look like terrorists" has led to discrimination against Muslims and others and barriers to their travel.[32] Muslim leaders in the United States, interviewed in September 2006, believe "American Muslims still face high levels of hatred and suspicion nearly 5 years after the September 11th attacks and political leaders and the news media are mostly to blame."[33]

CIVIL LIBERTIES ISSUES IN THE UNITED STATES

Since the discussion of civil liberties in the first printing of this book (Chapter 17), tensions between efforts to guard against another terrorist attack and threats to civil liberties have vastly expanded.[34] Adoption of the Homeland Security Act in 2003 and other federal actions of doubtful legality have expanded the power of the federal government. Examples include the tapping, without obtaining judicial warrant, of telephone calls made between the United States and other countries by the National Security Agency (NSA) and the request by the NSA to U.S. telephone companies to provide records of billions of domestic telephone calls made by U.S. residents.[36,37] The tapping of phone calls without warrants was, according to the NSA, intended to eavesdrop on conversations between people in the United States and members of terrorist groups in other countries. Access to the telephone records was, according to the NSA, intended to identify calling patterns that might uncover

planning of terrorist acts.[38] In August 2006, a U.S. district judge banned surveillance without warrants, ruling that the program broke federal law and violated the Constitution's prohibition on unreasonable searches; the ruling has
not been implemented, pending the results of a Justice Department appeal.

Furthermore, for the first time since the Civil War, the United States was,
in 2002, designated a military theater of operations—a radical change in the
role of the DoD and an erosion of the principle, in force since 1878, that the
U.S. military not be used for domestic law enforcement. In 2003, the Congress created the position of Undersecretary of Defense for Intelligence to
oversee the DoD intelligence agencies, including a new agency, the Coun-
terintelligence Field Activity (CIFA). The CIFA was ordered to maintain a
"domestic law-enforcement database" and it began collecting information on
U.S. citizens.[39]

An agreement with the European Union to provide 34 categories of personal information to U.S. authorities about airline passengers on flights to
the United States from 25 countries has been viewed as another infringement
of civil liberties. The personal data that were provided included names, addresses, phone numbers, itineraries, and payment information, including
credit card numbers. In 2006, the highest court of the European Union (EU)
ruled that the EU had overstepped its authority and that the agreement should
be renegotiated.[40]

WARS IN AFGHANISTAN AND IRAQ

In response to the 9/11 attacks, the United States initiated wars in Afghanistan
and Iraq. The war in Afghanistan, which began within a few weeks of 9/11,
was designed to topple the Taliban regime, which had supported Al Qaeda.
The war in Afghanistan brought down the Taliban regime, but, as of September 2006, Taliban forces were increasing their strength, especially in the
southern part of Afghanistan.[41]

The war in Iraq, which began in March 2003, was initiated to address alleged reports that the regime of Saddam Hussein had weapons of mass destruction and was harboring and supporting Al Qaeda terrorists. U.S.-led
Coalition forces failed to find weapons of mass destruction (WMDs) or ties
between the regime of Saddam Hussein and Al Qaeda. As of early September 2006, more than 2,800 Coalition forces had been killed and more than
19,000 wounded. In addition, there were at least 30,000—and perhaps considerably more than 100,000—fatalities among Iraqis.[42] In addition, many
Iraqis have been wounded. There has been widespread destruction to the
health-supporting infrastructure, such as health-care facilities and water treatment plants. Several hundred thousand Iraqis have been forced to flee their

homes and become internally displaced persons or refugees in other countries. There has been much environmental devastation, including widespread dispersion of unexploded ordnance and depleted uranium, a radioactive and toxic substance used to harden shell casings and armor.

INTERNATIONAL HUMAN RIGHTS ISSUES

There have been many human rights violations related to the wars in Afghanistan and Iraq as well as other parts of the "war on terror."[43,44] This has included torture and other forms of maltreatment of detainees, in violation of the Geneva Conventions, at Abu Ghraib and other prisons in Iraq and Afghanistan; the U.S. military base at Guantanamo Bay, Cuba;[45] and prisons in Central and Eastern Europe operated by the U.S. Central Intelligence Agency. In addition, in a program of "rendition," the United States has transferred detainees from these and other prisons to countries with poor human rights records, where these detainees may have been tortured or otherwise maltreated.[46]

Military interrogators at Guantanamo Bay have used aggressive measures in a systematic manner to pressure detainees to cooperate, including sleep deprivation, prolonged isolation, painful body positions, feigned suffocation, and beatings. The International Committee of the Red Cross and other organizations claim that such tactics constitute cruel and inhuman treatment, including torture. Health information on detainees has been routinely available to psychologists, other behavioral science consultants, and others who designed and implemented interrogation strategies. This situation has made health-care providers into accessories to the gathering of intelligence, which has undermined detainees' trust in physicians and has placed prisoners at increased risk of significant abuse.[47] In June 2006, three detainees at Guantanamo Bay committed suicide.[48] Also in June 2006, the Supreme Court, in a 5-to-3 decision, repudiated the plan of the Bush administration to place Guantanamo detainees on trial before military commissions, ruling that the commissions were not authorized by federal statue and that they also violated international law.[49]

In Iraq and at Guantanamo Bay, physicians and other health-care workers passed health information on detainees to military intelligence personnel. In addition, physicians helped to design interrogation strategies, such as sleep deprivation and other coercive methods, which were developed in relation to detainees' specific medical problems. Medical personnel also coached interrogators on their questioning techniques. The physicians who helped in planning the interrogations tended not to see these practices as being unethical. They claimed that they were not acting as physicians and were thus not bound by ethical principles oriented to patients. The Surgeon General of the U.S. Army is developing rules for health-care professionals working with detainees.[47]

There is a need for a systematic, transparent review of the behavior of physicians and other medical personnel in interrogating detainees in Iraq, at Guantanamo Bay, and elsewhere and the pressures that led to this behavior.[50] Had the Geneva Conventions been applied to Iraq, torture and other abuse of prisoners at Abu Ghraib probably would not have occurred. These conventions ban torture and humiliating and abusive treatment of prisoners, and also protect physicians who ethically report and refuse to participate in torture and abuse of prisoners.[51]

Leaders of Physicians for Human Rights and other organizations have stated that the efforts of U.S. military officials to develop ethical guidelines that enable physicians to participate in coercive interrogation practices are not consistent with international principles of medical ethics and could establish a dangerous precedent. In addition, they have stated that the duty of a physician to promote health and human dignity necessitates unity and action among physicians—both in and outside of the military—to maintain medical professional ethics and the trust of people served by physicians.[52,53]

In May 2006, a United Nations panel charged with monitoring compliance with the 1984 Convention Against Torture, which the United States had ratified, called on the United States to (a) close its prison at Guantanamo, (b) expressly ban controversial interrogation techniques, and (c) halt the transfer of detainees to countries with a history of abuse and torture.[54,55]

WEAPONS OF MASS DESTRUCTION

In previous wars, nation-states have used WMDs, usually defined as chemical, biological, and nuclear weapons. In contrast, the use of WMDs by individuals or groups has been extremely rare, in part because of the difficulties in obtaining or using such weapons. Nonetheless, the U.S. government has placed great emphasis on preparedness for a terrorist attack with WMDs as well as radiological weapons ("dirty bombs").

Access to biological agents that could be used in a terrorist attack remains a concern. In addition, the individual or group responsible for the dissemination of anthrax spores in the United States in 2001 has not yet been identified or apprehended. Based on follow-up of those individuals exposed to anthrax spores in 2001, prompt immunization combined with antibiotic treatment after exposure is effective in preventing death from anthrax.

There has been considerable concern about nuclear weapons, including: (a) the continuing possibility of their use by the countries that possess them; (b) the possibility of additional countries obtaining them; and (c) the possibility of nuclear weapons, or material to make them, being acquired by other individuals or groups. Negotiations between the United States and Russia, which have the world's largest stockpiles of nuclear weapons, have aimed at eliminating or reducing the number of weapons in both nations. These negotiations have not been very successful. However, they have concentrated on protecting nuclear stockpiles in Russia, which are less well guarded against transfer or theft than those in other nations. The Nunn-Lugar Cooperative Threat Reduction Program, which has been designed to safeguard or destroy these materials, has had some success.[56]

The Nuclear Nonproliferation Treaty of 1968 (NPT) had called for an agreement between the then-nuclear weapons states (the United States, the Soviet Union, Britain, France, and China) and all other nations to curb the spread of nuclear weapons. Each weapons state agreed not to transfer nuclear weapons to any non-weapons state or subnational group and not to assist any non-weapons state to acquire such weapons. All nations were to have full access to nuclear technology for peaceful purposes.

The weapons states offered to the non-weapons states, in return for their agreement not to develop nuclear weapons, a promise in Article VI of the NPT: "Each of the Parties to this Treaty undertakes to pursue negotiations in good faith on effective measures to cessation of the nuclear arms race at an early date and to nuclear disarmament, and on a Treaty on general and complete disarmament under strict and effective international control." Despite the advisory opinion of the International Court of Justice in 1996 calling on the weapons states to fulfill this obligation, little progress has been made.

In May 2006, the United States proposed to the 65-nation Conference on Disarmament, which meets regularly in Geneva, a draft treaty banning production of weapons-grade fissile material. The proposed Fissile Material Cutoff Treaty contained no verification measures and current stockpiles of fissile material would not have been affected.[57] In short, stockpiles of nuclear weapons and fissile materials remain vulnerable to transfer to, or theft by, individuals or groups.

Acknowledgments

We are grateful to Carrie Pedersen, Mariclaire Cloutier, and Regan Hofmann of Oxford University Press for facilitating the publication of this paperback edition of *Terrorism and Public Health* and to Robert Gould, Philip Landrigan, Mark Sidel, and Patrice Sutton for reviewing the Epilogue.

REFERENCES

1. U.S. Code, Title 22, Section 2656f(d).
2. National Counterterrorism Center. Country Reports on Terrorism 2005, Statistical Annex. Available at http://www.state.gov/documents/organization/65469.pdf. Accessed June 14, 2006.

3. Alison S. Moscow confirms siege gas based on fentanyl. *Reuters*, October 30, 2002. Available at http://www.cdi.org/russia/johnson/6523-1.cfm. Accessed September 2, 2006.

4. Brackbill RM, Thorpe LE, DiGrande L, et al. Surveillance for World Trade Center disaster health effects among survivors of collapsed and damaged buildings. *MMWR* 2006; 55(SS-2):1–18.

5. DePalma A. Tracing lung ailments that rose with 9/11 dust. *New York Times*, May 13, 2006, pp. A1, A16.

6. Prezant DJ, Weiden M, Banauch GI, et al. Cough and bronchial responsiveness in firefighters at the World Trade Center site. *N Engl J Med* 2002; 347:806–815.

7. Landrigan PJ, Lioy PJ, Thurston G, et al. Health and environmental consequences of the World Trade Center disaster. *Environ Health Perspect* 2004; 112:731–739.

8. Landrigan P. Health and environmental consequences of the World Trade Center disaster. Abstract submitted for the 134th Annual Meeting of the American Public Health Association, Boston, 2006.

9. Tapp LC, Baron S, Bernard B, et al. Physical and mental health symptoms among NYC transit workers seven and one-half months after the WTC attacks. *Am J Ind Med* 2005; 47:475–483.

10. Centers for Disease Control and Prevention. Injuries and illnesses among New York City Fire Department rescue workers after responding to the World Trade Center Attacks. *MMWR* 2002; 51:1–5.

11. Centers for Disease Control and Prevention. Physical health status of World Trade Center rescue and recovery workers and volunteers—New York City, July 2002–August 2004. *MMWR* 2004; 53:807–812.

12. DePalma A. Illness persisting in 9/11 workers, big study finds. *New York Times*, September 6, 2006, pp. A1, C13.

13. Lioy PJ, Weisel CP, Millette JR, et al. Characterization of the dust/smoke aerosol that settled east of the World Trade Center (WTC) in lower Manhattan after the collapse of the WTC 11 September 2001. *Environ Health Perspect* 2002; 110:703–714.

14. Lin S, Reibman J, Bowers JA, et al. Upper respiratory symptoms and other health effects among residents living near the World Trade Center site after September 11, 2001. *Am J Epidemiol* 2005; 162:499–507.

15. Centers for Disease Control and Prevention. Self-reported increase in asthma severity after the September 11 attacks on the World Trade Center—Manhattan, New York, 2001. *MMWR* 2002; 51:781–782.

16. Galea S, Ahern J, Resnick H, et al. Psychological sequelae of the September 11 terrorist attacks in New York City. *N Engl J Med* 2002; 346:982–987.

17. Galea S, Vlahov D, Resnick H, et al. Trends of probably post-traumatic stress disorder in New York City after the September 11 terrorist attacks. *Am J Epidemiol* 2003; 158:514–524.

18. Jordan NN, Hoge CW, Tobler SK, et al. Mental health impact of 9/11 Pentagon attack: validation of a rapid assessment tool. *Am J Prev Med* 2004; 26:284–293.

19. Lederman SA, Rauh V, Weiss L, et al. The effects of the World Trade Center event on birth outcomes among term deliveries at three lower Manhattan hospitals. *Environ Health Perspect* 2004; 112:1772–1778.

20. DePalma A. New York Health officials issue guide to 9/11 illnesses. *New York Times*, September 1, 2006.

21. Sidel VW, Levy VS. War, terrorism, and public health. *J Law Med Ethics* 2003; 31: 516–523.

22. Sidel VW. Bioshield, biosword. *Gene Watch* 2004; 17(5/6):3–7, 20.

23. Rosner D, Markowitz G. *Are We Ready? Public Health Since 9/11.* Berkeley, CA: University of California Press, 2006.
24. Gaskins M, Rumm PD, Cummings CE, Hu X. Terrorism preparedness two years after the Bioterrorism Preparedness Accountability Indicators Project, December 2005. *HSI Journal of Homeland Security.* Available at http://www.homelandsecurity.org/ newjournal/articles. Accessed May 17, 2006.
25. Eggen D, Sheridan MB. Anti-terror funding cut in D.C. and New York: homeland security criticized over grants. *Washington Post,* June 1, 2006.
26. Cardwell D, Baker A. Who divides antiterror money? That's a secret. *New York Times,* June 3, 2006.
27. Brundtland GH. World Health Organization announced updated guidance on smallpox vaccination. Available at http://www.who.int/inf-pr-2001/en/state2001-16.html. Accessed September 9, 2003.
28. Center for Disease Control and Prevention. Update: adverse events following civilian smallpox vaccination—United States, 2003. *MMWR* 2003; 53:106–107.
29. Cohen HW, Gould RM, Sidel VW. The pitfalls of bioterrorism preparedness: the anthrax and smallpox experiences. *Am J Public Health* 2004; 94:1667–1671.
30. Smith S. Anthrax vs. the flu. *Boston Globe,* July 29, 2003.
31. Siegel M. *False Alarm: The Truth About the Epidemic of Fear.* New York: Wiley, 2005.
32. MacFarquhar N. Terror fears hamper U.S. Muslims' travel. *New York Times,* June 1, 2006.
33. Muslim leaders bemoan "Islamophobia" since 9/11. *New York Times,* September 1, 2006.
34. Sidel M. *Antiterrorism Policy and Civil Liberties after September 11.* Ann Arbor: University of Michigan Press, 2004.
35. Lichtblau E, Risen J. Domestic surveillance, the program: spy agency mined vast data trove, officials report. *New York Times,* December 24, 2005.
36. Risen J, Lichtblau E. Bush lets U.S. spy on callers without courts. *New York Times,* December 16, 2005.
37. Markoff J. Questions raised for phone giant in spy data furor. *New York Times,* May 13, 2006.
38. Pincus W. Gonzales's rationale on phone data disputed. *Washington Post,* May 25, 2006.
39. Donohue LK. Battlefield: U.S. *Los Angeles Times,* May 18, 2006.
40. Clark N, Wald ML. Hurdle for U.S. in getting data on passengers. *New York Times,* May 31, 2006.
41. Afghanistan, unraveling (editorial). *New York Times,* June 1, 2006.
42. Roberts L, Lafta R, Garfield R, et al. Mortality before and after the 2003 invasion of Iraq: cluster sample survey. *Lancet* 2004; 364:1857–1864.
43. Cowell A. U.S. "thumbs its nose" at rights, amnesty says. *New York Times,* May 26, 2005.
44. Degrading America's image (editorial). *New York Times,* June 6, 2006.
45. Okie S. Glimpses of Guantanamo Bay: medical ethics and the war on terror. *N Engl J Med* 2005; 343:2529–2534.
46. Brinkley J. Rice is challenged in Europe over secret prisons. *New York Times,* December 7, 2005.
47. Bloche MG, Marks JH. Doctors and interrogators at Guantanamo Bay. *N Engl J Med* 2005; 353:6–8.
48. Three Guantanamo detainees committed suicide, military says. *New York Times,* June 10, 2006.

49. Greenhouse L. Supreme Court blocks Guantanamo tribunals. *New York Times,* June 29, 2006. Available at: http://www.nytimes.com. Accessed September 4, 2006.
50. Bloche MG, Marks JH. When doctors go to war. *N Engl J Med* 2005; 352:3–6.
51. Lifton RJ. Doctors and torture. *N Engl J Med* 2004; 351:415–416.
52. Annas GJ. Unspeakably cruel: torture, medical ethics, and the law. *N Engl J Med* 2005; 352:2127–2132.
53. Rubenstein L, Pross C, Davidoff F, Iacopino V. Coercive U.S. interrogation policies: a challenge to medical ethics. *JAMA* 2005; 294:1544–1549.
54. Lynch C. Military prison's closure is urged. *Washington Post,* May 20, 2006.
55. Golden T. U.S. should close prison in Cuba, U.N. panel says. *New York Times,* May 20, 2006.
56. Lugar R. Eliminating the obstacles to Nunn-Lugar. *Arms Control Today,* March 2004. Available at http://www.armscontrol.org/act/2004_3/lugar.asp. Accessed September 2, 2006.
57. Arms Control Association. U.S. fissile material production proposal flawed. May 10, 2006. Available at http://www.armscontrol.org/pressroom/2006/20060518_FMCT_proposal.asp. Accessed September 2, 2006.

INDEX